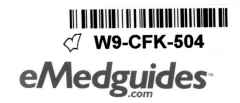

eMedguides™
.com

online and in-print Internet
directories in medicine

PSYCHIATRY
2000

AN INTERNET
RESOURCE GUIDE

CONSULTING EDITOR
Phillip R. Slavney, M.D.

Eugene Meyer III Professor of Psychiatry and Medicine
Johns Hopkins University School of Medicine

eMedguides.com, Inc., Princeton, New Jersey

For electronic browsing of this book, see
http://www.eMedguides.com

The publisher offers discounts on the eMedguides
series of books. For more information, contact

Sales Department
eMedguides.com, Inc.
P.O. Box 2331
Princeton, NJ 08543
tel   800-230-1481
fax   609-520-2023
e-mail sales@eMedguides.com

This book is set in Avenir, Gill Sans, and Sabon typefaces
and was printed and bound in the United States of America.

10 9 8 7 6 5 4 3 2 1

ISBN 0-9676811-2-X

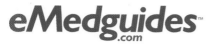

PSYCHIATRY 2000
AN INTERNET RESOURCE GUIDE

Daniel R. Goldenson
Editor-in-Chief

Phillip R. Slavney, M.D.
Consulting Editor,
Eugene Meyer III Professor of Psychiatry and Medicine,
Johns Hopkins University School of Medicine

Karen M. Albert, MLS
Consulting Medical Librarian,
Director of Library Services, Fox Chase Cancer Center

Adam T. Bromwich
Managing Editor

Rebecca L. Crane, MPH
Development Editor

Kristina Hasselbring
Alysa M. Wilson
Senior Research Editors

Daniela Maina, PhD
Senior Researcher

Sue Bannon
Designer

eMEDGUIDES.COM

Raymond C. Egan
Chairman of the Board

Daniel R. Goldenson
President

Adam T. Bromwich
Chief Operating Officer

Raymond Egan, Jr.
Marketing Director

P.O. Box 2331
Princeton, NJ 08543-2331
Book orders 800.230.1481
Facsimile   609.520.2023
E-mail   psychiatry@eMedguides.com

2000 ANNUAL EDITION

Anesthesiology & Pain Management

Arthritis & Rheumatology

Cardiology

Dental Medicine

Dermatology

Diet & Nutrition

Emergency Medicine

Endocrinology & Metabolism

Family Medicine

Gastroenterology

General Surgery

Infectious Diseases & Immunology

Internal Medicine

Neurology & Neuroscience

Obstetrics & Gynecology

Oncology & Hematology

Ophthalmology

Orthopedics & Sports Medicine

Otolaryngology

Pathology & Laboratory Medicine

Pediatrics

Physical Medicine & Rehabilitation

Plastic Surgery

Psychiatry

Radiology

Respiratory & Pulmonary Medicine

Urology & Nephrology

Veterinary Medicine

Disclaimer

eMedguides.com, Inc., hereafter referred to as the "publisher," has developed this book for informational purposes only, and not as a source of medical advice. The publisher does not guarantee the accuracy, adequacy, timeliness, or completeness of any information in this book and is not responsible for any errors or omissions or any consequences arising from the use of the information contained in this book. The material provided is general in nature and is in summary form. The content of this book is not intended in any way to be a substitute for professional medical advice. One should always seek the advice of a physician or other qualified health provider. Further, one should never disregard medical advice or delay in seeking it because of information found through an Internet Web site included in this book. The use of the eMedguides.com, Inc. book is at the reader's own risk.

All information contained in this book is subject to change. Mention of a specific product, company, organization, Web site URL address, treatment, therapy, or any other topic does not imply a recommendation or endorsement by the publisher.

Non-liability
The publisher does not assume any liability for the contents of this book or the contents of any material provided at the Internet sites, companies, and organizations reviewed in this book. Moreover, the publisher assumes no liability or responsibility for damage or injury to persons or property arising from the publication and use of this book; the use of those products, services, information, ideas, or instructions contained in the material provided at the third-party Internet Web sites, companies, and organizations listed in this book; or any loss of profit or commercial damage including but not limited to special, incidental, consequential, or any other damages in connection with or arising out of the publication and use of this book. Use of third-party Web sites is subject to the Terms and Conditions of use for such sites.

Copyright Protection
Information available over the Internet and other online locations may be subject to copyright and other rights owned by third parties. Online availability of text and images does not imply that they may be reused without the permission of rights holders. Care should be taken to ensure that all necessary rights are cleared prior to reusing material distributed over the Internet and other online locations.

Trademark Protection
The words in this book for which we have reason to believe trademark, service mark, or other proprietary rights may exist have been designated as such by use of initial capitalization. However, no attempt has been made to designate as trademarks or service marks all personal computer words or terms in which proprietary rights might exist. The inclusion, exclusion, or definition of a word or term is not intended to affect, or to express any judgment on, the validity or legal status of any proprietary right that may be claimed in that word or term.

VISIT US ON THE INTERNET

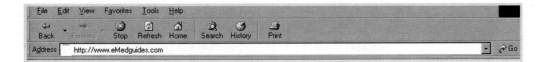

www.eMedguides.com

Instant access to all of our selected Web sites

Each print edition is online, *in its entirety*, so you can browse with your mouse, never typing in a single Web address. Simply visit www.eMedguides.com, click the appropriate specialty, enter your access code (printed in a circle on the title page), and you are presented with every site, listed by topic. Browse through the book online, or enter a keyword term to search the entire specialty.

Visit us often—our staff is continually adding new and interesting sites to each medical specialty database!

- ✪ Read the latest medical headlines each day in *your* specialty, as well as the top news in the medical field in general.

- ✪ Select a forthcoming conference, meeting, or CME program with a click of the mouse.

- ✪ Check out the latest issue of up to 100 medical journals in your field, and review abstracts and tables of contents without any charge.

- ✪ Review the newest drugs in your field, and the journal articles that discuss them.

- ✪ Use over 50 medical search engines to find any information in any field, just by typing in a keyword.

- ✪ Review the current bibliography of new books published in your field, organized topically for your convenience.

- ✪ Open up the world of the Internet. Find new and useful sites. Become Internet savvy!

Table of Contents

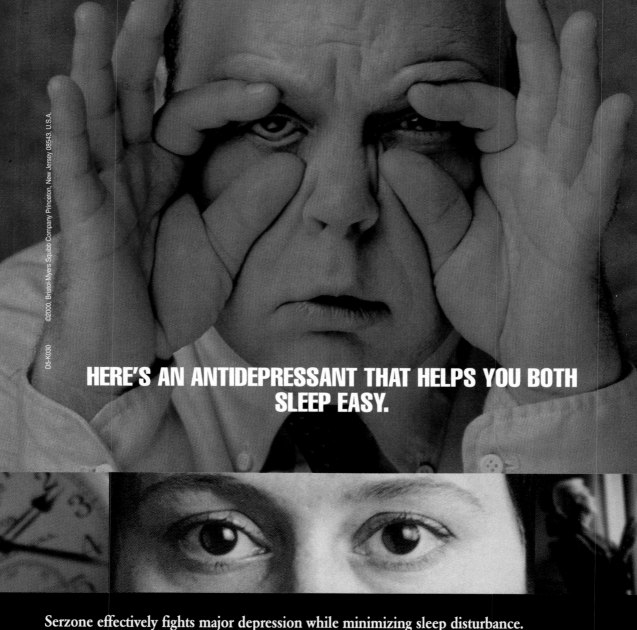

HERE'S AN ANTIDEPRESSANT THAT HELPS YOU BOTH SLEEP EASY.

Serzone effectively fights major depression while minimizing sleep disturbance.

Patients who are tired of being sick–and sick of being tired–may find that Serzone is right for them. It offers early improvement in sleep quality and minimal treatment-emergent sleep disturbance.[8-10] And comparable response rates on the HAM-D scale to SSRIs like fluoxetine, sertraline, and paroxetine.[1-3]

The most common adverse events (reported at ≥5% and significantly different from placebo in placebo-controlled trials) were dry mouth, somnolence, nausea, dizziness, constipation, asthenia, lightheadedness, blurred vision, confusion, and abnormal vision.

Coadministration of Serzone with terfenadine, astemizole, cisapride, or pimozide is contraindicated. Coadministration with monoamine oxidase inhibitors is not recommended. Coadministration with triazolam should be avoided for most patients, including the elderly.

See efficacy in a whole new light.

serzone®
nefazodone HCl
50, 100, 150, 200, 250 MG TABLETS

Please see references and brief summary of prescribing information in Appendix A.

FOR ANTIDEPRESSANTS, THE MOST DESIRABLE TREATMENT-EMERGENT EFFECT IS RELIEF.

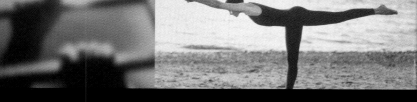

Serzone focuses on the treatment as well as the treatment-emergent.

Consider how Serzone effectively meets the challenge of major depression: It provides comparable response rates on the HAM-D scale to SSRIs such as fluoxetine, sertraline, and paroxetine.[1-3] It has proven efficacy, both in reducing relapse and for inpatients with moderate to severe depression.[4,5] And it shouldn't compromise sexual function, sleep, anxiety, and weight.[2,6,7]

The most common adverse events (reported at ≥5% and significantly different from placebo in placebo-controlled trials) were dry mouth, somnolence, nausea, dizziness, constipation, asthenia, lightheadedness, blurred vision, confusion, and abnormal vision.

Coadministration of Serzone with terfenadine, astemizole, cisapride, or pimozide is contraindicated. Coadministration with monoamine oxidase inhibitors is not recommended. Coadministration with triazolam should be avoided for most patients, including the elderly.

See efficacy in a whole new light.

serzone®
nefazodone HCl
50, 100, 150, 200, 250 MG TABLETS

Please see references and brief summary of prescribing information in Appendix A.

Coming May 2000

www.serzone.com

See Serzone
in a whole new light.

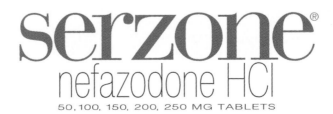

serzone®
nefazodone HCl
50, 100, 150, 200, 250 MG TABLETS

Foreword

The Information Age entered a new chapter when the Internet was established, and the field of medical information has been one of the fastest growing sectors of the World Wide Web. It is now estimated that 25% of Internet activity relates to medicine and health. Today's physicians and researchers have new search engines and databases available to them right from their offices or laboratories, making their desktop computers a *gateway* to instantaneous fact-finding, journal searches, medical planning, and clinical practice management.

As this "Internet World of Information" has grown exponentially, the need for organizational tools in each medical discipline has increased. It is impossible to grasp the extent and depth of information resources that now can be consulted on any topic, disease, therapy, drug protocol, procedure, or practice. While search engines are useful, they do not provide an orderly overview of a body of information, only a way to access it if one knows the objective in advance.

The field of Psychiatry can be explored in all its dimensions through the Internet, since every journal, association, medical school department, research program, and government agency dealing with the field has its own Web site. *Psychiatry 2000: An Internet Resource Guide* provides a detailed and fully-indexed guide to these resources. From articles that can be found using citation and full-text search tools to extensive data on individual disorders and clinical issues, the medical professional can locate any important fact or new development that may be useful in his or her clinical or research work.

For me, *Psychiatry 2000: An Internet Resource Guide* is designed to be helpful in two ways. It is like a mirror image of a textbook, providing all of the typical chapter topics and leading the reader to the appropriate Web sites for details. On a second level, it is like a yearbook, with professional information covering every aspect of the field in a timely fashion. There are daily news Web sites just for psychiatry, more electronic journals than any one library stocks, and dozens of associations with all of their activities, conferences, and research.

Perhaps even more important is the fact that this body of information is also available at a dedicated Web site, so that every item in the printed edition can be consulted with the click of a mouse.

Time is the professional's most valuable commodity. Allocating time for reading, conference participation, research, and clinical practice management is a more difficult job than ever. This new book, and its companion Web site offering the same information, can help manage this scarce resource more efficiently. It can enable a great deal of work to be performed through the Internet from any convenient location—the clinic, the laboratory, or from home, as long as a personal computer is at hand.

— Robert Hales, M.D.,
Professor and Chairman
Department of Psychiatry
University of California, Davis

I. INTRODUCTION

1.1 **Welcome to eMedguides**

Welcome to eMedguides, the newest and largest online and in-print Internet directories for physicians and other healthcare professionals, covering every major field in medicine!

As a user of this book, you now have a gateway to an extraordinary amount of information to help you find every possible, useful resource in your field, from electronic journals to selected Web sites on dozens of common and uncommon diseases and disorders.

We would like to thank our Consulting Medical Editor, Phillip R. Slavney, M.D., Eugene Meyer III Professor of Psychiatry and Medicine, Johns Hopkins University School of Medicine, for his valued assistance in this new project, and for his many organizational and topical suggestions. In addition, we wish to thank our Consulting Medical Librarian, Karen Albert, Director of Library Services for the Fox Chase Cancer Center, for her assistance in the development of this volume.

We have approached the compilation of this directory from the point of view of the professional practitioner and researcher, by organizing and heavily indexing topics and disorders, associations and government agencies, so that we lead you directly to the right destination on the Internet. Our medical compilers are trained professionals, and have written and rated Web sites in every category to let you know ahead of time what you can expect to find.

This book has been divided into sections, providing ease of access to material. The first part this book is devoted solely to psychiatry resources, including clinical information, disorder profiles, glossaries, current news sources, electronic journals, latest books, statistics, clinical studies, "supersites," therapies, and numerous topical resources.

The second part of the book is focused on the broad fields of medicine reference, clinical practice, and patient education. We have listed online databases and general medical resources, sources of current news and legislation, library access sites, government agencies in the health field, pharmaceutical data, student resources, and patient planning information.

Finally, a very extensive index is included, covering every topic, disorder, association, and Web site title, to make the fact-finding mission as efficient as possible.

How to Benefit Most from this Book

We realize that many physicians and other healthcare professionals may be over-whelmed by the extraordinary number of search engines to choose from, and the difficulty in finding very specific information that may only appear in a few locations on the Web. Our aim, therefore, has been to organize this book logically, topic by topic, giving descriptions of Web sites that we feel our readers will want to visit. To access a Web site, the user can type in the provided Web address (URL), or go straight to http://www.eMedguides.com where sites are listed just as they are in the book—but with "hot links" that merely require a mouse click. *The access code included on the title page of this volume provides access to our Web site.*

Physicians and researchers may want to examine several of the unique resources in this volume. We have provided a list of the most recent books published in the past year in the specialty, which are all available at http://www.amazon.com. Those readers who are interested in research can browse through our comprehensive journal section for access to thousands of articles and article abstracts every month. A further exploration can lead to medical libraries, university and nonprofit centers for research across the country, clinical studies currently underway in every phase, FDA trials of the latest drugs, and instant news sources for the latest breakthroughs.

Although much of the material in this book is intended for a professional, medical audience, key patient Web resources are also provided. Physicians may wish to refer patients to these sites. Many patient sites include up-to-date news and research and clear descriptions of diseases and their treatments.

Psychiatry 2000: An Internet Resource Guide is an annual volume, since so much information on the Web keeps changing, better sites and sources are assembled, hundreds of new books are published, new conferences are constantly scheduled, and major research progress is made every day.

The Benefits of Both Print and Online Editions

We feel that both the print and online editions of eMedguides can play an important role in the information gathering process, depending on the needs of the physician or health professional. The *print* edition is a "hands-on" tool, enabling the reader to thumb through a comprehensive directory, finding Web information and topical sources that are totally new and unexpected. Each page can provide discoveries of resources previously unknown to the reader that may never have been the subject of an online search. Without knowing what to expect, the reader can be introduced to useful Web site information just by glancing at the book at different times, looking through the detailed Table of Contents, or examining the extensive Index. This type of browsing is difficult to achieve online.

The *online* edition serves a different purpose. It provides "hot links" for each Web site, so the user can click on a topic and visit the destination instantaneously, without having to type the Web address into a browser. In addition, there are search features in this edition that can be used to find specific information quickly, and then the user can print out only what he or she wishes to use. The online edition will also have more frequent updates during the year. Articles are posted daily, giving recent news and updates on each specialty, allowing the user to stay up-to-date.

Accessing the Online Edition

We encourage our readers to visit our Web site, through which readers can access any of the included sites with a simple click of the mouse. Our Web address is http://www.eMedguides.com. You will need a special access code that is included on the title page of this volume. By simply clicking on a specialty and typing in this code, the entire contents of the book can be browsed and then used as an online Internet guide. We will continually update the information in this volume on our Web site. Information will be posted on new books published in the field, newly announced conferences, and of course additional Web resources that become available and are of interest to physicians. You can also submit the names of other Web sites that you have discovered by e-mailing us at psychiatry@eMedguides.com.

We hope you will find the print and online versions of this volume to be useful Internet companions, always on hand to consult.

Site Selection

Selection Criteria

Our medical research staff has carefully chosen the sites for this guide. We perform extensive searches for all of the topics listed in our table of contents, and then select only the sites that meet established criteria. The pertinence and depth of content, presentation, and usefulness for physician and advisory purposes are taken into account.

The sites in this physician guide contain detailed reference material, news, clinical data, and current research articles. We also include and appropriately label numerous sites that may be useful for patient reference. We focus primarily on government, university, medical association, and research organization sources and sponsors. Sites operated by private individuals or corporations are only included if they are content-rich and useful to the physician. In these cases, we clearly identify the operator in the title and/or description of the site.

Ratings Guide

Those sites that are selected based on these criteria are subsequently rated on a scale of one star (✿) to three stars (✿✿✿). This rating only applies to the pool of sites that are in the guide; therefore, a one star site is considered useful enough for inclusion but is not outstanding.

In addition, if a site requires a fee, some fees, or a free registration/disclosure of personal information, we indicate this information next to the rating.

Abbreviations

See "Medical Abbreviations and Acronyms" under "Reference Information and News Sources" in Part 2 for Web sites that provide acronym translation. Below are a few acronyms you will find throughout this volume:

APA	American Psychiatric Association
CME	Continuing Medical Education
FAQ	Frequently Asked Questions
NIH	National Institutes of Health
NIMH	National Institute of Mental Health
PDQ	Physician Data Query
URL	Uniform Resource Locator (the address of a Web site on the Internet)

1.2 Getting Online

The Internet is growing at a fantastic rate, but the vast majority of individuals are not yet online. What is preventing people from jumping on the "information highway"? There are many factors, but probably the most common factor is a general confusion about what the Internet is, how it works, and how to access it.

The following few pages are designed to clear up any confusion for readers who have not yet accessed the Internet. We will look at the process of getting onto and using the Internet, step by step. It is also helpful to consult other resources, such as the technical support department of the manufacturer or store where you bought your computer. Although assistance varies widely, most organizations provide startup assistance for new users and are experienced with guiding individuals onto the Internet. Books can also be of great assistance, as they provide a simple and clear view of how computers and the Internet work, and can be studied at your own pace.

What is the Internet?

The Internet is a large network of computers that are all connected to one another. A good analogy is to envision a neighborhood, with houses and storefronts, all connected to one another by streets and highways. Often the Internet is referred to as the "information superhighway" because of the vastness of this neighborhood.

The Internet was initially developed to allow people to share computers, that is, sublet part of their "house" to others. The ability to connect to so many other computers quickly and easily made this feasible. As computers proliferated, people used the Internet for sending information quickly from one computer to another.

For example, the most popular feature of the Internet is electronic mail (e-mail). Each computer has a mailbox, and an electronic letter can be sent instantly. People also use the Internet to post bulletins, or other information, for others to see. The process of sending e-mail or viewing this information is simple. A computer and a connection to the Internet are all you need to begin.

How is an Internet connection provided?

The Internet is accessed either through a "direct" connection, which is sometimes found in businesses and educational institutions, or through a phone line. Phone line connections are commonly used in small businesses and at home (although direct connections are becoming available for home use via cable and special phone lines). There are many complex options in this area; for the new user it is simplest to use an existing phone line to experience the Internet for the first time. After connecting a computer to a common phone jack, the computer can access the Internet. It will dial the number of an Internet provider, ask you for a user name and password, and give you access to the Internet. Keep in mind that while you are using the Internet, your phone line is tied up, and callers will hear a busy signal. Also, call waiting can sometimes interrupt an Internet connection and disconnect you from your provider.

Who provides an Internet connection?

There are many providers at both the local and national levels. One of the easiest ways to get online is with America Online (AOL). They provide software and a user-friendly environment through which to access the Internet. Because AOL manages both this environment and the actual connection, they can be of great assistance when you are starting out. America Online takes you to a menu of choices when you log in, and while using their software you can read and send e-mail, view Web pages, and chat with others.

Many other similar services exist, and most of them also provide an environment using Microsoft or Netscape products. These companies, such as the Microsoft Network (MSN), Mindspring, and Earthlink, also provide simple, easy-to-use access to the Internet. Their environment is more standard and not limited to the choices America Online provides.

Internet connections generally run from $10–$20 per month (depending on the length of commitment) in addition to telephone costs. Most national providers have local phone numbers all over the country that should eliminate any telephone charges. The monthly provider fee is the only charge for accessing the Internet.

How do I get on the Internet?

Once you've signed up with an Internet provider and installed their software (often only a matter of answering basic questions), your computer will be set up to access the Internet. By simply double-clicking on an icon, your computer will dial the phone number, log you in, and present you with a Web page (a "home" page).

What are some of the Internet's features?

From the initial Web page there are almost limitless possibilities of where you can go. The address at the top of the screen (identified by an "http://" in front) tells you where you are. You can also type the address of where you would like to go next. When typing a new address, you do not need to add the "http://". The computer adds this prefix automatically after you type in an address and press return. Once you press return, the Web site will appear in the browser window.

You can also navigate the Web by "surfing" from one site to another using links on a page. A Web page might say "Click here for weather." If you click on this underlined phrase, you will be taken to a different address, where weather information is provided.

The Internet has several other useful features. E-mail is an extremely popular and important service. It is free and messages are delivered instantly. Although you can access e-mail through a Web browser (AOL has this feature), many Internet services provide a separate e-mail program for reading, writing, and organizing your correspondence. These programs send and retrieve messages from the Internet.

Another area of the Internet offers chat rooms where users can hold round table discussions. In a chat room you can type messages and see the replies of other users around the world. There are chat rooms on virtually every topic, although the dialog certainly varies in this free-for-all forum. There are also newsgroups on the Internet, some of which we list in this book. A newsgroup is similar to a chat room but each message is a separate item and can be viewed in sequence at any time. For example, a user might post a question about Lyme disease. In the newsgroup you can read the question, and then read the answers that others have provided. You can also post your own comments. This forum is usually not managed or edited, particularly in the medical field. Do not take the advice of a chat room or newsgroup source without first consulting your physician.

How can I find things on the Internet?

Surfing the Internet, from site to site, is a popular activity. But if you have a focused mission, you will want to use a search engine. A search engine can scan lists of Web sites to look for a particular site. We provide a long list of medical search engines in this book.

Because the Internet is so large and unregulated, sites are often hard to find. In the physical world it is difficult to find good services, but you can turn to the yellow pages or other resources to get a comprehensive list. Physical proximity is also a major factor. On the Internet, none of this applies. Finding a reliable site takes time and patience, and can require sifting through hundreds of similar, yet irrelevant sites.

The most common way to find information on the Internet is to use a search engine. When you go to the Web page of a search engine, you will be presented with two distinct methods of searching: using links to topics, or using a keyword search. The links often represent the Web site staff's best effort to find quality sites. This method of searching is the core of the Yahoo! search engine (http://www.yahoo.com). By clicking on Healthcare, then Disorders, then Lung Cancer, you are provided with a list of sites the staff has found on the topic.

The keyword approach is definitely more daring. By typing in search terms, the engine looks through its list of Web sites for a match and returns the results. These engines typically only cover 15% of the Internet, so it is not a comprehensive process. They also usually return far too many choices. Typing lung cancer into a search engine box will return thousands of sites, including one entry for every site where someone used the words lung cancer on a personal Web page.

Where do eMedguides come in?

eMedguides are organized sources of information in each major medical specialty. Our team of editors continually scour the Net, searching for quality Web sites that relate to specific specialties, disorders, and research topics. More importantly, of the sites we find, we only include those that provide professional and useful content. eMedguides fill a critical gap in the Internet research process. Each guide provides more than 500 Web sites that focus on every aspect of a single medical discipline.

Other Internet companies that lack our medical and physician focus have teams of "surfers" who can only cover a subject on its surface. Search engines, even medical search engines, return far too many choices, requiring hours of time and patience to sift through. With an eMedguide in hand, you can quickly identify the sites worth visiting on the Internet and jump right to them. At our site, http://www. eMedguides.com, you can access the same listings as in this book, and can simply click on a site to go straight to it. In addition, we provide continual updates to the book through the site and annually in print. Our editors do the surfing for you, and do it professionally, making your Internet experience efficient and fulfilling.

Taking medical action must involve a physician

As interesting as the Internet is, the information that you will find is both objective and subjective. Our goal is to expose our readers to Web sites on hundreds of topics—for informational purposes only. If you are not a physician and become interested in the ideas, guidelines, recommendations, or experiences discussed online, bring these findings to a physician for personal evaluation. Medical needs vary considerably, and a medical approach or therapy for one individual could be entirely misguided for another. Final medical advice and a plan of action must come only from a physician.

PSYCHIATRY WEB RESOURCES

2. QUICK REFERENCE

2.1 Psychiatry Disorder Summaries

National Institute of Mental Health (NIMH): Public Resources ◎ ◎ ◎
http://www.nimh.nih.gov/publicat/index.cfm

This National Institute of Mental Health site for the public offers links to pages devoted to information on major mental disorders, including anxiety disorders, learning disorders, bipolar disorder, obsessive-compulsive disorder, depression, panic disorder, attention deficit hyperactivity disorder, phobias, autism, posttraumatic stress disorder, generalized anxiety disorder, and schizophrenia. Information on medications, mental disorders, and clinical trial resources are also available.

Internet Mental Health ◎ ◎ ◎
http://www.mentalhealth.com/fr20.html

Internet Mental Health offers fact sheets on 50 of the most common mental disorders. Information includes descriptions, diagnoses, treatments, current research information, and links to online brochures offering additional information on the disorders. Disorders are listed both alphabetically and categorically for easy reference.

Symptoms and Treatments of Mental Disorders ◎ ◎ ◎
http://www.grohol.com/sx.htm

Concise listings of symptoms and general treatment guidelines for 100 mental disorders are available at this Web site via summarized versions of official diagnostic criteria.

Medical College of Wisconsin
Health Link Neurological Disorders ◎ ◎ ◎
http://www.healthlink.mcw.edu/neurological-disorders

An A to Z listing of neurological disorder descriptions are presented at the Medical College of Wisconsin Physicians & Clinics Web site. Disease description information is provided by the National Institute of Neurological Disorders and Stroke of the National Institutes of Health. Links to relevant articles can be found.

Mentalwellness.com: Basic Information on Mental Disorders ◎ ◎ ◎
http://www.mentalwellness.com

A brief description of a variety of mental illnesses is available from this site, including anxiety disorders, bipolar disorder, clinical depression, dementia, schizoaffective disorder, and schizophrenia. Links are also available to fact sheets from the National Institute of Mental Health.

Neurological Disorders ⊙ ⊙ ⊙

http://chorus.rad.mcw.edu/index/1.html

Nearly 150 diseases are explained in terms of signs and symptoms and diagnostic considerations in the field of neurology. Associated disease processes and radiological findings are highlighted. This site is presented by the Medical College of Wisconsin.

2.2 Psychiatry Glossaries

Glossary of Mental Health Terms ⊙ ⊙

http://mirconnect.com/glossary/delusions.html

This online dictionary provides concise definitions of common mental health disorders, from agoraphobia to Tourette's disorder, as well as other related terms, such as behavior modification and separation anxiety.

Glossary Online: Psychiatry ⊙ ⊙ ⊙

http://www.pol-it.org/gloss.htm

This glossary provides brief but useful definitions of numerous psychiatric terms, and is designed for the general public. Though not comprehensive, the glossary addresses many specialized conditions that will be unfamiliar to many readers.

Mental Health Net: Managed Care Glossary ⊙ ⊙ ⊙

http://www.mentalhelp.net/articles/glossary.htm

This specialized glossary of common managed care vocabulary includes detailed definitions of more than 100 terms, such as adverse selection, capitation, risk sharing, and many highly specialized terms. Comments are available with some definitions, as well as links to other related terms.

American Academy of Child and Adolescent Psychiatry (AACAP): Teenage Mental Illness Glossary ⊙ ⊙ ⊙

http://www.aacap.org/Web/aacap/about/glossary/index.htm

The AACAP assists parents and families in understanding developmental, behavioral, emotional, and mental disorders affecting children and adolescents. A glossary of teenage mental illnesses lists approximately 20 disorders with full descriptions.

Glossary of Children's Mental Health Terms ⊙ ⊙ ⊙

http://www.mentalhealth.org/publications//allpubs/CA-0005/Glossary.htm

As a service of the Center for Mental Health Services (CMHS), this glossary contains terms frequently encountered when dealing with the mental health needs of children. Entries may include italicized words that have their own separate definitions. The terms included describe services that may or may not be available in all communities. Visitors are therefore encouraged to contact the CMHS National Mental Health Services Knowledge Exchange Network for details regarding grantees demonstrating services.

2.3 Psychiatry News and Headlines

Daily News from Mentalhelp ☺ ☺ ☺
http://www.mentalhelp.net/news/daily.htm

Collected from Johns Hopkins, Yahoo! Health, Science Daily, The National Alliance for the Mentally Ill, The National Institute of Mental Health, Psychotherapy Finances, and the American Psychiatric Association, this site offers daily updated mental health news and research findings. The subject areas included behavioral healthcare policy issues and technical findings and developments in the medical field.

Doctor's Guide: Psychiatry News ☺ ☺ ☺
http://www.docguide.com

Dozens of daily articles on new developments in psychiatry are provided at this useful Web site. For a review of medical news developments in different fields, the user can navigate to any topic of interest through http://www.docguide.com and by clicking on Explore All News, and then selecting the appropriate specialty.

Medscape: Psychiatry News ☺ ☺ ☺
http://aids.medscape.com/Home/Topics/psychiatry/directories/dir-PSY.News.html

Medscape offers psychiatry news from Reuters and other sources at this site, with articles mainly related to therapy, treatment guidelines, research, and pharmaceutical advances. General medical news is provided under clinical, regulatory, professional, epidemiology, legal, science, public health, and managed care headings. General health news for non-professionals is also available under the heading, "What Your Patients are Reading."

Mental Health News on the Net ☺ ☺ ☺
http://www.mentalhealth.org/newsroom/index.htm

Operated by the Center for Mental Health Services, a federal agency, this site provides important daily articles from numerous newspapers, news organizations, journals, and other sources of interest to the mental health community. It is one of the best such sources of current news on the Internet.

Psychiatric Times ☺ ☺ ☺
http://www.mhsource.com/psychiatrictimes.html

This site provides visitors with monthly articles related to psychiatric therapy, pharmaceuticals, and other psychiatry topics. Articles can be accessed by author,

Continuing Medical Education (CME) credit, title, and topic. Articles are available each month for CME credit. Visitors can also access subscription information and writers' guidelines.

2.4 Conferences in Psychiatry

Introduction

A number of key Web sites that offer event calendars along with details of conference programs and locations are provided here. Although a comprehensive conference calendar is provided by the PSL Group's *Doctor's Guide,* (our first listing), the other listed sites have valuable additional listings. Taken together, this group provides an overall source of conference scheduling information for the year.

Forward Conference Calendar ⊙ ⊙ ⊙

http://www.pslgroup.com/dg/psychiatry.htm

This partial listing of conferences and meetings for the year 2000 is compiled by the *Doctor's Guide to Medical Conferences and Meetings.* Dates, places, and other details are located at the main Web site. Upon visiting this site, the reader can click on any conference listing for additional information. The conference list is continually updated and should be consulted frequently.

Medical Conferences & Meetings: Psychiatry ⊙ ⊙ ⊙

http://www.medicalconferences.com/scripts/search_new.pl

Medical Conferences is an excellent source of information on forthcoming conferences and meetings. This site provides a search engine, enabling the visitor to type in "psychiatry" or other topics into the keyword space in order to receive a lengthy listing of conferences to be held over the next 12 months or longer. Each conference is an active link in itself, further permitting the visitor to obtain more detailed information about the event. There are over 150 meetings in the database for psychiatry, and more are added on a regular basis.

MediConf Online: Psychiatry Forthcoming Meetings ⊙ ⊙ ⊙

http://www.mediconf.com/online.html

MediConf Online provides an excellent directory of forthcoming meetings and conferences in every major medical specialty. The menu at this site enables the visitor to select the field of choice. For each meeting there is a listing including the dates, the contact telephone number, the contact e-mail address, and a link to the city where the visitor can learn about accommodations, weather, and other information.

Professional Events Calendar by Month for Mental Health ◎ ◎ ◎
http://www.mentalhealth.org/calendar/searchcal.cfm

A service of the Center for Mental Health Services, the site offers visitors a chance to search for meetings, conferences, and conventions nationwide. Users may search by month of event or event topic. The search engine returns a list of upcoming events with brief descriptions, location, and contact information for each. E-mail and Web addresses are provided where applicable.

2.5 Mental Health Statistics

Statistics: A Service of the Center for Mental Health Services ◎ ◎ ◎
http://www.mentalhealth.org/cmhs/mentalhealthstatistics/statistics.htm

This site contains links to the National Institute of Mental Health (NIMH) where recent study results can be accessed. Study results are provided by the World Health Organization, the World Bank, and Harvard University on the most common mental health disorders and estimated economic cost to society. Additional articles cover the complex behavior of suicide with its age, gender, and racial differences, information on older persons from the Administration on Aging, and statistics on the national indicators of child well-being, including detailed tables and limitations of data.

Numbers Count: Mental Illness in America ◎ ◎ ◎
http://www.nimh.nih.gov/publicat/numbers.cfm

The National Institute of Mental Health offers statistics on depression, bipolar illness, suicide, schizophrenia, anxiety disorders, panic disorder, obsessive-compulsive disorder, posttraumatic stress disorder, social phobia, attention-deficit/hyperactivity disorder, and autism in this informative fact sheet.

FedStats: One Stop Shopping for Federal Statistics ◎ ◎ ◎
http://www.fedstats.gov

FedStats, maintained by the Federal Interagency Council on Statistical Policy, serves as a comprehensive directory of statistical resources of interest to the public. The site offers an alphabetical index of materials, a site search engine, and a "Fast Facts" section for the latest economic and social indicators. Also available are data access tools for locating specific statistics from federal agency databases, links to federal agencies supplying statistical resources, resources for kids, press releases, and links to sources of demographic statistics. Regional topics covered include agriculture, demographics and economics, crime, education, energy and the environment, health, labor, and national accounts.

National Center for Health Statistics (NCHS): FASTATS Statistical Rolodex ◉ ◉ ◉

http://www.cdc.gov/nchs/fastats/fastats.htm

FASTATS is a service of the National Center for Health Statistics, providing state and national statistics on health-related topics. Specific topics include accidents/unintentional injuries, diseases, alcohol use, births, deaths, dental/oral health, diet and nutrition, disability/impairments, divorces, drug use (illegal and therapeutic), exercise/physical activity, health insurance coverage, immunization, life expectancy, minority health, occupational safety and health, vitamins, and numerous other related topics.

2.6 Topical Searches

Search Engine at NIMH ◉ ◉ ◉

http://www.nimh.nih.gov/search/search_form.cfm

The National Institute of Mental Health offers its own search engine to gain access to information by disorder or topic. This page explains the use of the search tool which draws upon a vast database of mental health articles, summaries, definitions, research laboratories, and other vital resources.

At Health.com Mental Health Topics ◉ ◉ ◉

http://www.athealth.com/topics.html

To view basic information about specific mental health topics, simply click on the preferred category of over 35 mental health sections. This At Health Web site provides unique topic coverage including such subjects as written expression disorder and amnesia. Should the user need further information, the site directs visitors to a mental health professional database of specialists in the specified area as well as to bookstore, medication, and Q&A links.

Health Sciences Library Psychiatric Resources Arranged by Topic ◉ ◉

http://www.hsls.pitt.edu/intres/mental/psyreso.html

This continuously updated page contains a listing of some of the best mental health resources pertaining to particular subjects or providing general mental health information. Twenty-eight subjects range from addictions to violence. Subtopics may be included within each section heading.

MEDLINEplus: Health Information
Mental Health and Behavior Topics ⊙ ⊙ ⊙

http://www.nlm.nih.gov/medlineplus/mentalhealthandbehavior.html

Selected by the National Library of Medicine, this topical index leads the visitor to comprehensive resource listings for each mental health disorder. Related categories, National Library of Medicine/National Institute of Health resources, governmental resources, basic research, clinical trials, diagnosis, and information in Spanish are included for each disorder. Related organizations, treatment information, and material regarding the disorder in special populations can also be found.

Mental Health InfoSource ⊙ ⊙ ⊙

http://www.mhsource.com

At the new and improved Mental Health Infosource home page, users can find a symptom/disorder list leading to complete information on over 39 mental health topics including bipolar disorder, dissociation, fear, eating disorders, obsessive-compulsive disorder, and seasonal affective disorder. General disorder information as well as diagnostics, home study courses, and conference information are accessible for each topic listed. Separate "Ask the Expert" sections are contributed for both consumer and professional questions. Additional links and authoritative articles make this topical search engine all-inclusive.

Mental Health Links ⊙ ⊙ ⊙

http://www.mentalhealth.org/links/KENLINKS.htm

The links provided by the Center for Mental Health Services (CMHS) cover a broad range of over 50 mental health divisions and lead the visitor to a colorful main page link specific to each disorder or topic. The connections offered at each of the over 50 CMHS Web sites provide some of the most comprehensive, interesting, and unique information on the World Wide Web in the area of mental health.

Mental Health Net: Topical Search ⊙ ⊙

http://mentalhelp.net/dxtx.htm

Listed in alphabetical order are not only the most common mental health problems and disorders as well as links to treatment information, but also a wide variety of other health and medical issues where support and information resources may be valuable and informative to visitors. The Quick Index allows easy access to an impressive collection of major subject headings. A popular resource section includes connections to information on alcohol and substance abuse, attention-deficit/hyperactivity disorder, sleep disorders, personality disorders, eating disorders, depression, anxiety, and schizophrenia resources.

National Voice on Mental Illness Link Manager   ⊙ ⊙ ⊙

http://www.apollonian.com/namilocals/linkmgr/linkmgr.asp

The National Voice on Mental Illness (NAMI) Link Manager provides its users with links to a multitude of informative Web pages on mental illness. Visitors can select among a list of 29 mental health categories ranging from advocacy to youth and everything in between. Most mental illnesses are included in addition to governmental, research, and international sections.

Online Dictionary of Mental Health   ⊙ ⊙ ⊙

http://www.human-nature.com/odmh/index.html

The Online Dictionary of Mental Health is brought to you by Human-Nature.com as a global information resource and research tool, compiled by and for Internet mental health resource users. A large assortment of disciplines contributing to the understanding of mental health are covered, and links to many sites offer varying viewpoints on mental health issues. A mental health search engine provides the ability to search over 100 major information resources, including many organizations that do not have their own internal search engines. Interesting discussion Web groups, such as a debate on the validity of modern psychoanalysis, are accessible.

2.7 Clinical Studies and Trials

All Trials

Centerwatch: Clinical Trials Listing Service (by disorder)   ⊙ ⊙ ⊙

http://www.centerwatch.com/studies/listing.htm

Designed for both patients and healthcare professionals, this site provides an extensive listing of therapeutic clinical trials organized by disorder, and sponsored by both industry and government. Over 50 psychiatry disorders are arranged alphabetically by type. It is international in scope and provides data on more than 5,200 clinical trials that are actively recruiting patients. Keyword search accessible, it also covers information on new FDA-approved drug therapies. Trials are listed by geographical region within each disorder.

NIH Clinical Trials

Centerwatch: NIH Trials Listing (by disease) ⊙ ⊙ ⊙
http://www.centerwatch.com/nih/index.htm

Centerwatch provides a convenient resource for accessing information on clinical trials at the NIH. These are clinical trials publicized by the NIH, located at the Warren Grant Magnuson Clinical Center in Bethesda, Maryland. Trials are organized by disorder and have short descriptions.

2.8 Drug Pipeline: Approved and Developmental Drugs

Centerwatch: FDA Drug Approvals ⊙ ⊙ ⊙
http://www.centerwatch.com/drugs/druglist.htm

This clinical trials listing service provides a cataloguing and descriptive profile of each new drug approved by the FDA in the last five years. Drugs are organized by year and by specialty.

Medicines in Development for Mental Illnesses ⊙ ⊙ ⊙
http://www.phrma.org/charts/archive/1998/m_c98.html

For current pharmaceutical trends, the complete text and charts of this publication as well as an additional file for neurological disorders are downloadable from the Web site and readily available in Adobe Acrobat PDF format. Acrobat Reader 3.0 can easily be installed, free-of-charge, from the site if necessary. Product name, company, indications, and developmental status are found within the documents. Additionally available is the article, "Pharmaceutical Companies are Developing 85 Medicines to Treat Mental Illness," outlining the current research and pharmaceutical therapy in mental illness.

Neurology and Neuroscience Drugs Under Development ⊙ ⊙ ⊙
http://www.phrma.org/charts/neurochart99.html

More than 350 new drugs are under development in all major neurology and neuroscience areas. This Web site is a detailed source providing the product names, pharmaceutical company developers, indications, and status.

Mental Health InfoSource: Approved Drugs ⊙ ⊙
http://www.mhsource.com/resource/approved.html

More than 100 pharmaceutical drugs currently approved by the Food and Drug Administration for the treatment of psychiatric disorders are listed at this site.

Information includes generic and brand names, a general description of the drug's action, and a list of approved indications.

Internet Mental Health: Medication Research ❂ ❂ ❂
http://www.mentalhealth.com/drugrs/index.html

Visitors to this site can conduct searches of PubMed for citations related to specific drug research. Over 150 drug names are listed at the site. Users can also limit searches to specific subtopics, including administration and dosage, adverse effects, chemistry, comparative studies, metabolism, pharmacokinetics, and many other subjects.

3. JOURNALS, ARTICLES, AND 1999 BOOKS

3.1 Abstract, Citation, and Full-text Search Tools

MEDLINE/PubMed at the National Library of Medicine (NLM) ◎ ◎ ◎
http://www.ncbi.nlm.nih.gov/PubMed

PubMed is a free MEDLINE search service providing access to 11 million citations with links to the full text of articles of participating journals. Probably the most heavily used and reputable free MEDLINE site, PubMed permits advanced searching by subject, author, journal title, and many other fields. It includes an easy-to-use "citation matcher" for completing and identifying references, and its PreMEDLINE database provides journal citations before they are indexed, making this version of MEDLINE more up-to-date than most.

3.2 Psychiatry Newsgroups

Internet newsgroups are places where individuals can post messages on a common site for others to read. Many newsgroups are devoted to medical topics, and these groups are listed below. To access these groups you can either use a newsreader program (often part of an e-mail program), or search and browse using a Web site (one popular site is http://www.deja.com).

Since newsgroups are mostly unmoderated, there is no editorial process or restrictions on postings. The information at these groups is therefore neither authoritative nor based on any set of standards.

sci.med.psychobiology
alt.support.anxiety-panic
alt.support.attn-deficit
alt.support.cerebral-palsy
alt.support.depression
alt.support.depression.manic
alt.support.depression.seasonal
alt.support.eating-disord
alt.support.epilepsy

alt.support.mult-sclerosis
alt.support.musc-dystrophy
alt.support.obesity
alt.support.schizophrenia
alt.support.sleep-disorder
alt.support.survivors.prozac
alt.support.tinnitus
alt.support.tourette

3.3 Journals and Articles on the Internet: Psychiatry

Directories of Electronic Journals

Mental Health Net: Links to Journals ⊙ ⊙ ⊙
http://mentalhelp.net/journals

This site allows users to search over 1,600 journals for relevant publications. Users can specify type of journal (electronic journals, journals providing table of contents, abstracts, or full-text articles online), a journal language (English, Dutch, French, German, or Spanish), and subject matter. Users can also search by keyword. Links to journal sites include a description of resources at the site and publishing information.

Selected Psychiatry Articles

Behavioral and Mental Disorder Reviews for Primary Care Providers ⊙ ⊙ ⊙
http://library.mcphu.edu/resources/reviews/psych.htm

As a service of MCP Hahnemann University Libraries, this comprehensive listing provides references and complete citations to 33 indexed review articles in the field of psychiatry with topics divided into the categories of behavioral disorders, mood disorders, psychotic disorders, dementia, substance abuse and addictive disorders, and anxiety and stress-related disorders. Links to primary care journals available on the Internet, as well as the psychiatry chapter of the University of Iowa's Family Practice Handbook may be accessed.

Menninger Articles on Mental Health ⊙ ⊙
http://www.menninger.edu/tmc_info_articles.html

This Web site lists links to online articles on various psychiatric disorders, such as addiction, eating disorders, personality disorders, sleep, anxiety, schizophrenia, and more. In addition, links to the Menninger Institute's different programs, reference materials, a telephone directory, a bulletin, services for adults, children, and corporations, and a referral service are present. General information about the Institute is also listed.

Mental Health InfoSource: Psychiatric Times ⊙ ⊙ ⊙
http://www.mhsource.com/psychiatrictimes.html

This online list of articles published in various journals on all aspects of the field of psychiatry has a large number of links. Articles can be searched by title, author, date, or CME credit. Articles on disorders, managed care, substance abuse, children and adolescents, careers, general mental health, and other psychiatry-related fields and topics are present.

PharmInfoNet's Mental Health Information Center ○ ○ ○

http://pharminfo.com/disease/mental.html

This division of PharmInfoNet provides an extensive compilation of links to articles and drug information related to mental health, neurological, and CNS disorders. Information from reputable sources, such as the National Institute of Neurological Disorders and Stroke, material on specific neurological disease-states, and article archives from professionally indexed medical publications are all accessible. PharmInfoNet's acclaimed Drug Information Database and plenty of other interesting connections can be found, including newsgroups, e-mail lists, and related Web site links.

Skeptical Psychiatrist ○ ○

http://home.gci.net/~dougs

At this site, professionals and consumers can read about current research articles and reviews, including a variety of articles discussing disorders and their treatment effects. There are a number of article reviews for schizophrenia, genetics, suicide, and alcoholism, as well as pharmacologics used in treating psychiatric illnesses, and other assorted topics.

Individual Journal Web Sites

Introduction

The following journals may be accessed on the Internet. Our table of information for each journal identifies content that is accessible free-of-charge or with a free registration, and also identifies content that requires a password and fee for access. We have also indicated if back issues are accessible. Journals are listed in alphabetical order by title.

Academic Psychiatry

http://ap.psychiatryonline.org

Publisher	American Association of Directors of Psychiatric Residency Training and the Association for Academic Psychiatry
Free resources	Table of Contents, Abstracts, Articles
Pay resources	None

Addiction
http://www.tandf.co.uk/journals/alphalist.html

Publisher	Taylor & Francis Group
Free resources	Table of Contents
Pay resources	Abstracts, Articles

Advances in Psychiatric Treatment
http://www.rcpsych.ac.uk/pub/apt.htm

Publisher	Royal College of Pharmacists
Free resources	Table of Contents
Pay resources	Abstracts, Articles

Age and Aging
http://www3.oup.co.uk/jnls/list/ageing

Publisher	Oxford University Press
Free resources	Table of contents, Abstracts
Pay resources	Articles

Alzheimer's Disease Review
http://www.coa.uky.edu/ADReview

Publisher	Sanders-Brown Center on Aging
Free resources	Table of Contents, Abstracts, Articles
Pay resources	None

American Journal of Family Therapy
http://www.tandfdc.com/JNLS/AFT.htm

Publisher	Brunner/Mazel
Free resources	Table of Contents
Pay resources	Articles

American Journal of Geriatric Psychiatry
http://ajgp.psychiatryonline.org

Publisher	American Association for Geriatric Psychiatry, HighWire Press
Free resources	Table of Contents, Abstracts, Articles
Pay resources	None

American Journal of Geriatric Psychiatry
http://ajgp.psychiatryonline.org

Publisher	American Association for Geriatric Psychiatry
Free resources	Table of Contents, Abstracts, Articles
Pay resources	None

American Journal of Occupational Therapy
http://www.aota.org/nonmembers/area7/links/LINK03.asp

Publisher	American Occupational Therapy Association
Free resources	None
Pay resources	Articles

American Journal of Psychiatry
http://ajp.psychiatryonline.org

Publisher	American Psychiatric Association
Free resources	Table of Contents, Abstracts, Articles
Pay resources	None

American Journal of Psychoanalysis
http://www.wkap.nl/journalhome.htm/0002-9548

Publisher	Kluwer Academic Publishers
Free resources	Table of Contents
Pay resources	Articles

American Journal on Mental Retardation
http://www.aamr.org/Periodicals/periodicals.html

Publisher	American Association on Mental Retardation
Free resources	Table of Contents, Abstracts
Pay resources	Articles

Annals of Clinical Psychiatry
http://www.aacp.com/annals.html

Publisher	Kluwer Academic/Plenum Publishing Corporation
Free resources	Table of Contents
Pay resources	Abstracts, Articles

Archive of Suicide Research

http://kapis.www.wkap.nl/kapis/CGI-BIN/WORLD/journalhome.htm?1381-1118

Publisher	Kluwer Academic/Plenum Publishing Corporation
Free resources	Table of Contents
Pay resources	Abstracts, Articles

Archives of Clinical Neuropsychology

http://www.elsevier.nl/inca/publications/store/8/0/2

Publisher	Elsevier
Free resources	Table of Contents
Pay resources	Articles

Archives of General Psychiatry

http://archpsyc.ama-assn.org

Publisher	American Medical Association
Free resources	Table of Contents, Abstracts
Pay resources	Articles

Archives of Women's Mental Health

http://link.springer.de/link/service/journals/00737/index.htm

Publisher	Springer Wien New York
Free resources	Table of Contents, Abstracts
Pay resources	Articles

Behavioral and Brain Sciences

http://www.cup.cam.ac.uk/journals/jnlscat/bbs/bbs.html

Publisher	Cambridge University Press
Free resources	Table of Contents
Pay resources	Abstracts, Articles

Behavioral and Cognitive Psychotherapy

http://www.cup.cam.ac.uk/scripts/webjrn1.asp?mnemonic=bcp

Publisher	Cambridge University Press
Free resources	Registration required to access Table of Contents and Abstracts
Pay resources	Articles

Behavioural Pharmacology
http://www.behaviouralpharm.com

Publisher	Lippincott, Williams, and Wilkins
Free resources	Table of Contents
Pay resources	Abstracts, Articles

Biological Psychiatry
http://www-east.elsevier.com/bps/bpsline.htm

Publisher	Elsevier Science Inc.
Free resources	Table of Contents
Pay resources	Abstracts, Articles

Bipolar Disorders
http://www.munksgaarddirect.dk/usr/munksgaard/tidsskrifter.nsf/Alfabetisk?OpenView

Publisher	Munksgaard International Publishers
Free resources	Table of Contents
Pay resources	Abstracts, Articles

Brain
http://brain.oupjournals.org

Publisher	Oxford University Press
Free resources	Table of Contents, Abstracts
Pay resources	Articles

Brain and Cognition
http://www.academicpress.com/www/journal/br.htm

Publisher	Academic Press
Free resources	Table of Contents, Abstracts
Pay resources	Articles

British Journal of Clinical and Social Psychiatry
http://www.scpnet.com/journ.htm

Publisher	Society of Clinical Psychiatrists
Free resources	Table of Contents, Abstracts, Articles
Pay resources	None

Canadian Journal of Psychiatry

http://www.cpa-apc.org/cjp-toc-98.html

Publisher	Canadian Psychiatric Association
Free resources	Articles, Abstracts, Table of Contents
Pay resources	None

Child and Adolescent Psychiatry Online

http://www.priory.com/psychild.htm

Publisher	Priory Lodge Education, Ltd.
Free resources	Articles, Abstracts, Table of Contents
Pay resources	None

Child Psychiatry and Human Development

http://www.wkap.nl/journalhome.htm/0009-398X

Publisher	Kluwer Academic/Plenum Publishing Corporation
Free resources	Table of Contents
Pay resources	Abstracts, Articles

Child Psychology and Psychiatry Review

http://www.cup.cam.ac.uk/scripts/webjrn1.asp?mnemonic=cpr

Publisher	Cambridge University Press
Free resources	Registration required to access Table of Contents and Abstracts
Pay resources	Articles

Clinical Child Psychology and Psychiatry

http://www.sagepub.co.uk/journals/details/j0063.html

Publisher	SAGE Publications
Free resources	Table of Contents, Abstracts
Pay resources	Articles

Clinical Psychiatry News

http://www.medscape.com/IMNG/ClinPsychNews/public/journal.ClinPsychNews.html

Publisher	The International Medical News Group
Free resources	Table of Contents, Abstracts, Articles
Pay resources	None

Clinical Psychology and Psychotherapy

http://www.interscience.wiley.com/jpages/1063-3995

Publisher	Wiley
Free resources	Registration required to access Table of Contents and Abstracts
Pay resources	Articles

Cognitive Science

http://www.umich.edu/~cogsci/about.html

Publisher	Cognitive Science Society, Inc.
Free resources	Table of Contents, Abstracts
Pay resources	Articles

Cognitive Therapy and Research

http://www.sci.sdsu.edu/CAL/CTR/CTR.html

Publisher	Plenum Press
Free resources	Table of Contents
Pay resources	Abstracts, Articles

Community Mental Health Journal

http://www.wkap.nl/journalhome.htm/0010-3853

Publisher	Kluwer Academic Publishers
Free resources	Table of Contents
Pay resources	Articles

Comprehensive Psychiatry

http://167.208.232.26/catalog/wbs-prod.pl?0010-440X

Publisher	W.B. Sauders Company
Free resources	None
Pay resources	Articles

Crisis: The Journal of Crisis Intervention and Suicide Prevention

http://www.hhpub.com/journals/crisis/index.html

Publisher	Hogrefe & Huber Publishers
Free resources	Table of Contents, Abstracts, Editorials
Pay resources	Articles

Culture, Medicine, and Psychiatry
http://kapis.www.wkap.nl/kapis/CGI-BIN/WORLD/journalhome.htm?0165-005X

Publisher	Kluwer
Free resources	Table of Contents
Pay resources	Abstracts, Articles

Current Therapeutics Online
http://www.ctonline.com.au

Publisher	Adis International Pty Ltd.
Free resources	Table of Contents, Selected Abstracts & Articles
Pay resources	Articles

Dementia and Geriatric Cognitive Disorders
http://www.karger.com/journals/dem

Publisher	S. Karger AG, Basel
Free resources	Table of Contents, Abstracts
Pay resources	Articles

Depression and Anxiety
http://www.interscience.wiley.com/jpages/1091-4269

Publisher	Wiley
Free resources	Registration required to access Table of Contents and Abstracts
Pay resources	Articles

Development and Psychopathology
http://www.cup.cam.ac.uk/journals/jnlscat/dpp/dpp.html

Publisher	Cambridge University Press
Free resources	Table of Contents
Pay resources	Articles

Drug and Alcohol Review
http://www.tandf.co.uk/journals/carfax/09595236.html

Publisher	Carfax Publishing
Free resources	Table of Contents
Pay resources	Articles

ECT Online

http://www.priory.co.uk/psych/ectol.htm

Publisher	Priory Lodge Education, Ltd.
Free resources	Articles, Table of Contents
Pay resources	None

Evidence-Based Mental Health

http://cebmh.warne.ox.ac.uk/cebmh/journal

Publisher	Centre for Evidence-Based Mental Health, Oxford
Free resources	Table of Contents, Abstracts, Articles
Pay resources	None

Experimental and Clinical Psychopharmocology

http://www.apa.org/journals/pha.html

Publisher	American Psychological Association
Free resources	Table of Contents, Abstracts
Pay resources	Articles

Forensic Psychiatry Online

http://www.priory.com/forpsy.htm

Publisher	Priory Lodge Education, Ltd.
Free resources	Table of Contents, Abstracts, Articles
Pay resources	None

General Hospital Psychiatry

http://www.elsevier.nl/inca/publications/store/5/0/5/7/6/1

Publisher	Elsevier Science. Inc.
Free resources	Table of Contents
Pay resources	Abstracts, Articles

Geriatrics

http://209.240.227.143

Publisher	Advanstar Communications, Inc.
Free resources	Table of Contents, Abstracts
Pay resources	Articles

German Journal Of Psychiatry
http://www.gwdg.de/~bbandel/gjp-homepage.htm

Publisher	German Journal of Psychiatry
Free resources	Table of Contents, Abstracts, Articles
Pay resources	None

Gerontologist
http://www-cpr.maxwell.syr.edu/gerontologist/gerontologist.html

Publisher	Gerontological Society of America
Free resources	Table of Contents
Pay resources	Abstracts, Articles

Gerontology
http://www.karger.ch/journals/ger/ger_jh.htm

Publisher	S. Karger AG
Free resources	Table of Contents, Abstracts
Pay resources	Articles

Harvard Mental Health Letter
http://www.health.harvard.edu/newsletters/mtltext.html

Publisher	HMS Harvard Health Publications
Free resources	Topic Highlights
Pay resources	Articles

Harvard Review of Psychiatry
http://www3.oup.co.uk/harrev/contents

Publisher	Oxford University Press
Free resources	Table of Contents, Abstracts
Pay resources	Articles

Human Psychopharmocology
http://www.interscience.wiley.com/jpages/0885-6222

Publisher	Wiley
Free resources	Registration required to access Table of Contents and Abstracts
Pay resources	Articles

Infant Mental Health Journal
http://www.interscience.wiley.com/jpages/0163-9641

Publisher	Wiley
Free resources	Registration required to access Table of Contents and Abstracts
Pay resources	Articles

International Clinical Psychopharmacology
http://www.intclinpsychopharm.com

Publisher	Lippincott Williams & Wilkins
Free resources	Table of Contents
Pay resources	Abstracts, Articles

International Forum of Psychoanalysis
http://www.scup.no/journals/en/j-449.html

Publisher	Scandinavian University Press
Free resources	Table of Contents
Pay resources	Abstracts, Articles

International Journal of Clinical and Experimental Hypnosis
http://sunsite.utk.edu/IJCEH/ijcehframes.htm

Publisher	Sage Publications
Free resources	Table of Contents, Abstracts
Pay resources	Articles

International Journal of Eating Disorders
http://www.interscience.wiley.com/jpages/0276-3478

Publisher	John Wiley & Sons, Inc.
Free resources	Users must register to view Table of Contents and Abstracts
Pay resources	Articles

International Journal of Geriatric Psychiatry
http://www.interscience.wiley.com/jpages/0885-6230

Publisher	John Wiley & Sons, Inc.
Free resources	Users must register to view Table of Contents and Abstracts
Pay resources	Articles

International Journal of Group Psychotherapy
http://www.groupsinc.org/pubs/IJGPindex.html

Publisher	Guilford Publications
Free resources	Table of Contents
Pay resources	Abstracts, Articles

International Journal of Law and Psychiatry
http://www.elsevier.nl:80/inca/publications/store/2/9/5

Publisher	Elsevier Science Inc.
Free resources	Table of Contents
Pay resources	Abstracts, Articles

International Journal of Obesity and Related Metabolic Disorders
http://www.stockton-press.co.uk/ijo/index.html

Publisher	Nature Publishing Group
Free resources	Table of Contents
Pay resources	Articles

International Journal of Psychiatry in Medicine
http://www.dartmouth.edu/~ijpm

Publisher	Baywood Publishing Company
Free resources	Table of Contents, Abstracts
Pay resources	Articles

International Journal of Psychoanalysis
http://www.ijpa.org

Publisher	Institute of Psychoanalysis, London
Free resources	Users must register with CatchWord Journal Service to view Table of Contents, Abstracts, and Articles.
Pay resources	None

International Journal of Psychosocial Rehabilitation
http://www.psychosocial.com

Publisher	The Southern Development Group
Free resources	Table of Contents, Articles
Pay resources	None

International Journal of Short-Term Psychotherapy

http://www.interscience.wiley.com/jpages/1096-7028

Publisher	Wiley
Free resources	Registration required to access Table of Contents and Abstracts
Pay resources	Articles

International Review of Psychiatry

http://www.tandf.co.uk/journals/carfax/09540261.html

Publisher	Carfax Publishing
Free resources	Table of Contents
Pay resources	Articles

JAMA

http://jama.ama-assn.org

Publisher	American Medical Association
Free resources	Articles, Abstracts, Table of Contents
Pay resources	None

Journal of Abnormal Psychology

http://www.apa.org/journals/abn.html

Publisher	American Psychological Association
Free resources	Table of Contents, Abstracts
Pay resources	Articles

Journal of Adolescence

http://www.academicpress.com/www/journal/adnojs.htm

Publisher	Academic Press
Free resources	Table of Contents, Abstracts
Pay resources	Articles

Journal of Affective Disorders

http://www.elsevier.nl:80/inca/publications/store/5/0/6/0/7/7

Publisher	Elsevier Science Inc.
Free resources	Table of Contents
Pay resources	Abstracts, Articles

Journal of Anxiety Disorders
http://www.elsevier.nl:80/inca/publications/store/8/0/1

Publisher	Elsevier Science Inc.
Free resources	Table of Contents
Pay resources	Abstracts, Articles

Journal of Applied Behavior Analysis
http://www.envmed.rochester.edu/wwwrap/behavior/jaba/jabahome.htm

Publisher	Society for the Experimental Analysis of Behavior, Inc.
Free resources	Table of Contents, Abstracts
Pay resources	Articles

Journal of Attention Disorders
http://www.mhs.com/jad

Publisher	Multi Health Systems, Inc
Free resources	Table of Contents, Abstracts
Pay resources	Articles

Journal of Behavior Therapy and Experimental Psychiatry
http://www.elsevier.nl:80/inca/publications/store/3/3/9

Publisher	Elsevier Science, Inc.
Free resources	Table of Contents
Pay resources	Abstracts, Articles

Journal of Behavioral Medicine
http://www.wkap.nl/journalhome.htm/0160-7715

Publisher	Kluwer Academic Publishers
Free resources	Table of Contents
Pay resources	Articles

Journal of Child Psychology and Psychiatry and Allied Disciplines
http://www.cup.cam.ac.uk/journals/jnlscat/cpp/cpp.html

Publisher	Cambridge University Press
Free resources	Table of Contents
Pay resources	Articles

Journal of Clinical and Experimental Neuropsychology

http://sun.swets.nl/sps/journals/jcen.html

Publisher	Swets & Zeitlinger Publishers
Free resources	Table of Contents, Abstracts
Pay resources	Articles

Journal of Clinical Psychiatry

http://www.psychiatrist.com

Publisher	Physicians Postgraduate Press
Free resources	Table of Contents
Pay resources	Abstracts, Articles

Journal of Clinical Psychoanalysis

http://plaza.interport.net/nypsan/jcp.html

Publisher	International Universities Press, Inc.
Free resources	Table of Contents, Abstracts, Articles
Pay resources	None

Journal of Clinical Psychopharmacology

http://www.psychopharmacology.com

Publisher	Lippincott, Williams & Wilkinson
Free resources	Table of Contents
Pay resources	Articles

Journal of Cognitive Rehabilitation

http://www.neuroscience.cnter.com/jcr/NSP/Default.htm

Publisher	NeuroScience Publishers
Free resources	None
Pay resources	Articles

Journal of Consulting and Clinical Psychology

http://www.apa.org/journals/ccp.html

Publisher	American Psychological Association
Free resources	Table of Contents, Selected Articles
Pay resources	Articles

Journal of Contemporary Neurology

http://mitpress.mit.edu/e-journals/CONE

Publisher	MIT Press
Free resources	Table of Contents, Articles
Pay resources	Articles

Journal of Developmental and Behavioral Pediatrics

http://lww.com/DBP

Publisher	Lippincott Williams & Wilkins
Free resources	Table of Contents, Abstracts
Pay resources	Articles

Journal of ECT

http://www.ectjournal.com

Publisher	Lippincott, Williams & Wilkinson
Free resources	Table of Contents
Pay resources	Articles

Journal of Family Therapy

http://www.blackwell-science.com/products/journals/jnltitle.htm

Publisher	Blackwell Publishers
Free resources	Table of Contents, Abstracts
Pay resources	Articles

Journal of Marital and Family Therapy

http://www.aamft.org/resources/jmft_menu.htm

Publisher	American Association for Marriage and Family Therapy
Free resources	None
Pay resources	Articles

Journal of Nervous and Mental Disease

http://www.wwilkins.com/NMD

Publisher	Lippincott, Williams & Wilkins
Free resources	None
Pay resources	Articles

Journal of Neurology, Neurosurgery, and Psychiatry
http://jnnp.bmjjournals.com

Publisher	BMJ Publishing
Free resources	Table of Contents, Abstracts
Pay resources	Articles

Journal of Neuropsychiatry and Clinical Neurosciences
http://neuro.psychiatryonline.org

Publisher	American Neuropsychiatric Association, HighWire Press
Free resources	Table of Contents, Abstracts, Articles
Pay resources	None

Journal of Personality and Social Psychology
http://www.apa.org/journals/psp.html

Publisher	American Psychological Association
Free resources	Table of Contents, Selected Articles
Pay resources	Articles

Journal of Practical Psychiatry and Behavioral Health
http://www.practicalpsychiatry.com

Publisher	Lippincott Williams & Wilkins
Free resources	Table of Contents, Abstracts
Pay resources	Articles

Journal of Psychiatric and Mental Health Nursing
http://www.blacksci.co.uk/~cgilib/jnlpage.bin?Journal=JPMHN&File=JPMHN&Page=aims

Publisher	Blackwell Science Ltd.
Free resources	Table of Contents
Pay resources	Articles

Journal of Psychiatric Research
http://www.elsevier.com/inca/publications/store/2/4/1

Publisher	Elsevier Science Inc.
Free resources	Table of Contents
Pay resources	Abstracts, Articles

Journal of Psychiatry

http://www.CCSPublishing.com/j_psych.htm

Publisher	CSS Publishing
Free resources	Table of Contents
Pay resources	Abstracts, Articles

Journal of Psychiatry and Neuroscience

http://www.cma.ca/jpn/index.htm

Publisher	Canadian Medical Association
Free resources	Table of Contents, Abstracts
Pay resources	Articles

Journal of Psychosomatic Research

http://www.elsevier.nl:80/inca/publications/store/5/2/5/4/7/4

Publisher	Elsevier Science Inc.
Free resources	Table of Contents
Pay resources	Abstracts, Articles

Journal of Psychotherapy Practice and Research

http://jppr.psychiatryonline.org

Publisher	American Psychiatric Association
Free resources	Table of Contents, Abstracts, Articles
Pay resources	None

Journal of Sex Research

http://www.ssc.wisc.edu/ssss/jsr.htm

Publisher	Society for the Scientific Study of Sexuality
Free resources	Table of Contents
Pay resources	Abstracts, Articles

Journal of Sleep

http://www.stanford.edu/dept/sleep/journal

Publisher	American Sleep Disorders Association
Free resources	Table Of Contents, Abstracts
Pay resources	Articles

Journal of the Academy of Psychiatry and the Law

http://www.cc.emory.edu/AAPL/journal.htm

Publisher	American Academy of Psychiatry and the Law
Free resources	Table of Contents, Abstracts
Pay resources	Articles

Journal of the American Academy of Child and Adolescent Psychiatry

http://www.aacap.org/publications/journal/index.htm

Publisher	Lippincott Williams & Wilkins
Free resources	Table of Contents, Abstracts
Pay resources	Articles

Journal of the American Academy of Child and Adolescent Psychiatry

http://www.aacap.org/journal/journal.htm

Publisher	Lippincott, Williams & Wilkins
Free resources	Table of Contents, Abstracts
Pay resources	Articles

Journal of the American Academy of Psychiatry and the Law

http://www.cc.emory.edu/AAPL/journal.htm

Publisher	American Academy of Psychiatry and the Law
Free resources	Table of Contents, Abstracts
Pay resources	Articles

Journal of the American Academy of Psychoanalysis

http://aapsa.org/jaap.html

Publisher	American Academy of Psychoanalysis
Free resources	Table of Contents
Pay resources	None

Journal of the American Geriatrics Society

http://www.amgeriatrics.com

Publisher	Lippincott Williams & Wilkins
Free resources	Table of Contents, Abstracts
Pay resources	Articles

Journal of the American Psychoanalytic Association

http://apsa.org/japa/index.htm

Publisher	American Psychoanalytic Association
Free resources	Table of Contents, Abstracts
Pay resources	Articles

Journal of the Experimental Analysis of Behavior

http://www.envmed.rochester.edu/wwwrap/behavior/jeab/jeabhome.htm

Publisher	Society for the Experimental Analysis of Behavior, Inc.
Free resources	Table of Contents, Abstracts
Pay resources	Articles

Journal of the International Neuropsychological Society

http://www.cup.cam.ac.uk/journals/jnlscat/ins/ins.html

Publisher	Cambridge University Press
Free resources	Registration required to access Table of Contents and Abstracts
Pay resources	Articles

Journal of Traumatic Stress

http://www.wkap.nl/journalhome.htm/0894-9867

Publisher	Kluwer Academic Publishers
Free resources	None
Pay resources	Articles

Mental Retardation

http://www.aamr.org/Periodicals/periodicals.html

Publisher	American Association on Mental Retardation
Free resources	Table of Contents, Abstracts
Pay resources	Articles

Molecular Psychiatry

http://www.stockton-press.co.uk/mp/index.html

Publisher	Stockton Press
Free resources	Table of Contents, Abstracts
Pay resources	Articles

Narcolepsy & Sleep Disorders Newsletter
http://www.narcolepsy.com

Publisher	WebSciences, Brain Information Service
Free resources	Articles
Pay resources	None

Neurocase
http://www3.oup.co.uk/neucas/contents

Publisher	Oxford University Press
Free resources	Table of Contents, Abstracts
Pay resources	Articles

Neurogenetics
http://link.springer.de/link/service/journals/10048/index.htm

Publisher	Springer-Verlag
Free resources	Table of Contents, Abstracts
Pay resources	Articles

Neuropsychologia
http://www.elsevier.nl/inca/publications/store/2/4/7

Publisher	Elsevier Science
Free resources	Table of Contents
Pay resources	Articles

Neuropsychology
http://www.apa.org/journals/neu.html

Publisher	American Psychological Association
Free resources	Table of Contents, Abstracts
Pay resources	Articles

Neuropsychopharmacology
http://www.elsevier.nl:80/inca/publications/store/5/0/5/7/7/8

Publisher	Elsevier Science, Inc.
Free resources	Table of Contents
Pay resources	Abstracts, Articles

New Directions for Mental Health Services
http://www.jbp.com/JBJournals/ndmhs.html

Publisher	Jossey-Bass
Free resources	Table of Contents
Pay resources	Articles

New England Journal of Medicine
http://www.nejm.org/content/index.asp

Publisher	New England Journal of Medicine
Free resources	Table of Contents
Pay resources	Articles, Abstracts

Nordic Journal of Psychiatry
http://www.scup.no/journals/en/j-223.html

Publisher	Scandinavian University Press
Free resources	Table of Contents
Pay resources	Abstracts, Articles

Perspectives: A Mental Health Journal
http://mentalhelp.net/perspectives

Publisher	Mental Health Net
Free resources	Table of Contents, Articles
Pay resources	None

Perspectives in Psychiatric Care
http://www.nursecominc.com/html/ppc.html

Publisher	Nursecom Inc.
Free resources	Table of Contents
Pay resources	Articles

Pharmabulletin
http://www.mhri.edu.au/pda/Bulletin3.html

Publisher	Mental Health Research Institute
Free resources	None
Pay resources	Articles

Pharmacopsychiatry
http://www.thieme.com/cgi-win/thieme.exe/onGJDIMAHEKEJI/display/771

Publisher	Thieme
Free resources	Selected forthcoming topics
Pay resources	Articles

Philosophy, Psychiatry, and Psychology
http://muse.jhu.edu/journals/philosophy_psychiatry_and_psychology

Publisher	John Hopkins University Press
Free resources	Table of Contents, Abstracts
Pay resources	Articles

Prevention and Treatment
http://journals.apa.org/prevention

Publisher	American Psychological Association
Free resources	Table of Contents, Abstracts
Pay resources	Articles

Progress in Neuropsychopharmacology and Biological Psychiatry
http://www.elsevier.com/inca/publications/store/5/2/5/4/8/8

Publisher	Elsevier Science
Free resources	Table of Contents, Abstracts
Pay resources	Articles

PSYCHE
http://psyche.cs.monash.edu.au

Publisher	Association for the Scientific Study of Consciousness
Free resources	Articles, Table of Contents
Pay resources	None

Psychiatric Care
http://www.stockton-press.co.uk/pc/index.html

Publisher	Stockton Press
Free resources	Table of Contents, Abstracts
Pay resources	Articles

Psychiatric News

http://www.psych.org/pnews

Publisher	American Psychiatric Association
Free resources	Table of Contents, Articles
Pay resources	None

Psychiatric Quarterly

http://www.wkap.nl/journalhome.htm/0033-2720

Publisher	Kluwer Academic Publishers
Free resources	None
Pay resources	Articles

Psychiatric Services

http://psychservices.psychiatryonline.org

Publisher	American Psychiatric Association
Free resources	Table of Contents, Abstracts
Pay resources	Articles

Psychiatric Times

http://www.mhsource.com/psychiatrictimes.html

Publisher	CME Incorporated
Free resources	Articles, Table of Contents
Pay resources	None

Psychiatry and Clinical Neurosciences

http://www.blacksci.co.uk/products/journals/xpcn.htm

Publisher	Blackwell Science
Free resources	Table of Contents
Pay resources	Abstracts, Articles

Psychiatry Online

http://www.priory.co.uk/psych.htm

Publisher	Priory Lodge Education Ltd.
Free resources	Table of Contents, Abstracts, Articles
Pay resources	None

Psychiatry, Psychology, and Law

http://www.australianacademicpress.com.au/Publications/ppl/ppl1.html

Publisher	Australian Academic Press
Free resources	Table of Contents, Abstracts
Pay resources	Articles

Psycho-Oncology

http://www.interscience.wiley.com/jpages/1057-9249

Publisher	Wiley
Free resources	Registration required to access Table of Contents and Abstracts
Pay resources	Articles

Psychological Assessment

http://www.apa.org:80/journals/pas.html

Publisher	American Psychological Association
Free resources	Table of Contents, Abstracts
Pay resources	Articles

Psychological Bulletin

http://www.apa.org/journals/bul.html

Publisher	American Psychological Association
Free resources	Table of Contents, Abstracts
Pay resources	Articles

Psychological Medicine

http://www.cup.cam.ac.uk/journals/jnlscat/psm/psm.html

Publisher	Cambridge University Press
Free resources	Table of Contents
Pay resources	Articles

Psychological Review

http://www.apa.org/journals/rev.html

Publisher	American Psychological Association
Free resources	Table of Contents, Abstracts
Pay resources	Articles

Psychology of Addictive Behaviors

http://www.apa.org/journals/adb.html

Publisher	American Psychological Association
Free resources	Table of Contents, Abstracts
Pay resources	Articles

Psychoneuroendocrinology

http://www.elsevier.nl:80/inca/publications/store/4/7/3

Publisher	Elsevier Science Inc.
Free resources	Table of Contents
Pay resources	Abstracts, Articles

Psychopathology

http://www.karger.ch/journals/psp/psp_jh.htm

Publisher	S. Karger AG
Free resources	Table of Contents, Abstracts
Pay resources	Articles

Psychopharmacology

http://link.springer.de/link/service/journals/00213/index.htm

Publisher	Springer-Verlag
Free resources	Table of Contents, Abstracts
Pay resources	Articles

Psychosomatic Medicine

http://www.psychosomatic.org/pm.html

Publisher	Lippincott Williams & Wilkins
Free resources	Table of Contents, Abstracts
Pay resources	Articles

Psychosomatics

http://psy.psychiatryonline.org

Publisher	Academy of Psychosomatic Medicine
Free resources	Table of Contents, Abstracts
Pay resources	Articles

Psychotherapy and Psychosomatics

http://www.karger.ch/journals/pps/pps_jh.htm

Publisher	S. Karger AG
Free resources	Table of Contents, Abstracts
Pay resources	Articles

Psychotherapy Patient

http://bubl.ac.uk/journals/soc/psypat

Publisher	Haworth Press
Free resources	Table of Contents, Abstracts
Pay resources	Articles

Psychotherapy Research

http://ted.educ.sfu.ca/Society/Journal

Publisher	Society for Psychotherapy Research
Free resources	Table of Contents
Pay resources	Abstracts, Articles

Scandinavian Journal Of Behavior Therapy

http://www.scup.no/journals/en/j-493.html

Publisher	Scandinavian University Press
Free resources	Table of Contents
Pay resources	Abstracts, Articles

Sexual Dysfunction

http://www.blackwell-science.com/products/journals/jnltitle.htm

Publisher	Blackwell Science
Free resources	Table of Contents
Pay resources	Abstracts, Articles

Social Psychiatry

http://link.springer.de/link/service/journals/00127/index.htm

Publisher	Springer–Verlag
Free resources	Table of Contents, Abstracts
Pay resources	Articles

Social Psychiatry and Psychiatric Epidemiology
http://link.springer.de/link/service/journals/00127/index.htm

Publisher	Springer–Verlag
Free resources	Table of Contents, Abstracts
Pay resources	Articles

Stress Medicine
http://www.interscience.wiley.com/jpages/0748-8386

Publisher	John Wiley & Sons, Inc.
Free resources	Users must register to view Table of Contents and Abstracts
Pay resources	Articles

The Therapist
http://www.the-therapist.ltd.uk

Publisher	European Therapy Studies Institute
Free resources	Table of Contents, Abstracts
Pay resources	Articles

Transactional Analysis Journal
http://www.tajnet.org

Publisher	International Transactional Analysis Association
Free resources	Table of Contents, Articles
Pay resources	None

Transcultural Psychiatry
http://www.sagepub.co.uk/journals/details/j0183.html

Publisher	SAGE
Free resources	Table of Contents, Abstracts
Pay resources	Articles

Traumatology
http://www.fsu.edu/~trauma

Publisher	Green Cross Foundation
Free resources	Articles, Table of Contents, Abstracts
Pay resources	None

World Federation for Mental Health
http://www.wfmh.org/newsletter.htm

Publisher	World Federation for Mental Health
Free resources	Articles, Table of Contents, Abstracts
Pay resources	None

3.4 **Books on Psychiatry Published in 1999**

Introduction

The following listing contains books published during the past 12 months in the field of Psychiatry. We have categorized the books under major topics, although many of the books contain material that extends beyond the highlighted subject. All of these books may be purchased through Amazon at http://www.amazon.com.

General Psychiatry Books

1999 Year Book of Psychiatry (Year Book of Psychiatry and Applied Mental Health), John A. Talbott, James C. Ballenger, Richard J. Frances, H. Meltzer. Mosby-Year Book, 1999, ISBN: 0815197349.

A Handbook for the Study of Mental Health: Social Contexts, Theories, and Systems, Allan V. Horwitz (Editor). Cambridge University Press (Short), 1999, ISBN: 0521561337.

Black Psychiatrists and American Psychiatry, Jeanne Spurlock (Editor). Amer Psychiatric Press, 1999, ISBN: 089042411X.

Desktop Neurology and Psychiatry, Patrick F. Bray. Lippincott Williams & Wilkins Publishers, 1999, ISBN: 068330657X.

Difficult Clinical Problems in Psychiatry, Malcolm Lader, Dieter Naber. Dunitz Martin Ltd, 1999, ISBN: 1853175501.

Enter the Super Mind, Maurie Pressman. CeShore Publishing Company, 1999, ISBN: 1585010030.

Examination Notes in Psychiatry—Basic Sciences: A Postgraduate Text, Gin S. Malhi. Butterworth-Heinemann, 1999, ISBN: 075064088X.

Handbook of Psychiatric Education and Faculty Development, Jerald Kay (Editor), Edward K. Silberman (Editor), Linda Pessar (Editor). Amer Psychiatric Press 1999, ISBN: 0880487801.

Handbook of the Sociology of Mental Health, Carol S. Aneshensel (Editor), Jo C. Phelan (Editor). Kluwer Academic Publishers, 1999, ISBN: 0306460696.

Kaplan & Sadock's Comprehensive Textbook of Psychiatry/VII, Benjamin J. Sadock (Editor), Harold I. Kaplan (Editor). Lippincott Williams & Wilkins Publishers, 1999, ISBN: 0683301284.

Learning from the Patient, Patrick J. Casement, Robert S. Wallerstein, M.D. Guilford Press, 1999, ISBN: 0898621577.

Let's Talk Facts About Choosing a Psychiatrist, The American Psychiatric Association Division of Public Affairs. Amer Psychiatric Press, 1999, ISBN: 089042361X.

One World, One Language: Paving the Way to Better Perspectives for Mental Health: Proceedings of the X World Congress of Psychiatry, Madrid, Spain, Juan J. Lopez-Ibor (Editor), Felice Lieh-Mak (Editor), Harold M. Visotsky (Editor). Hogrefe & Huber Pub, 1999, ISBN: 0889372144.

Psychiatric Care of the Medical Patient, Barry Fogel (Editor), Donna Greenberg (Editor). Oxford University Press, 1999, ISBN: 0195124529.

Psychiatry and the Cinema, Glen O. Gabbard, Krin Gabbard. Amer Psychiatric Press, 1999, ISBN: 0880488263.

Psychiatry (House Officer Series), David A. Tomb. Lippincott Williams & Wilkins, 1999, ISBN: 0683306340.

Psychiatry in the New Millennium, Sidney H. Weissman (Editor), Melvin Sabshin (Editor), Harold Eist (Editor). Amer Psychiatric Press, 1999, ISBN: 0880489383.

The American Psychiatric Press Textbook of Psychiatry, Robert E. Hales (Editor), Stuart C. Yudofsky (Editor), John A. Talbott (Editor). Amer Psychiatric Press, 1999, ISBN: 0880488190.

The Harvard Guide to Psychiatry, Armand M. Nicholi (Editor). Belknap Press, 1999, ISBN: 067437570X.

The Healing Brain, Robert Ornstein, David S. Sobel. Malor Books, 1999, ISBN: 1883536170.

The Massachusetts General Hospital Comprehensive Psychiatry Update and Review, Theodore Stern, John Herman. Appleton & Lange, 1999, ISBN: 0071354352.

The Recognition and Management of Early Psychosis: A Preventive Approach, Patrick D. McGorry (Editor), Henry J. Jackson (Editor). Cambridge University Press (Trade), 1999, ISBN: 0521553830.

What Is Clinical Psychology? (Oxford Medical Publications), John S. Marzillier (Editor), John Hall (Editor). Oxford University Press, 1999, ISBN: 019262928X.

Abnormal Psychology

Abnormal Psychology and Modern Life, Robert C. Carson, James Neal Butcher, Susan Mineka. Addison-Wesley Pub Company (Net), 1999, ISBN: 0321034309.

Abnormal Psychology in a Changing World, Jeffrey S. Nevid, Spencer A. Rathus, Beverly Greene. Prentice Hall, 1999, ISBN: 0130300055.

Abuse and Neglect

Dangerous Sex Offenders: A Task Force Report of the American Psychiatric Association,. Amer Psychiatric Press, 1999, ISBN: 089042280X.

Psychodynamic Perspectives on Abuse: The Cost of Fear, Una McCluskey (Editor), Carol-Ann Hooper (Editor). Jessica Kingsley Pub, 1999, ISBN: 1853026867.

Reducing Spouse/Partner Abuse: A Psychoeducational Approach for Individuals & Couples, Robert Geffner, Carol Mantooth. Springer Pub Company, 1999, ISBN: 0826112692.

The Healing Power of Play: Working With Abused Children, Eliana Gil. Guilford Press, 1999, ISBN: 0898624673.

Academic

The Mind and Its Discontents: An Essay in Discursive Psychiatry,. Oxford University Press, 1999, ISBN: 0198523130.

Addiction and Substance Abuse

Addictions: A Comprehensive Guidebook, Barbara S. McCrady (Editor), Elizabeth E. Epstein (Editor). Oxford University Press, 1999, ISBN: 0195114892.

Community Treatment of Drug Misuse: More than Methadone, Nicholas Seivewright. Cambridge University Press, 1999, ISBN: 0521665620.

Dual Diagnosis: Counseling the Mentally Ill Substance Abuser, Katie Evans, Michael Sullivan. Guilford Press, 1999, ISBN: 0898624509.

The American Psychiatric Press Textbook of Substance Abuse Treatment (American Psychiatric Press Textbook of Substance Abuse Treatment, 2nd Ed.), Marc Galanter (Editor), Herbert D. Kleber (Editor). Amer Psychiatric Press 1999, ISBN: 0880488204.

Treating Addiction As a Human Process (Library of Substance Abuse and Addiction Treatment), Edward J. Khantzian. Jason Aronson, 1999, ISBN: 0765701863.

Adolescent Psychiatry

Adolescent Psychiatry (Serial), Aaron H. Esman (Editor). Analytic Press, 1999, ISBN: 0881631981.

Alternative Medicine

The Embrace of Spirit a Woman's Guide to Mind/Body Healing, Marcy A. Witkin-Lupo. Four Seasons Pub, 1999, ISBN: 0965681130.

Assessment

Assessment Scales in Old Age Psychiatry, Alistair Burns, Brian Lawlor, Sarah Craig. Dunitz Martin Ltd, 1999, ISBN: 1853175625.

Assessments in Occupational Therapy Mental Health: An Integrative Approach, Barbara J. Hemphill-Pearson (Editor). Slack Inc, 1999, ISBN: 1556422660.

Complete McQ's in Psychiatry: Self-Assessment for Parts 1 & 2 of the Mrcpsych, Basant K. Puri, Anne D. Hall. Edward Arnold, 1999, ISBN: 0340740353.

Conducting Insanity Evaluations, Second Edition, Richard Rogers, Daniel W. Shuman. Guilford Press Cassettes, 1999, ISBN: 1572305215.

Current Psychiatric Diagnosis & Treatment, Lewis R. Baxter (Editor), Robert O. Friedel (Editor). Current Medicine, 1999, ISBN: 068330772X.

Functional Analysis of Problem Behavior: From Effective Assessment to Effective Support (The Wadsworth Special Educator Series), Alan C. Repp (Editor), Robert H. Horner (Editor). Wadsworth Pub Company, 1999, ISBN: 0534348505.

Functional Needs Assessment: Program for Chronic Psychiatric Patients, Lynn Blewett Dombrowski. Psychological Corp, 1999, ISBN: 0761642307.

Handbook of Assessment in Clinical Gerontology (Wiley Series on Adulthood and Aging), Peter A. Lichtenberg (Editor). John Wiley & Sons, 1999, ISBN: 0471283002.

Handbook of Multi-Cultural Mental Health: Assessment and Treatment of Diverse Populations, Israel Cuellar, Freddy A. Paniagua. Academic Press, 1999, ISBN: 0121993701.

Handbook of Polysomnogram Interpretation, Mark Pressman. Butterworth-Heinemann Medical, 1999, ISBN: 0750697822.

Psychiatric Self-Assessment & Review (Psa-R: American Psychiatric Association). Amer Psychiatric Press, 1999, ISBN: 0890422869.

Self Psychology and Diagnostic Assessment: Identifying Selfobject Functions Through Psychological Testing (Personality and Clinical Psychology series), Marshall L. Silverstein. Lawrence Erlbaum Assoc, 1999, ISBN: 0805822801.

The Mental Status Examination in Neurology, Richard L. Strub, F. William Black. F A Davis Company, 1999, ISBN: 0803604270.

The Use of Psychological Testing for Treatment Planning and Outcome Assessment, Mark Edward Maruish (Editor). Lawrence Erlbaum Assoc, 1999, ISBN: 0805827617.

Training Manual for the Children's Interview for Psychiatric Syndromes, Chips, Marijo Teare Rooney (Editor). Amer Psychiatric Press, 1999, ISBN: 0880488492.

Behavioral Analysis

Behavioral Science (Board Review Series), Barbara Fadem. Lippincott, Williams & Wilkins, 1999, ISBN: 0683306812.

Clinical Behavior Analysis, Mike Dougher (Editor). Context Press, 1999, ISBN: 1878978381.

Cognitive Aspects of Chronic Illness in Children, Ronald T. Brown (Editor). The Guilford Press, 1999, ISBN: 1572304685.

Biofeedback

Introduction to Quantitative EEG and Neurofeedback, James R. Evans (Editor), Andrew Abarbanel (Editor). Academic Press, 1999, ISBN: 012243790X.

Child Psychiatry

Advancing Mental Health and Primary Care Collaboration in the Public Sector (New Directions for Mental Health Services, 81), David A. Pollack (Editor), Rupert Goetz (Editor). Jossey-Bass Publishers, 1999, ISBN: 0787914282.

Child Focused Practice: A Collaborative Systemic Approach, Jim Wilson. Karnac Books, 1999, ISBN: 1855752042.

Children & Disasters (Series in Trauma and Loss), Norma S. Gordon, Norman L. Farberow, Carl A. Maida. Brunner/Mazel, 1999, ISBN: 0876309325.

Handbook of Infant Mental Health, Joy D. Osofsky (Editor), Hiram E. Fitzgerald (Editor), World Association for Infant Mental Health (WAIMH). John Wiley & Sons, 1999, ISBN: 0471189413.

Handbook of Psychosocial Characteristics of Exceptional Children (Plenum Series on Human Exceptionality), Vicki L. Schwean (Editor), Donald H. Saklofske (Editor). Kluwer Academic Publishers, 1999, ISBN: 0306460637.

Improving Treatment Compliance: Counseling and Systems Strategies for Substance Abuse and Dual Disorders, Dennis C. Daley, Allan Zuckoff. Hazelden Information Education, 1999, ISBN: 1568382812.

Independent Practice for the Mental Health Professional: Growing a Private Practice for the 21st Century, Dorothy Barnes, Joan K. Beigel, Ralph H. Earle. Brunner/Mazel, 1999, ISBN: 0876308388.

Making Collaborative Connections With Medical Providers: A Guide for Mental Health Professionals, L. Kevin Hamberger, Christopher R. Ovide, Eric L. Weiner. Springer Pub Company, 1999, ISBN: 0826112587.

Managing Mental Health Services (Health Services Management), Amanda Reynolds, Graham Thornicroft. Open University Press, 1999, ISBN: 0335198333.

Protecting the Emotional Development of the Ill Child: The Essence of the Child Life Profession, Evelyn K. Oremland (Editor), Jerome D. Oremland (Editor). Psychosocial Press, 1999, ISBN: 1887841202.

The Therapist's Workbook: Self-Assessment, Self-Care, and Self-Improvement Exercises for Mental Health Professionals, Jeffrey A. Kottler. Jossey-Bass Publishers, 1999, ISBN: 0787945234.

Training and Professional Development Strategy for Dementia Care Settings, Anthea Innes. Jessica Kingsley Pub, 1999, ISBN: 1853027618.

Clinical Practice

Challenges in Clinical Practice: Pharmacologic and Psychosocial Strategies, Mark H. Pollack (Editor), Michael W. Otto (Editor), J. F. Rosenbaum (Editor). Guilford Press, 1999, ISBN: 1572300671.

City of One: A Memoir, Francine Cournos. W W Norton & Company, 1999, ISBN: 0393047318.

Classification of Endogenous Psychoses and Their Differentiated Etiology, H. Beckmann (Editor), Karl Leonhard, Charles H. Cahn. Springer-Verlag, Vienna, 1999, ISBN: 3211832599.

Clinical Applications of Music Therapy in Psychiatry, Tony Wigram (Editor), Jos De Backer (Editor). Jessica Kingsley Pub, 1999, ISBN: 1853027332.

Clinical Decision Making in Psychiatry, Siegfried Kasper, Joseph Zohar. Dunitz Martin Ltd, 1999, ISBN: 1853175943.

Clinical Research in Psychiatry: A Practical Guide, Stephen Curran, Christopher Williams. Butterworth-Heinemann Medical, 1999, ISBN: 0750640731.

Cognitive Case Conceptualization: A Guidebook for Practitioners (Lea Series in Personality and Clinical Psychology), Lawrence D. Needleman. Lawrence Erlbaum Assoc, 1999, ISBN: 0805819088.

Concise Guide to Psychiatry for Primary Care Practitioners (Concise Guides), Michael F. Gliatto (Editor), Stanley N. Caroff (Editor), Robert M. Kaiser. Amer Psychiatric Press, 1999, ISBN: 0880483458.

Concise Guide to the Psychiatric Interview of Children and Adolescents (Concise Guides), Caludio Cepeda (Editor). Amer Psychiatric Press, 1999, ISBN: 088048330X.

Essentials of Clinical Psychiatry: Based on the American Psychiatric Press Textbook of Psychiatry, Robert E. Hales (Editor), Stuart C. Yudofsky (Editor). Amer Psychiatric Press, 1999, ISBN: 0880488484.

Essentials of Consultation-Liaison Psychiatry: Based on the American Psychiatric Press Textbook of Consulta-tion-Liaison Psychiatry, James R. Rundell (Editor), Michael G. Wise (Editor). Amer Psychiatric Press, 1999, ISBN: 0880488018.

Goodness of Fit: Clinical Applications from Infancy Through Adult Life, Stella Chess, Thomas Alexander, M.D. Brunner/Mazel, 1999, ISBN: 0876308930.

Handbook of Research Methods in Clinical Psychology, Philip C. Kendall (Editor), James N. Butcher (Editor), Grayson N. Holmbeck (Editor). John Wiley & Sons, 1999, ISBN: 0471295094.

Practical Guide to DSM-IV Diagnosis & Treatment, Carol Joy Cole. Technical Book Company, 1999, ISBN: 1890961035.

Privacy and Confidentiality in Mental Health Care, John J. Gates (Editor), Bernard S. Arons (Editor). Paul H Brookes Pub Company, 1999, ISBN: 1557664269.

Psychiatric Care of the Medical Patient, Barry Fogel (Editor), Donna Greenberg (Editor). Oxford University Press, 1999, ISBN: 0195124529.

Psychiatric Home Care: Clinical and Economic Dimensions, Alan Menikoff (Editor). Academic Press 1999, ISBN: 012490940X.

Psychiatry: Behavioral Sciences and Clinical Essentials, Jerald Kay, Jeffrey A. Lieberman, Allan Tasman. W B Saunders Company, 1999, ISBN: 0721658466.

Psychotherapy and Managed Care: Reconciling Research and Reality, Catherine Hartl Chambliss. Allyn & Bacon, 1999, ISBN: 0205279503.

The Clinical Documentation Sourcebook: A Comprehensive Collection of Mental Practice Forms, Handouts, and Records (Practice Planners), Donald E. Wiger. John Wiley & Sons, 1999, ISBN: 0471326925.

The Couple and Family Clinical Documentation Sourcebook: A Comprehensive Collection of Mental Health Practice Forms, Handouts, and Records, Terence Patterson, Terry Michael McClanahan. John Wiley & Sons, 1999, ISBN: 0471326925.

Traumatic and Nontraumatic Loss and Bereavement: Clinical Theory and Practice, Ruth Malkinson (Editor), Simon Shimshon Rubin (Editor), Eliezer Witztum. Psychosocial Press, 1999, ISBN: 188784130X.

Community Health

Creating Health Behavior Change: How to Develop Community-Wide Programs for Youth (Developmental Clinical Psychology and Psychiatry (Paper), Vol 43), Cheryl Perry. Altamira Press, 1999, ISBN: 0761912274.

Managing Mental Health Care in the Community: Chaos and Containment, Angela Foster (Editor), Vega Zagier Roberts (Editor). Routledge, 1999, ISBN: 0415167965.

MMPI-2 Correlates for Outpatient Community Mental Health Settings, John R. Graham, Yossef S. Ben-Porath, John L. McNulty. Univ of Minnesota Press (Txt), 1999, ISBN: 0816625646.

Neuropsychotherapy and Community Integration: Brain Illness, Emotions, and Behavior (Critical Issues in Neuropsychology), Tedd Judd. Plenum Pub Corp, 1999, ISBN: 0306461706.

Research in Community and Mental Health 1999: Coercion in Mental Health Services-International Perspectives (Vol 10), Joseph Morrissey (Editor), John Monahan (Editor). JAI Press, 1999, ISBN: 0762304820.

The Community Mental Health Treatment Planner, Arthur E. Jongsma, David J. Berghuis, Kellye Slaggert. John Wiley & Sons, 1999, ISBN: 0471359459.

Conferences

Proceedings of the X World Congress of Psychiatry, Madrid, Spain, August 23-28, 1996, Juan J. Lopez-Ibor, World Congress of Psychiatry, 1996, Madrid, Spain. Hogrefe & Huber Pub, 1999, ISBN: 0889372144.

Disorders

Anorexia Nervosa and Related Eating Disorders in Childhood and Adolescence, Bryan Lask (Editor), Rachel Bryant-Waugh (Editor). Lawrence Erlbaum Assoc, 1999, ISBN: 0863778038.

Bipolar Disorders: A Guide to Helping Children and Adolescents, Mitzi Waltz. O'Reilly & Associates, 1999, ISBN: 1565926560.

Caring for Depression (Rand Study), Kenneth B. Wells, Roland Sturm, Cathy D. Sherbourne, Lisa Meredith. Harvard University Press, 1999, ISBN: 0674097300.

Challenging Behavior of Persons With Mental Health Disorders and Severe Disabilities, Norman Anthony Wieseler (Editor), Ronald Halton Hanson (Editor). Amer Assn Mental Retardation, 1999, ISBN: 0940898667.

Chronic Fatigue Syndrome: An Integrative Approach to Evaluation and Treatment, Mark A. Demitrack (Editor), Susan E. Abbey (Editor), Stephen E. Straus. Guilford Press, 1999, ISBN: 1572304995.

Common Mental Disorders in Primary Care: Essays in Honour of Professor Sir David Goldberg, Michele Tansella (Editor), Graham Thornicroft (Editor). Routledge, 1999, ISBN: 0415205727.

Coping With HIV Infection: Psychological and Existential Responses in Gay Men (AIDS Prevention and Mental Health), Lena Nilsson Schonnesson, Michael W. Ross. Plenum Pub Corp, 1999, ISBN: 0306462206.

Coping With Self-Mutilation: A Helping Book for Teens Who Hurt Themselves (Coping Library), Alicia Clarke, Carolyn Simpson. Rosen Publishing Group, 1999, ISBN: 0823925595.

Delusional Disorder: Paranoia and Related Illnesses, Alistair Munro. Cambridge University Press (Short), 1999, ISBN: 052158180X.

Dementia Handbook, Richard J. Harvey, Nick C. Fox, Martin N. Rossor. Blackwell Science Inc, 1999, ISBN: 1853177539.

Depression, Kasper. Blackwell Science Inc, 1999, ISBN: 1853176567.

Developmental Disability and Behaviour, Christopher Gillberg, Gregory O'Brien. Cambridge University Press (Trd), 1999, ISBN: 1898683182.

Disabilities Sourcebook: Basic Consumer Health Information About Physical and Psychiatric Disabilities, Including Descriptions of Major Causes, Dawn D. Matthews (Editor). Omnigraphics, Inc., 1999, ISBN: 0780803892.

Disordered Personalities, David, J. Robinson. Rapid Psychler Press, 1999, ISBN: 0968209440.

Disruptive Behavior Disorders in Children and Adolescents (Review of Psychiatry Series, Vol 18, No 2), Robert L. Hendren (Editor). Amer Psychiatric Press, 1999, ISBN: 088048960X.

Emotional Illness and Creativity: A Psychoanalytic and Phenomenologic Study, Richard D. Chessick. Psychosocial Press, 1999, ISBN: 0823616657.

Encyclopedia of Stress, F. J. McGuigan. Prentice Hall, 1999, ISBN: 0205178766.

Extreme Fear, Shyness, and Social Phobia: Origins, Biological Mechanisms, and Clinical Outcomes (Series in Affective Science), Louis A. Schmidt (Editor), Jay Schulkin (Editor). Oxford University Press, 1999, ISBN: 0195118871.

Fear of Intimacy, Robert Firestone, Joyce Catlett. Amer Psychological Assn, 1999, ISBN: 1557986053.

Field Guide to Personality Disorders, David J. Robinson. Rapid Psychler Press, 1999, ISBN: 096803246X.

First Episode Psychosis, Kathy J. Aitchison, Karena Meehan, Robin M. Murray. Blackwell Science Inc, 1999, ISBN: 1853174351.

Functional Somatic Syndromes: Etiology, Diagnosis and Treatment, Peter Manu (Editor). Cambridge University Press (Short), 1999, ISBN: 0521591309.

Gender Differences in Mood and Anxiety Disorders: From Bench to Bedside (Review of Psychiatry Series, Vol 18), Ellen Leibenluft (Editor). Amer Psychiatric Press, 1999, ISBN: 0880489588.

Gender Loving Care: A Guide to Counseling Gender-Variant Clients, Randi Ettner, George R. Brown. W W Norton & Company, 1999, ISBN: 0393703045.

Generalized Anxiety Disorder: Diagnosis, Treatment and Its Relationship to Other Anxiety Disorders, David Nutt, Spilios Argyropoulos, Sam Forshall. Blackwell Science Inc, 1999, ISBN: 1853176591.

Handbook of Psychosomatic Medicine (Stress and Health Series, Monograph 9), G. A. Fava (Editor), H. Freyberger (Editor). International University Press, 1999, ISBN: 0823623025.

Healing Depression: A Holistic Guide, Catherine Carrigan, William G. Crook. Marlowe & Company, 1999, ISBN: 1569246564.

Interface Between Dementia and Depression, Steven P. Roose, D. P. Devanand. Dunitz Martin Ltd, 1999, ISBN: 1853176583.

Late Onset Schizophrenia, Robert Howard (Editor), Peter V. Rabins (Editor), David J. Castle (Editor). Wrightson Biomedical Pub Ltd, 1999, ISBN: 1871816394.

Mental Health and HIV Infection: Psychological and Psychiatric Aspects (Social Aspect of AIDS Series), Jose Catalan (Editor). UCL Press, 1999, ISBN: 1857281705.

Montgomery: Obsessive Compulsive Disorders. Blackwell Science Inc, 1999, ISBN: 1853173878.

Munchausen Syndrome by Proxy-Fabricated Illness in Children: A Handbook for Professional, D. Mary Eminson, Robert J. Postlethwaite. Butterworth-Heinemann, 1999, ISBN: 0029286064.

Obsessive-Compulsive and Related Disorders in Adults: A Comprehensive Clinical Guide, Lorrin M. Koran. Cambridge University Press(Short), 1999, ISBN: 0521559758.

Overcoming Anxiety, Panic, and Depression: New Ways to Regain Your Confidence, James, Gardner, M.D., Art Bell, Ph.D. Career Press, 1999, ISBN: 1564144356.

Overcoming Depression: Using Cognitive Therapy for Taming the Depression BEAST, Mark Gilson, Arthur Freeman. Mass Market Paperback, 1999, ISBN: 0158131681.

Panic Disorder: Assessment and Treatment Through a Wide-Angled Lens, Frank M. Dattilio, Jesus A. Salas-Auvert. Zeig Tucker & Company Inc, 1999, ISBN: 1891944355.

Personality Disorder and Serious Offending: A Practitioner's Guide to Treatment and Care, Clive Meux, Chris Newrith, Pamela J. Taylor. Butterworth-Heinemann, 1999, ISBN: 0750638400.

Personality Disorders in Older Adults: Emerging Issues in Diagnosis and Treatment (Lea Series in Personality and Clinical Psychology), Erlene Rosowsky (Editor), Robert Abrams (Editor), Richard A. Zweig (Editor). Lawrence Erlbaum Assoc, 1999, ISBN: 0805826831.

Pervasive Developmental Disorders: Finding a Diagnosis and Getting Help (Patient-Centered Guides), Mitzi Waltz (Preface). O'Reilly & Associates, 1999, ISBN: 1565925300.

Postpartum Depression and Child Development, Lynne Murray (Editor), Peter J. Cooper (Editor), Michael Rutter, E. S. Paykel. Guilford Press, 1999, ISBN: 1572305177.

Practical Dementia Care, Peter Rabins, Constantine G. Lyketsos, Cynthia Steele, Pete Rabins. Oxford University Press, 1999, ISBN: 0195106253.

Prozac Nation: Young and Depressed in America, Elizabeth Wurtzel. Replica Books, 1999, ISBN: 073510137X.

Psychiatric and Behavioural Disorders in Developmental Disabilities and Mental Retardation, Nick Bouras (Editor). Cambridge University Press(Short), 1999, ISBN: 0521643953.

Psychoneuroimmunology: Stress, Mental Disorders, and Health (Progress in Psychiatry Series, No 59), Karl Goodkin (Editor), Adrian Philip Visser (Editor). Amer Psychiatric Press, 1999, ISBN: 0880481714.

Schizophrenia and Mood Disorders: The New Drug Therapies in Clinical Practice, Peter E. Buckley (Editor), John L. Waddington (Editor). Butterworth-Heinemann, 1999, ISBN: 0750640960.

Schizophrenia: Concepts and Clinical Management, Eve C. Johnstone, Martin S. Humphreys, Fiona H. Lang, Stephen M. Lawrie. Cambridge University Press (Short), 1999, ISBN: 0521580846.

Schizophrenia in a Molecular Age (Review of Psychiatry, 18), Carol A. Tamminga (Editor). Amer Psychiatric Press, 1999, ISBN: 0880489618.

Search for the Causes of Schizophrenia, W. F. Gattaz, H. Hafner. Springer-Verlag, 1999, ISBN: 3798511721.

Sexual Addiction: An Integrated Approach, Aviel Goodman. International University Press, 1999, ISBN: 082366063X.

Smart but Stuck: What Every Therapist Needs to Know About Learning Disabilities and Imprisoned Intelligence, Myrna Orenstein. Haworth Press 1999, ISBN: 078900853X.

Stress and Anxiety: Practical Ways to Restore Health Using Complementary Medicine (Help Yourself to Health), Adrian White. Sterling Publications, 1999, ISBN: 0806931345.

Stress, Coping, and Development: An Integrative Perspective, Carolyn M. Aldwin, Richard S. Lazarus. Guilford Press, 1999, ISBN: 0898622611.

The Antidepressant Era, David Healy. Harvard University Press, 1999, ISBN: 0674039580.

The Boy Who Couldn't Stop Washing: The Experience and Treatment of Obsessive-Compulsive Disorder, Judith L Rapaport. Plume, 1999, ISBN: 0452263654.

The Condition of Madness, Brian W. Grant. University Press of America, 1999, ISBN: 0761814442.

The Hatherleigh Guide to Psychiatric Disorders, Part II, Hatherleigh Editorial Board (Editor), Hatherleigh. Hatherleigh Press 1999, ISBN: 157826023X.

The Management of Stress and Anxiety in Medical Disorders, David I. Mostofsky (Editor), David H. Barlow (Editor). Allyn & Bacon, 1999, ISBN: 0205287042.

The Pain Behind the Mask: Overcoming Masculine Depression, John Lynch, Christopher T. Kilmartin. Haworth, 1999, ISBN: 0789005581.

Treating Emotional Disorder in Gay Men, Martin Kantor. Praeger Pub Text, 1999, ISBN: 0275963330.

Treatment of Schizophrenia: Status and Emerging Trends, H.D. Brenner (Editor), W. Boker (Editor), R. Genner (Editor). Hogrefe & Huber Pub, 1999, ISBN: 0889371954.

Win the Battle: The 3-Step Lifesaving Formula to Conquer Depression and Bipolar Disorder, Bob Olson, Melissa Olson (Contributor). Chandler House Press, 1999, ISBN: 1886284318.

Drugs

The Antidepressant Era, David Healy. Harvard University Press, 1999, ISBN: 0674039580.

Education

Multiple Choice Questions for the Mrcpsych: Sciences Basic to Psychiatry, Gin S. Malhi. Butterworth-Heinemann, 1999, ISBN: 0750640898.

Postgraduate Psychiatry: Clinical and Scientific Foundations, Tim Amos, Helen Barker, Helen Forshaw, Louis Appleby. Butterworth-Heinemann Medical, 1999, ISBN: 0750635037.

Psychiatry: Key Questions Answered (Key Questions Answered Series), Alan Doris (Editor), Deborah Nelson (Editor), Mark Taylor (Editor). Oxford University Press, 1999, ISBN: 0192630334.

Psychoanalysis and the Philosophy of Science: Collected Papers of Benjamin B. Rubinstein (Psychological Issues, Monograph No 62-63), Benjamin B. Rubinstein, Robert R. Holt (Editor), Morris N. Eagle (Introduction). International University Press, 1999, ISBN: 0823652459.

Study Guide to the American Psychiatric Press Textbook of Consultation-Liaison Psychiatry, Jude Berman, James R. Rundell, Michael G. Wise. Amer Psychiatric Press, 1999, ISBN: 0880488050.

Electroconvulsive Therapy (ECT)

ELECTROSHOCK: Restoring the Mind, Max Fink. Oxford University Press (Trade), 1999, ISBN: 0195119568.

Emotions

Expressing Emotion: Myths, Realities, and Theraupeutic Strategies, Eileen Kennedy-Moore, Jeanne C. Watson, Jeremy D. Safran. The Guilford Press, 1999, ISBN: 1572304731.

Ethics

Ethics in Psychiatric Research: A Resource Manual for Human Subjects Protection, Harold Alan Pincus (Editor), Jeffrey A. Lieberman (Editor), Sandy Ferris. Amer Psychiatric Press, 1999, ISBN: 0890422818.

Psychiatric Ethics (Oxford Medical Publications), Sidney Bloch (Editor), Paul Chodoff (Editor), Stephen Green (Editor). Oxford University Press, 1999, ISBN: 0192628992.

Family Psychiatry

Marriage, Divorce, and Children's Adjustment (Developmental Clinical Psychology and Psychiatry (Cloth), Vol 14), Robert E. Emery. Sage Pubns, 1999, ISBN: 0761902511.

One Couple, Four Realities: Multiple Perspectives on Couple Therapy, Richard Chasin (Editor), Henry Grunebaum (Editor), Margaret Herzig (Editor), Ric Chasin (Editor). Guilford Press, 1999, ISBN: 0898620295.

Sibling Rivalry: Relational Problems Involving Brothers and Sister (Encyclopedia of Psychological Disorders), Elizabeth Russel Connelly, Carol C. Nadelson (Editor), Claire E. Reinburg, Ann Holmes. Chelsea House Pub (Library), 1999, ISBN: 0791049523.

Forensic Psychiatry

Adolescent Forensic Psychiatry, Susan Bailey, Mairead Dolan. Butterworth-Heinemann, 1999, ISBN: 0750640901.

Forensic Assessment With the Millon Inventories, Joseph T. McCann, Frank Dyer (Contributor). Guilford Press, 1999, ISBN: 1572300558.

Forensic Mental Health Nursing: Policy, Strategy, and Implementation, Paul Tarbuck (Editor), Philip Burnard (Editor). Whurr Pub Ltd, 1999, ISBN: 1861561288.

Handbook of Couples and Family Forensic Issues (Wiley Series in Couples and Family Dynamics and Treatment), Florence Whiteman Kaslow (Editor). John Wiley & Sons, 1999, ISBN: 0471191299.

Law & Mental Health Professionals: Minnesota: 1999 Supplement, Eric S. Janus, Ruth Mickelsen, Sheva Sanders. Amer Psychological Assn, 1999, ISBN: 1557985480.

Law & Mental Health Professionals: Pennsylvania (Law & Mental Health Professionals Series), Donald N. Bersoff (Editor), Stephen Anderer (Editor), Robert Field (Editor). Amer Psychological Assn, 1999, ISBN: 1557985553.

Legal and Ethical Dimensions for Mental Health Professionals, Patrick Brendan Malley, Eileen Petty Deklewa, Eileen Petty Reilly. Accelerated Development, 1999, ISBN: 1560326875.

Mental Health Services in Criminal Justice System Settings, Rodney Van Whitlock, Bernard Lubin (Compiler). Greenwood Publishing Group, 1999, ISBN: 0313301867.

Psychiatric Aspects of Justification, Excuse and Mitigation: The Jurisprudence of Mental Abnormality in Anglo-American Criminal Law (Forensic Focus,), Alec Buchanan. Jessica Kingsley Pub, 1999, ISBN: 1853027979.

Psychopathia Sexualis—A Clinical-Forensic Study, Richard Von Krafft-Ebing, Brian King (Editor). Bloat Books, 1999, ISBN: 0965032418.

Race, Culture and Ethnicity in Psychiatric Practice: Working With Difference (Forensic Focus, 13), Charles Kaye (Editor), Tony Lingiah (Editor). Jessica Kingsley Pub, 1999, ISBN: 1853026964.

Reforming the Law: Impact of Child Development Research (Guilford Law and Behavior Series), Gary B. Melton (Editor). Guilford Press, 1999, ISBN: 0898622786.

The Monotheistic Religions and Forensic Psychiatry (Forensic Focus, 11), Harvey Gordon (Editor). Jessica Kingsley Pub, 1999, ISBN: 1853026077.

Gender

Gender and Mental Health, Pauline M. Pressor. New York University Press, 1999, ISBN: 0814766749.

Psychotherapy With Women: Feminist Perspectives, Marilyn Lawrence (Editor), Marie Maguire (Editor), Jo Campling (Editor). Routledge, 1999, ISBN: 0415922658.

Women and Self-Harm: Understanding, Coping, and Healing from Self-Mutilation, Gerrilyn Smith, Dee Cox, Jacqui Saradjian. Routledge, 1999, ISBN: 0415924111.

Women and Stress: A Practical Approach to Managing Tension, Jean Lush, Pamela W. Vredevelt (Contributor). Fleming H Revell Company, 1999, ISBN: 0800756177.

Women in Context: Toward a Feminist Reconstruction of Psychotherapy, Marsha Pravder Mirkin (Editor), Monica McGoldrick. Guilford Press, 1999, ISBN: 0898620953.

Genetics

Genetics of Mental Disorders: A Guide for Students, Clinicians, and Researchers, Stephen V. Faraone, Ming T. Tsuang, Debby W. Tsuang. The Guilford Press, 1999, ISBN: 1572304790.

Geriatric Psychiatry

Aging and Mental Health (Understanding Aging), Michael A. Smyer, Sara H. Qualls. Blackwell Pub, 1999, ISBN: 1557865566.

Everything You Need to Know About Old Age Psychiatry, Robert Howard (Editor). Wrightson Biomedical Pub Ltd, 1999, ISBN: 1871816386.

Psychological Problems of Ageing: Assessment, Treatment and Care (Wiley Series in Clinical Psychology), Robert T. Woods (Editor). John Wiley & Sons, 1999, ISBN: 047197434X.

History

Care of the Psyche: A History of Psychological Healing, Stanley W. Jackson. Yale University Press, 1999, ISBN: 0300076711.

Masters of Bedlam: The Transformation of the Mad-Doctoring Trade, Andrew Scull, Charlotte MacKenzie, Nicholas Hervey. Princeton University Press, 1999, ISBN: 0691002517.

Revels in Madness: Insanity in Medicine and Literature (Corporealities), Allen Thiher. Univ of Michigan Press, 1999, ISBN: 0472110357.

Sex, Religion, and the Making of Modern Madness: The Eberbach Asylum and German Society, 1815-1849, Ann Goldberg. Oxford University Press, 1999, ISBN: 0195125819.

The Klein-Lacan Dialogue, Bernard Burgoyne (Editor), E. Mary Sullivan (Editor). Other Press, LLC, 1999, ISBN: 1892746166.

The Life Work of Dr. Elisabeth Kubler-Ross and Its Impact on the Death Awareness Movement (Symposium Series [Edwin Mellen Press], V 49), Michele Chaban. Edwin Mellen Press, 1999, ISBN: 0773483020.

Hypnotherapy

Hypnosis: A Jungian Perspective (Guilford Clinical and Experimental Hypnosis Series), James A. Hall. Guilford Press, 1999, ISBN: 0898623820.

Legal

Psychological Consultation in Parental Rights Cases, Frank J. Dyer. The Guilford Press, 1999, ISBN: 157230474X.

Social Work, Psychiatry and the Law, Norman N. Pringle, Paul J. Thompson. Ashgate Publishing Company, 1999, ISBN: 1857424166.

The Scientific Basis of Child Custody Decisions, Robert M. Galatzer-Levy (Editor), Louis Kraus (Editor). John Wiley & Sons, 1999, ISBN: 0471174785.

Loss and Bereavement

Grief As a Family Process: A Developmental Approach to Clinical Practice, Ester R. Shapiro. Guilford Press, 1999, ISBN: 0898621968.

Traumatic and Nontraumatic Loss and Bereavement: Clinical Theory and Practice, Ruth Malkinson (Editor), Simon Shimshon Rubin (Editor), Eliezer Witztum (Editor). Psychosocial Press, 1999, ISBN: 188784130X.

Memory

Memory: A Guide for Professionals, Alan Parkin. John Wiley & Sons, 1999, ISBN: 0471983012.

Mental Health

A Handbook for the Study of Mental Health: Social Contexts, Theories, and Systems, Allan V. Horwitz (Editor). Cambridge University Press (Short), 1999, ISBN: 0521561337.

A Sociology of Mental Health and Illness, David Pilgrim (Preface), Anne Rogers (Preface). Open University Press, 1999, ISBN: 0335203477.

A Sociology of Mental Illness, Mark Tausig, Janet Michello, Sree Subedi. Prentice Hall, 1999, ISBN: 0134596374.

ABC of Mental Health, Craig Davies. B M J Books, 1999, ISBN: 0727912208.

Al-Junun: Mental Illness in the Islamic World, Ihsan Al-Issa (Editor). Psychosocial Press, 1999, ISBN: 0823633373.

Insider's Guide to Mental Health: Resources Online, 1999 Edition (The Clinician's Toolbox), John M. Grohol, Edward L. Zuckerman. Guilford Press, 1999, ISBN: 1572304529.

Molecules and Mental Illness, Samuel H. Barondes. W H Freeman & Company, 1999, ISBN: 0716760339.

Organized Religion and Seniors' Mental Health, Anthony J. Blasi. University Press of America, 1999, ISBN: 0761813489.

Telling Is Risky Business: The Experience of Mental Illness Stigma, Otto F. Wahl. Rutgers University Press, 1999, ISBN: 0813527244.

Your Mental Health: A Layman's Guide to the Psychiatrist's Bible, Allen Frances, Michael B. First. Scribner, 1999, ISBN: 068483720X.

Multicultural, General

Asian Americans: Personality Patterns, Identity, and Mental Health, Laura Uba. Guilford Press, 1999, ISBN: 0898623723.

Culture & Mental Health: A Southern African View, Leslie Swartz. Oxford University Press, 1999, ISBN: 0195709810.

Psychosocial Wellness of Refugees: Issues in Qualitative and Quantitative Research (Studies in Forced Migration, V. 7), Frederick L. Ahearn (Editor). Berghahn Books, 1999, ISBN: 1571812040.

Using Race and Culture in Counseling and Psychotherapy: Theory and Process, Janet E. Helms, Donelda A. Cook. Allyn & Bacon, 1999, ISBN: 0205285651.

Neuropsychiatry

Neuropsychiatry and Mental Health Services, Fred Ovsiew (Editor). Amer Psychiatric Press 1999, ISBN: 0880487305.

Synopsis of Neuropsychiatry, Barry S. Fogel (Editor), Stephen M. Rao (Editor). Lippincott Williams & Wilkins, 1999, ISBN: 0683306995.

The Fundamentals of Clinical Neuropsychiatry, Michael Alan Taylor. Oxford University Press, 1999, ISBN: 0195130375.

The Neuropsychology of Emotion, Joan Borod. Oxford University Press, 1999, ISBN: 0195114647.

Using CNS Tissue in Psychiatric Research: A Practical Guide, Brian Dean (Editor), Joel E. Kleinman (Editor), Thomas M. Hyde. Harwood Academic Pub, 1999, ISBN: 9057022982.

Nutrition

Nutritional Influences on Mental Illness 2nd edition, Melvyn R. Werbach. Third Line Press, 1999, ISBN: 0961855088.

Organ Transplant

The Transplant Patient: Biological, Psychiatric, and Ethical Issues in Organ Transplantation (Psychiatry and Medicine Series), Andrea Dimartini (Editor), Paula T. Trzepacz (Editor). Cambridge University Press (Short), 1999, ISBN: 0521553547.

Psychiatric Rehabilitation

Multicultural Issues in Occupational Therapy, Zeenat Meghani-Wise (Editor). Taylor & Francis, 1999, ISBN: 1853024740.

Psychiatric Rehabilitation, Carlos Pratt, Nora Barrett, Melissa Roberts, Kenneth D. Gill. Academic Press, 1999, ISBN: 0125642458.

Psychoanalysis

A Mind of One's Own: A Kleinian View of Self and Object (New Library of Psychoanalysis, 32), Robert Caper. Routledge, 1999, ISBN: 0415199115.

Approaching Psychoanalysis: An Introductory Course, David L. Smith. Karnac Books, 1999, ISBN: 1855751577.

The Emergent Ego: Complexity and Coevolution in the Psychoanalytic Process, Stanley R. Palombo, Stuart Kauffman. International University Press, 1999, ISBN: 0823616665.

Psychopathology

Basic Issues in Psychopathology, Charles G. Costello (Editor). Guilford Press, 1999, ISBN: 0898621399.

Psychopathology: Contemporary Jungian Perspectives, Andrew Samuels (Editor). Guilford Press, 1999, ISBN: 0898624738.

Psychopharmacology

Antidepressant Therapy: At the Dawn of the Third Millennium, Mike Briley, Stuart Montgomery. Dunitz Martin Ltd, 1999, ISBN: 1853177253.

Atlas of Psychiatric Pharmacotherapy, Roni Shiloh, David Nutt, Abraham Weizman. Dunitz Martin Ltd, 1999, ISBN: 1853176303.

Breakthroughs in Antipsychotic Medicines: A Guide for Consumers, Families, and Clinicians, Peter J. Weiden. W W Norton & Company, 1999, ISBN: 0393703037.

Caffeine and Behavior: Current Views and Research Trends, B. S. Gupta, Uma G. Gupta. CRC Press, 1999, ISBN: 0849311667.

Cocaine: A Clinician's Handbook, Arnold M. Washton, Mark S. Gold. Guilford Press, 1999, ISBN: 0898627257.

Drug Treatments and Dementia (Bradford Dementia Group), Stephen Hopker. Jessica Kingsley Pub, 1999, ISBN: 185302760X.

Handbook of Psychopharmacotherapy, Philip G. Janicak. Lippincott, Williams & Wilkins, 1999, ISBN: 0683307223.

Herbal Medicines for Neuropsychiatric Diseases: Current Developments and Research, Shigenobu Kanba (Editor), Elliott Richelson (Editor). Brunner/Mazel, 1999, ISBN: 0876308043.

Medicating Schizophrenia: A History, Sheldon Gelman. Rutgers University Press, 1999, ISBN: 0813526434.

Methadone Treatment for Opioid Dependence, Eric C. Strain, Maxine L. Stitzer. Johns Hopkins University Press, 1999, ISBN: 0801861373.

Practice Guideline for the Treatment of Patients With Delirium, American Psychiatric Association. Amer Psychiatric Press, 1999, ISBN: 089042313X.

Psychiatric Treatment of the Medically Ill (Medical Psychiatry, 13), Robert G. Robinson, William R. Yates. Marcel Dekker, 1999, ISBN: 0824719581.

Psychologists' Neuropsychotropic Drug Reference, Louis A. Pagliaro, Ann M. Pagliaro. Brunner/Mazel, 1999, ISBN: 0876309562.

Psychopharmacology and Psychotherapy: A Collaborative Approach, Michelle B. Riba, M.D., Richard Balon, M.D. Amer Psychiatric Press, 1999, ISBN: 0880489138.

Psychopharmacology of Antipsychotics, Stephen M. Stahl. Dunitz Martin Ltd, 1999, ISBN: 185317601X.

Psychotherapist's Resource on Psychiatric Medications: Issues of Treatment and Referral, George Buelow, Suzanne Hebert. 1999, ISBN: 0534357032.

Recognition and Treatment of Psychiatric Disorders: A Psychopharmacology Handbook for Primary Care, Charles B. Nemeroff, Alan F. Schatzberg. Amer Psychiatric Press, 1999, ISBN: 0880489901.

Textbook of Treatment Algorithms in Psychopharmacology, Jan Fawcett. John Wiley & Sons, 1999, ISBN: 0471981095.

The Antidepressant Era, David Healy. Harvard University Press, 1999, ISBN: 0674039580.

The Behavioral Medicine Treatment Planner (Practice Planners), Douglas E. Degood. John Wiley & Sons, 1999, ISBN: 0471319236.

The Feeling Good Handbook, David D. Burns. Plume, 1999, ISBN: 0452281326.

The Hatherleigh Guide to Psychopharmacology, Frederic Flach. Hatherleigh Press, 1999, ISBN: 1578260221.

The Psychopharmacology Sourcebook, Mark Zetin. Lowell House, 1999, ISBN: 0737302666.

The Road To Eleusis: Unveiling the Secret of the Mysteries, R. Gordon Wasson. William Dailey Antiquarian, 1999, ISBN: 091514820X.

Zoloft, Paxil, Luvox and Prozac: All New Information to Help You Choose the Right Antidepressant, Donald L. Sullivan, Craig Williams. Avon, 1999, ISBN: 0380795183.

Psychotherapy

Basics of Group Psychotherapy, Harold S. Bernard (Editor), K. Roy MacKenzie (Editor). Guilford Press, 1999, ISBN: 0898621178.

Carl Rogers' Helping System: Journey and Substance, Godfrey T. Barrett-Lennard. Altamira Press, 1999, ISBN: 0761956778.

Cognitive Behavioral Therapies for Persons With Disabilities, Cynthia Radnitz. Jason Aronson, 1999, ISBN: 076570238X.

College Psychotherapy, Paul A. Grayson (Editor), Kate Cauley (Editor). Guilford Press, 1999, ISBN: 0898627478.

Counseling and Psychotherapy: An Integrated, Individual Psychology Approach, Don C. Dinkmeyer, Len Sperry, Don Dinkmeyer, Sr. Prentice Hall, 1999, ISBN: 0023296712.

Countertransference Issues in Psychiatric Treatment (Review of Psychiatry, Vol 18), Glen O. Gabbard (Editor). Amer Psychiatric Press 1999, ISBN: 0880489596.

Deleuze and Guattari's Anti-Oedipus: Introduction to Schizoanalysis, Eugene W. Holland. Routledge, 1999, ISBN: 0415113180.

Foundations and Applications of Group Psychotherapy: A Sphere of Influence (International Library of Group Analysis, 10), Mark F. Ettin. Jessica Kingsley Pub, 1999, ISBN: 1853027952.

Group Psychotherapy With Adult Children of Alcoholics: Treatment Techniques and Countertransference Considerations, Marsha Vannicelli. Guilford Press, 1999, ISBN: 0898625335.

Handbook of Counseling and Psychotherapy With Older Adults (Wiley Series in Adulthood and Aging), Michael Duffy (Editor). John Wiley & Sons, 1999, ISBN: 0471254614.

Healing Stories: Narrative in Psychiatry and Psychotherapy, Glenn Roberts (Editor), Jeremy Holmes (Editor). Oxford University Press, 1999, ISBN: 0192628275.

Intercultural Therapy: Themes, Interpretations, and Practice, Jafar Kareem (Editor), Roland Littlewood (Editor). Blackwell Science Inc, 1999, ISBN: 0632052244.

International Handbook of Cognitive and Behavioural Treatments for Psychological Disorders, V. E. Caballo (Editor). Pergamon Press, 1999, ISBN: 0080434339.

Journey from Anxiety to Freedom: Moving Beyond Panic and Phobias and Learning to Trust Yourself, Mani Feniger. Prima Pub (Pbk), 1999, ISBN: 0761508600.

Normal Family Processes (Guilford Family Therapy Series), Froma Walsh (Editor), Norma Walsh. Guilford Press, 1999, ISBN: 0898620902.

One Couple, Four Realities: Multiple Perspectives on Couple Therapy, Richard Chasin (Editor), Henry Grunebaum (Editor), Margaret Herzig (Editor), Eric Chasin. Guilford Press, 1999, ISBN: 0898620295.

Play Therapy With Children in Crisis: A Casebook for Practitioners, Nancy Boyd Webb (Editor). Guilford Press, 1999, ISBN: 0898627605.

Psychoanalytic Case Formulation, Nancy McWilliams. Guilford Press, 1999, ISBN: 1572304626.

Psychodynamic Group Psychotherapy, J. Scott Rutan (Editor), Walter N. Stone (Editor). Guilford Press, 1999, ISBN: 0898620961.

Reducing Spouse/Partner Abuse: A Psychoeducational Approach for Individuals & Couples, Robert Geffner, Carol Mantooth. Springer Pub Company, 1999, ISBN: 0826112692.

Supervision and Dramatherapy, Elektra Tselikas-Portmann (Editor). Jessica Kingsley Pub, 1999, ISBN: 1853027383.

The Collapse of the Self: And Its Therapeutic Restoration, Rochelle G. K. Kainer. Analytic Press, 1999, ISBN: 0881631671.

The Gay and Lesbian Psychotherapy Treatment Planner (Practice Planners), Arthur E. Jongsma, Michael Avriette. John Wiley & Sons, 1999, ISBN: 047135080X.

The Group Therapy Treatment Planner (Practice Planners.), Kim Paleg, Arthur E. Jongsma, Arthur Freeman, David Castro-Blanco. John Wiley & Sons, 1999, ISBN: 0471254681.

The Heart & Soul of Change: What Works in Therapy, Mark A. Hubble (Editor), Barry L. Duncan (Editor), Scott D. Miller (Editor). Amer Psychological Assn, 1999, ISBN: 155798557X.

The Older Adult Psychotherapy Treatment Planner (Practice Planners), Deborah W. Frazer, Arthur E. Jongsma, Jr. John Wiley & Sons, 1999, ISBN: 0471295744.

The Primary Triangle: A Developmental Systems View of Mothers, Fathers, and Infants, Antoinette Corboz-Warnery, Elizabeth Fivaz-Depeur. Basic Books, 1999, ISBN: 0465095828.

The Psychotherapy Documentation Primer (Practice Planners), Donald E. Wiger. John Wiley & Sons, 1999, ISBN: 0471289906.

The Therapeutic Purposes of Reminiscence, Mike Bender, Paulette Bauckham, Andrew Norris. Sage Pubns, 1999, ISBN: 0803976429.

Therapeutic Communities (Therapeutic Communities, No 2), Rex Haigh (Editor), Penelope Campling (Editor). Jessica Kingsley Pub, 1999, ISBN: 1853026263.

Therapy's Delusions: The Myth of the Unconscious and the Exploitation of Today's Walking Worried, Ethan Watters, Richard Ofshe. Simon & Schuster, 1999, ISBN: 0684835843.

What Psychotherapists Should Know about Disability, Rhoda Olkin, Ph.D. Guilford Press Cassettes, 1999, ISBN: 1572302275.

Women and Psychotherapy: An Assessment Research and Practice, Annette M. Brodsky (Editor), Rachel Hare-Mustin (Editor). Guilford Press, 1999, ISBN: 0898629098.

Religion

Integrating Spirituality into Treatment: Resources for Practitioners, William R. Miller (Editor). Amer Psychological Assn, 1999, ISBN: 1557985812.

Organized Religion and Seniors' Mental Health, Anthony J. Blasi. University Press of America, 1999, ISBN: 0761813489.

Sleep

Sleep: Evolution and Disorders, I. G. Karmanova, Genrikh A. Oganesyan, L. N. Smirnova (Translator). University Press of America, 1999, ISBN: 0761813748.

Sleep Medicine (Contemporary Neurology Series, 53), Michael S. Aldrich. Oxford University Press, 1999, ISBN: 0195129571.

Sports Psychiatry

Counseling in Sports Medicine, Richard Ray (Editor), Diane M. Wiese-Bjornstal (Editor). Human Kinetics Pub, 1999, ISBN: 0880115270.

Sport Psychiatry: Theory and Practice, Daniel Begel (Editor), Robert Burton (Editor). W W Norton & Company, 1999, ISBN: 0393702952.

Suicide

Review of Suicidology, 2000, Ronald W. Maris (Editor), Silvia Sara Canetto (Editor), John L. McIntosh (Editor), Morton M. Silverman (Editor). Guilford Press, 1999, ISBN: 1572305037.

Risk Management with Suicidal Patients, Bruce Bongar (Editor), Alan L. Berman (Editor), Ronald W. Maris (Editor), Eric A. Harris (Editor), Wendy L. Packman (Editor), Morton M. Silverman. Guilford Press, 1999, ISBN: 1572304987.

4. CONTINUING MEDICAL EDUCATION (CME)

4.1 Continuing Medical Education Resources

Accredited Council for Continuing Medical Education (ACCME) ⊙ ⊙ ⊙
http://www.accme.org

The Accredited Council for Continuing Medical Education offers voluntary accreditation to providers of continuing medical education who are interested in being recognized further for their high standards and quality. At the ACCME Web site visitors will discover necessary information regarding all aspects of the accreditation process, as well as the current activities of the organization regarding communications and quality control protocols.

American Medical Association (AMA): CME Locator ⊙ ⊙ ⊙
http://www.ama-assn.org/iwcf/iwcfmgr206/cme

The AMA CME Locator is a database of over 2,000 AMA Physician Recognition Award (PRA) Category I activities sponsored by CME providers accredited by the Accreditation Council for Continuing Medical Education or approved by the AMA. This site also lists conferences, seminars, workshops, and home study programs in the United States, Canada, and internationally.

American Medical Association (AMA): Online Continuing Medical Education (CME) ⊙ ⊙ ⊙
http://www.ama-assn.org/cmeselec/cmeselec.htm

This site provides online courses and the opportunity to earn credit by reviewing the available material and answering test questions. A CME certificate is mailed or faxed within three to four weeks after the completion of the course.

AudioPsych Online Continuing Medical Education in Mental Health ⊙ ⊙ ⊙ (some features fee-based)
http://audiopsych.com/courses

Audiopsych's continuing medical education online for mental health professionals has never been easier or more interactive. In the privacy of your home, users, after checking out minimal computer requirements, are encouraged to view online demonstrations of courses and register for the complete course thereafter. Course descriptions, demonstrations and information, credit hours per course, and total cost of these psychotherapy, assessment, and treatment approach course offerings are all conveniently listed.

CME at Physician's Guide ⊙ ⊙ ⊙
http://www.physiciansguide.com/cme.html

The Physician's Guide to the Internet offers links to Continuing Medical Education resources at this site. Examples include links to information on the MMWR *(Morbidity and Mortality Weekly Report)* Continuing Education Program and the American Medical Association's CME Locator. A short description of each link is provided.

CME Calendar 2000, APA ⊙ ⊙ ⊙
http://www.psych.org/pract_of_psych/cme_calendar.html

The APA provides a very useful calendar of CME courses organized by month at this location. A large number of course offerings are provided offering diversity and convenience.

CME Conferences ⊙ ⊙ ⊙ (some features fee-based)
http://www.mhsource.com/conf

Descriptions and information on CME, Inc.'s weekend conferences, held in the eastern and western U.S. and Canada, may be accessed by clicking on the registration buttons appearing next to each conference description. Agenda, credit, and tuition information are available for each entry. Conferences are also indexed by date and topic for convenience, and a Java-based, interactive calendar for basic and in-depth event information is provided. Orders may be placed at the CME InfoStore, by phone, or e-mail request.

CME Courses Online from Medical Matrix ⊙ ⊙ ⊙ (some features fee-based)
http://www.medmatrix.org

Medical Matrix's CME Courses Online is a one-stop resource for excellence in continuing medical education on the World Wide Web, with 39 accessible CME credit listing sites. General learning modules are available via Virtual Lecture Hall Health Professionals CME, HealthGate CME Courses, and Medscape's Online Articles for CME Reviews. The Cleveland Clinic Foundation, the National Institutes of Health, and Virtual Hospital Online all provide opportunities to access Internet-based CME courses, often with immediate feedback on performance. A multitude of top-rated CME modules and interesting feature sites include The Interactive Patient, which provides users with the ability to view a simulated online patient, request history, perform exams, and review diagnostic data. Credit fees vary by organization site.

CME PsychScapes WorldWide, Inc. ⊙ ⊙ ⊙
http://www.mental-health.com/mhwr.html

An extraordinarily extensive registry of workshops, CME programs, and conferences in the field of mental health are cycled through this site annual, providing "the largest such registry" on the Internet.

CME Resources ◎ ◎ ◎ (some features fee-based)
http://www.slis.ua.edu/cdlp/cme/UAB

From the University of Alabama comes this comprehensive listing of continuing medical education opportunities. Listings are available from a wide variety of sources including the American Medical Association, the American Academy of Family Physicians, the American College of Physicians, other medical associations, and CME conference Web pages. Registration and organization membership may be required for access to online course information and material.

CME Reviews: 1999 Guide to Psychotropic Drug Interactions ◎ ◎ ◎
http://mblcommunications.com/PP699_DeVane.html

CME Reviews offers online Continuing Medical Education courses for psychiatrists, neurologists, and primary care physicians. Professionals can read this full-text article with tables and graphs presenting data, review educational objectives, and take a quiz at the end of the article. Resources in the article include a table of generic and trade names of major psychotropic drugs, and tables presenting known interactions with benzodiazepine, buproprion, buspirone, arbamazepine, clozapine, haloperidol, lamotrigine, lithium, MAOI, methadone, methylphenidate, mirtazapine, netazodone, olanzapine, phenothiazine, quetiapine, risperidone, selected anoretic/anti-obesity, selected cholinesterase inhibitor, SSRIs, topiramate, valproate, venlaxafine, and zolpidem drugs.

CME Sites from Medical Computing Today ◎ ◎ ◎ (some features fee-based)
http://www.medicalcomputingtoday.com/0listcme.html

This Web site of Medical Computing Today presents an alphabetical listing of currently available category I CME credit offerings listed by the Accredited Council for Continuing Medical Education (ACCME). Principal areas of specialty covered at each of 85 sites are listed and directions for searching the text via Netscape Navigator are viewable. Alphabetical navigation bars throughout the text also enable visitors the opportunity to successfully locate educational materials of their choosing. CME descriptions, credits, and associated costs are included in CME entries. Registration for CME credit may be done at the individual, online sites.

CME Unlimited ◎ ◎ ◎
http://www.landesslezak.com/cgi-bin/start.cgi/cmeu/index.htm

This nonprofit division of Audio-Digest Foundation, specializes in producing audio CME programs for delivery to physicians and allied healthcare professionals on a subscription basis, providing high-quality selection of over 6,000 continuing medical education products from medical associations, institutions, and societies via audio, video, and CD-ROM. The offerings at this Web site include 13 specialty series and two jointly sponsored activities, with audio materials of medical symposia, review courses, and specialty meetings readily available. Each course listing includes its description, sponsor, target audience, accreditation, objectives, and faculty in addition to a list of currently available formats.

CMECourses.com ☉ ☉ ☉
http://www.cmesearch.com/search.asp?specialty=P

This free, searchable database yields over four pages of CME courses in the field of mental health. Conference dates, prices, activities, and contact information are here, along with links to further program details and registration information.

CMEWeb ☉ ☉ ☉
http://www.cmeweb.com/#pdr

Through CMEWeb, physicians can register through an online process, take electronic CME tests over the Internet, and receive feedback and credit. The questions on these tests are pulled from the American Health Consultants publications corresponding to the particular testing areas.

Continuing Education from the National
Institutes of Health (NIH) Consensus Development Program ☉ ☉ ☉
http://text.nlm.nih.gov/nih/upload-v3/Continuing_Education/cme.html

This continuing medical education site, sponsored by NIH and the Foundation for Advanced Education in the Sciences, invites users to participate in an online experiment in distance learning. CME credits may be earned upon successful completion of testing materials. Further offerings are scheduled to be added to the Web site, including past NIH Consensus Development Conference reviews.

Current CME Reviews: Psychiatry ☉ ☉ ☉ (some features fee-based)
http://www.cme-reviews.com

At this Web page, Current CME Reviews offers user-friendly, educational opportunities for the practicing psychiatrist, neurologist, and primary care provider. Courses presented here, offered in conjunction with the Mt. Sinai School of Medicine, offer numerous opportunities for professionals to test their knowledge of clinical educational materials prepared by noted experts in the field. Educational modules in alcoholism, depression, neuropsychiatry, and serotonin subsystems constitute a good portion of the opportunities available. CME certificates are mailed to physicians upon completion of online material and acceptance.

Cyberounds ☉ ☉ ☉
http://www.cyberounds.com/links/home.html

Cyberounds is an online, interactive forum moderated by distinguished professionals, and is available for use by physicians, medical students, and other selected healthcare professionals. All users must register to access resources at the site. Registration is free-of-charge but restricted to healthcare professionals. Continuing Medical Education opportunities, an online bookstore, links to quality sites relevant to a variety of specialties, and additional educational resources are available at the site.

Ed Credits ◎ ◎ ◎
http://www.edcredits.com

Ed Credits offers opportunities for Continuing Medical Education credits for medical and other professionals. Registration is available for an annual fee, and any number of courses can be taken within this time. Material for the courses is available for free on the Web site, but registration is necessary to take the tests and to receive certificates.

InterPsych ◎ ◎
http://www.shef.ac.uk/~psysc/InterPsych/inter.html

This site provides a large list of links to psychiatry-related online forums for professionals and other interested parties. Included are forums for major psychiatric disorders, psychotherapy, research design, telehealth, and computers in mental health. The scope of each forum is summarized, and information on the leader, membership, and other statistics are provided. The bylaws of the association and information regarding affiliation with InterPsych are present.

MedPharm ◎ ◎ ◎
http://www.medfarm.unito.it:80/education/psychiat.html

This site provides psychiatry-related learning modules for continuous education. Links are included to extensive references for psychiatric disorders, practice and treatment guidelines for depression, psychopharmacology information, screening practices for mental disorders and substance abuse, and clinical assessment in neuropsychiatry schedules.

MegaPsych Home Page ◎ ◎ ◎
http://www.tulsa.oklahoma.net/~jnichols/megapsych.html

MegaPsych was created by John Nichols in part from the publication, *Addresses of Note for Psychology Faculty and Students*, which is a list of discussion forums for both professionals and students. Also included are links to an online bookstore, a list of relevant online journals, articles on various psychological topics and links to additional articles, updated information, and a large list of psychology-related Web sites, including associations and research institutes.

MindText ◎ ◎
http://www.cortext.com/index.shtml

This site provides professionals and other interested persons with information on psychiatry and psychology related seminars within and outside of the United States, as well as the latest scientific reports on mental health issues. There are also literature and home education resources, training information, and information about the organizations that host this site.

National Medical Society Journal of
Psychiatry Continuing Medical Education ⊙ ⊙ ⊙ (fee-based)
http://www.ccspublishing.com/j_psych.htm

Continuing Medical Education resources specific to 39 psychiatric conditions and topics are available to paid, registered subscribers to this online journal. Representative topics include acute stress disorder, anorexia nervosa, antidepressant drug therapy, clinical evaluation of the psychiatric patient, delirium, hypochondriasis, major depressive episodes, mental disorders due to a medical condition, substance-related disorders, obsessive-compulsive disorder, and posttraumatic stress disorder.

New York University
Department of Psychiatry: Interactive Testing in Psychiatry ⊙ ⊙
http://www.med.nyu.edu/Psych/itp.html

The New York University Department of Psychiatry offers continuing education resources for psychiatrists and related professionals at this address. Professionals can complete up to seven modules, comprised of 30 questions each, and receive Continuing Medical Education credits from the University. Instant scoring and feedback are provided.

Newpromises.com ⊙ ⊙
http://www.caso.com/home/home.phtml

NewPromises.com, founded by Harvard University and MIT professors, is an online education program working closely with accredited institutions of higher learning to offer courses in a variety of fields including health topics. The site offers information on registration, financial aid, career advice, links to research material, textbook resources, and degree and certificate details.

5. PSYCHIATRY OVERVIEW SITES

5.1 Supersites

About.com: Mental Health Resources ⊙ ⊙ ⊙

http://mentalhealth.about.com/health/mentalhealth

This site provides current news on mental health issues, online forums devoted to mental health, and links to bulletin boards and online newsletters. Links are also included to additional resources, including academic psychology, associations and institutes, colleges and universities, consumer sites, information on various mental health disorders, journals and publications, managed care, men's and women's resources, professional resources, self-help resources, trauma, and stress management.

American Psychiatric Association (APA) ⊙ ⊙ ⊙

http://www.psych.org

The American Psychiatric Association is a national and international association of psychiatric physicians. The site includes updates, public policy and advocacy information, clinical and research resources, membership information, medical education, related organizations, governance, library and publications, events schedule, psychiatric news, APA catalog, and a link to APPI (APA Press Inc.).

Internet Mental Health: Resources ⊙ ⊙ ⊙

http://Freenet.msp.mn.us/ip/stockley/mental_health.html

The Twin Cities Freenet provides an extensive listing of links to academic, clinical, and commercial sites at this address. Sites are divided into sections and are listed in alphabetical order. Sections include disorder/disease, field of study (such as cognitive psychology, psychotherapy, etc.), mailing lists, libraries, drugs, collaboration information, organizations, statistical information, and other relevant categories.

MedMark: Psychiatry ⊙ ⊙ ⊙

http://www.medmark.org/psy

Medmark, offering extensive listings of medical resources by specialty, serves as a valuable online directory for psychiatric resources worldwide. A sidebar table of contents makes finding direct connections to psychiatric organizations, institutions, and information a fast and simple procedure. Visitors can scroll down the listings of associations, hospitals, laboratories, governmental sites, journals, publications, programs, and projects related to psychiatry, or, alternatively, can click on the sidebar menu to jump directly to the desired section. Medmark's one-stop psychiatry resource also presents connections to a variety of therapy and treatment information sources as well as hundreds of pages of interesting, consumer-oriented information.

MedNets ○ ○ ○

http://www.Internets.com/mednets/spsychia.htm

Provided by the MedNets Community, professionals and the public will find links to numerous searchable psychiatry databases and Web sites. The Web sites are divided into sections including clinical information, diseases, news and research, subspecialty and esoteric fields, centers of excellence, and miscellaneous links (such as general psychiatry links and various sites provided by the British Medical Journal). There is also a section devoted to patient information that lists Web sites and databases relating to psychiatry and mental health.

Medscape: Psychiatry ○ ○ ○ (free registration)

http://psychiatry.medscape.com/home/misc/redirHost.cfm?/psychiatry.medscape.com

Medscape's psychiatry division includes extensive links and information on treatment updates, conference summaries and schedules, news, practice guidelines, journals and books, patient resources, and other links relevant to the practice of psychiatry.

Mental Health Links ○ ○ ○

http://www.mentalhealth.org/links/KENLINKS.htm

Organized alphabetically, this important Web resource provides a listing of more than 50 subject areas related to mental health, each of which is a link to a listing of further in-depth resources. It has been assembled by the Center for Mental Health Services, a division of the Mental Health Services Administration. Topics include abuse, advocacy, accessibility, aging, alternative treatment, Alzheimer's disease, anxiety, and dozens of others.

Mental Health Matters ○ ○ ○

http://www.mental-health-matters.com/resources.html

Mental Health Matters is designed to provide online resources for psychiatric professionals, students, and mental health consumers, and their families. Links are included to mental health research sites, organized according to disorder, statistics, workshops and notices, mental health law, psychiatric libraries, professional societies, searchable databases, and a list of speakers providing seminars on mental health. Also, a list of mental health meetings and conferences, and numerous links to psychophar-macology, assessment and diagnostic tools, case management and clinical resources, grant and funding sources, managed care, rehabilitation, and education resources, and a list of general psychiatry-related links are found at the site.

Mental Health Net ○ ○ ○

http://mentalhelp.net

Mental Health Net, an award-winning Web site, provides professionals with informa-tive links to resources on assessment issues, associations and organizations, therapy and diagnostic listings, grant information, medication, neuropsychology, psychiatry and law, academic departments, journals and newsgroups, employment opportunities, continuing education, government departments, and mental health-related products (books, software, etc.). Services for professionals listed at the site include conferences and workshop links, clinical yellow pages, and links to journal articles. Also, links to managed health care information, news, and online forums are provided. Public resources include free online books, chat rooms, therapist listings, disorders and treatment links, and a link for online psychiatric advice.

MentalHealthSource.com Directory ⚙ ⚙ ⚙

http://www.mhsource.com/hy/links.html

Organized alphabetically by topic area, the user-friendly MentalHealthSource.com Directory provides over 20 CNS disorder categories, 12 mental health-related topic divisions, journals and news, treatment approaches and literature, and continuing medical education links. An academic department connects the user with top-ranked psychology and psychiatry university programs, and the assessment grouping provides a worthy source of screening and diagnostic tools for the healthcare provider and patient alike. A comprehensive listing of links to most major mental health organizations is provided. Here, physician and patient users will find ample information and resources on virtually all aspects of the mental health field.

Neurosciences on the Internet ⚙ ⚙ ⚙

http://www.neuroguide.com

This site contains a large searchable index of neuroscience resources. Links are included to clinical departments and centers, databases, diseases, exams and tutorials, neuroscience Internet guides, images, journals, mailing lists, online forums, associations, software, and general information about the World Wide Web for new users.

Online Psych ⚙ ⚙

http://www.allhealth.com/onlinepsych

Online Psych provides links to articles, fact sheets, Web sites, forums, reference materials, and general information on major psychiatric and mental health disorders. Additional resources include an online bookstore for psychiatry-related materials and a searchable therapist directory.

Psychiatry Online ⚙ ⚙ ⚙

http://www.priory.com/psych.htm

Based in Great Britain, this address provides brief and case reports, an archive of professional documents, crosscultural mental health resources, news, a bulletin board, links to resources specific to child and adolescent psychiatry, forensic psychiatry resources, current research articles, Continuing Medical Education (CME) materials, a forum for students, a side-effect registry, and links to worldwide psychiatry resources and other related sites. Links are also provided to similar resources produced from Italy and Brazil. Users can search the site for specific information and order books and other products at the site. Similar resources are available through links at this site in the areas of chest medicine, general practice, lifestyle issues, family practice, and pharmacy. This site is supported by an unrestricted educational grant from AstraZeneca.

PSYweb.com ⊙ ⊙ ⊙

http://www.psyweb.com

PSYweb.com serves as a database of information on all aspects of psychiatry. Informative links are divided into sections on physiology, the brain, drugs, and mental health. Physiology links include a glossary of terms in physiological psychology, and the brain section provides anatomical information. Information under the drugs subheading is indexed according to trade, generic, and Canadian name, and provides links to in-depth fact sheets on the pharmaceutical profile and use of the drug. Information on drug indications in treating psychiatric diseases is also included. The mental health section is indexed according to clinical or cognitive disorders, common names, mental retardation, or personality disorder. Comprehensive disorder information includes a definition, diagnostic criteria, treatments, and other relevant information. Case studies, a glossary, reference lists, axis/disorder flow charts, mental disorder diagnosis sheets, specific disorder treatment plans, downloadable demonstrations, IQ testing, and other related links are present.

5.2 General Resources for Psychiatry

Ascend ⊙ ⊙ ⊙

http://members.tripod.com/~ascend2/index.html

This site has links to information, support, organizations, case studies, and other sites related to depression, grief, eating disorders, anxiety, personality disorders, stress disorders, psychoses, attention-deficit/hyperactivity disorder, children's topics, treatment, and other relevant subjects. Books and other reference materials, as well as professional training information, can be found.

At Health, Inc. ⊙ ⊙ ⊙

http://www.athealth.com

The professional resources available at this Web site include newsletters regarding mental health information, treatment centers, a directory of mental health professionals, continuing education and medication information, a reference list, online articles, an extensive list of information about mental health disorders, and practice tools. This Web site also has directories of licensed mental health therapists and treatment centers, a list of books, and an online bookstore. The resources section has numerous links to information about disorders and treatments, support groups and organizations related to mental health. Topics links provide general information about common mental health disorders. Guest articles from mental health professionals and medication information is also readily available.

CyberPsychLink ◎ ◎

http://cctr.umkc.edu/user/dmartin/psych2.html

This resource inventory of sites related to psychology and psychiatry provides links to databases, newsletters and online journals, employment and funding information, listservers, organizations, psychology software, a link to sites on teaching, and the history of psychology. In addition, there are links to self-help pages, general and specific psychology sites, and library catalogs.

Doctor's Guide: the Internet—Psychiatry ◎ ◎ ◎

http://www.pslgroup.com

This easily searchable medical news and conference database provides links to the latest information about psychiatry and related mental illness topics, including diagnosis and treatment of a variety of psychiatric disorders, as well as comprehensive conference and meeting details.

Health Education Board for Scotland (HEBS) Web: Mental Health ◎ ◎

http://www.hebs.scot.nhs.uk/menus/mental.htm

This site contains links to comprehensive fact sheets on common mental health disorders such as anxiety, grief, depression, eating disorders, phobias, stress, and schizophrenia. The fact sheets contain information on causes, treatment, and other topics. Also, there is a list of mental health related journal articles, information on leaflet ordering, mental health statistics, and support organizations.

Leicester University Library— Major Information Sources for Psychiatry ◎ ◎ ◎

http://www.le.ac.uk/library/sources/subject8/lisupsic.html

Links to major online databases, including MEDLINE, PSYCHInfo, BIDS-EMBASE, and the Cochrane Library are available at this site, including a paragraph summarizing the resources. Links to more general databases, institutes, and societies are also listed at the site.

MedExplorer: Mental Health ◎ ◎ ◎

http://www.medexplorer.com/category.dbm?category=Mental%5FHealth

As a service of MedExplorer's megasite, this innovative, mental health section offers an extensive resource listing with over 80 links to some unique subjects in the field of psychology and psychiatry. Included are the topics of dreams and nightmares, software to eradicate emotions, who's who in mental health, ultra-sensitive people, and a host of other distinctive subjects not found elsewhere. Basic mental health links are also included, as is a powerful site search engine. Over 250 health/medical newsgroups may be searched and MedExplorer Chat lets the user log in and chat with other like-minded users.

MedInfoSource ⊚ ⊚

http://www.medinfosource.com

This comprehensive Web site allows access to online articles from Medicine and Behavior, and has links to the latest medical psychiatric news, an interactive conference calendar, information on continuing education and an "ask the expert" section for consumers. In addition, users can search a classified section for practice opportunities, products, residencies, and fellowships. The site also contains a number of other resources, including links to related mailing lists, association meetings, professional practices, drug development process and manufacturers, managed care companies, practice guidelines, medical and mental health association addresses, and treatment centers.

Medscout: Mental Health ⊚ ⊚ ⊚

http://www.medscout.com/mental_health/index.htm

This Web site hosts a great number of links to mental health organizations, associations, mental health disorders information, position papers, national institutes and centers, and many links to general mental health information on the Internet. In addition, the site is searchable and contains links to clinical news, reference materials and products, alternative medicine, education, government issues, practice guidelines, hospitals and management, pharmaceutical information, research information, and telemedicine.

Mental Health InfoSource ⊚ ⊚ ⊚

http://www.mhsource.com

Resources available for professionals at this site include mental health news, conference calendars, chat forums, question and answer forums, employment listings, pharmaceutical drug information, physician directories, association links, and managed care contact details. Continuing Medical Education resources are available through an online store. Patients and caregivers are offered articles, support resources, and information on specific disorders. Specific disorder sections presenting answers to consumer and professional questions, articles, current research updates, links to related sites, conference listings, and other resources are available for schizophrenia, bipolar disorders, AD/HD, depression, and many other topics. The site also offers a search engine and quick directory of resources.

Mental Health Internet Resources ◎ ◎

http://www.mirconnect.com/index.html

This site serves as a home of mental health resources on the Internet. There is a directory of psychiatric therapists in the Chicago area, hotlines to local and national mental health organizations, a list of mental health terms and fact sheets, links to medical publication search engines, and a professional network.

Mental Help ◎ ◎ ◎

http://www.mentalhelp.com/Mental_Help_wellcome.htm

Within this internationally based Web site, links to information on the major psychiatric illnesses, including diagnosis and treatment are available. Professionals can organize clinical discussions online and access a doctor referral database, a variety of psychiatry-related journals and other publications, and a large list of other mental health-related Web sites.

Multimedia Medical Reference Library: Psychiatry ◎ ◎

http://www.med-library.com/medlibrary/Medical_Reference_Library/Psychiatry

This useful site provides links to documents, articles, Web sites, images and other Internet resources on common psychiatry topics, including diseases and disorders, therapeutic drugs, psychological therapies, support and professional organizations, newsgroups, and discussion lists.

Planet Psych ◎ ◎

http://www.planetpsych.com/index.htm

Primarily for consumers, this site offers online counseling, a searchable therapist directory, self-help exercises and information, a newsletter, bulletin board, and chat room. Links are available to mental disorders fact sheets and related sites, arranged according to diagnostic classifications defined by *DSM-IV*. Included are fact sheets on related mental health issues, such as anger management, substance abuse, parenting, behavioral health, relationship and sexuality issues, cyberpsychology, child development and other issues, as well as basic information on psychiatric and psychological treatments.

Psychiatric Disorder Info Center ◎ ◎ ◎

http://www.neuroland.com/psychiat.htm

As part of Neuroland's information for medical professionals, this Web page has links to information on diagnosis, assessment, and treatment for various disorders, such as anxiety disorders, depression, bipolar disorders, delirium, and somatic syndromes. There are links to information on various treatments and drugs, such as neuroleptics, antidepressants, and other treatments. In addition, there are links to virtual hospitals (which provide clinical practice guidelines) specializing in anxiety, mood disorders, and psychiatric emergencies.

ShakeyNet Mental Health Resources ○ ○ ○

http://www.shakey.net

This nonprofit organization provides mental health information on disorders, treatment, professionals, and other topics. For each disorder listed there are a number of links available. In addition, there are many sites listed providing information on medications, treatments, and psychopharmacology, consumer resources, home pages, professional resources, and other links.

Virtual Hospital: Patient Information
by Organ System: Neurological/Psychiatric ○ ○ ○

http://www.vh.org/Patients/IHB/OrgSys/NeuroPsych.html

This Web site has lists to patient education reference materials on a variety of topics including common psychiatric disorders, such as depression and attention-deficit/hyperactivity disorder, and neurological problems, such as facial nerve and brain injury. Additional resources are included on various assessment tests and techniques, hearing-related issues, pain clinics, Tourette's disorder, Trichotillomania, and sleep disorders.

Who's Who in Mental Health on the Web ○ ○

http://www.idealist.com/wwmhw

Professionals and consumers can obtain informative profiles of mental health professionals listed by state, country, or view all profiles. Professionals can add their own profile, and this site also contains links to related Web sites.

5.3 General Resources for Psychology

Academy of Psychological Clinical Science ○ ○

http://w3.arizona.edu/~psych/apcs/apcs.html

The Academy of Psychological Clinical Science is an alliance of leading and scientifi-cally-oriented doctoral training programs in clinical and health psychology in the United States and Canada. The site includes links to the various academic members, a list of officers, a mission statement, membership information, a history of the Academy and a link to related Web sites.

American Academy of Doctors of Psychology ◎ ◎ ◎

http://www.doctorsofpsychology.org

This site allows access to a directory of psychologists in the United States, and a large number of links to information about psychology and psychological disorders and treatment. In addition, there are links of interest to doctors, including specialties, media and literature information, as well as academy membership information. Graduates and students will find links to related organizations, as well as license, training, and employment information. Selected articles from the *Psychological Letter* are available online. Numerous online services, such as newsgroups and other listservers are present.

American Psychological Association (APA) ◎ ◎ ◎ (fee-based)

http://www.apa.org

The American Psychological Association Web site provides numerous links including reference materials, publications, national and international research sites, education, conferences, government information, and help centers. Comprehensive information regarding the Association itself is present.

American Psychological Society (APS) ◎ ◎ ◎

http://www.psychologicalscience.org

The American Psychological Society aims to provide a forum for research and application to the science of psychology. The site offers information regarding membership, current news, conventions, and APS publications. Updates on funding opportunities and legislative events relevant to psychology are provided.

Community Psychology Net ◎ ◎

http://www.cmmtypsych.net

This award-winning Web site serves both consumers and professionals with several links to sites and information on discussion lists, professional societies, education information, grant information, reference materials, including courses, and employment. There are links for students and others interested in graduate school, conferences, books, career choices, or the latest news. A bulletin board and library are also present.

Health Psychology and Rehabilitation ◎ ◎ ◎

http://www.healthpsych.com/index.html

This site provides resources relating to the practice of psychology in medical and rehabilitation settings. There is online access to articles, viewpoints, and general information about health psychology, practice and research information, a reference list and bookstore, information about disorders and treatment, Batter for Health Improvement (BHI) news and information, and links to mailing lists of interest. In addition, there is a section of links regarding psychologists as primary healthcare providers.

Health Psychology on the Net   ◉ ◉

http://www.pitt.edu/~tawst14/healthpsy.htm

This site provides links to resources on doctoral programs in health psychology, news updates in the field of health psychology, related organizations, education and training opportunities, journals, library databases, funding opportunities, employment resources, an online forum, and links to general psychology sites.

NetPsychology   ◉ ◉ ◉

http://www.netpsych.com

This database of information and links provides professionals and consumers with the opportunity to access Internet information relating to psychology. Included are links to relevant articles, including mental health disorders and treatments, general information on psychological disorders, and other topics of interest to professionals. There are lists of newsgroups, discussion groups, links to alternative or non-mainstream sites related to psychology, as well as a search feature.

Psych Net Mental Health   ◉ ◉

http://members.tripod.com/~Psycat/PsychNet.html

Summaries of the description, symptoms, treatment, and support information for various mental health issues, such as abuse, eating disorders, personality disorders, and suicide can be found at this site. In addition, there are links to hotline directories and related Web pages.

Psychology Information Online   ◉ ◉ ◉

http://www.psychologyinfo.com

Created by a licensed psychologist, this site serves as a clearinghouse of resources, including links to sites and very informative and detailed fact sheets on various topics in psychology. Included is a national directory of psychologists, practice information, an extensive amount of resources on psychological disorders, information about psychologists and psychiatrists, answers to frequently asked questions (FAQs) on psychological treatments, forensic psychology resources, a list of self-help books, and information on psychological treatments in general. The information presented within this site can by viewed by descriptive links, general links, or by using a topic index.

PsychREF: Resources in Psychology on the Internet   ◉ ◉ ◉

http://maple.lemoyne.edu/~hevern/psychref.html

The homepage lists resources to search engines, journals, professional associations related to psychology, as well as providing a large amount of information on educational materials, research information, conferences, online courses, and jobs. In addition, there are links to resources in clinical psychology, pharmacology, disorders, neuropsychology, developmental psychology, and many other topics.

Psychweb ⊙ ⊙ ⊙
http://www.psychweb.com

This very informative site hosts an extensive amount of psychology related resources, divided into topics such as depression, behavior, biofeedback, cognition, disorders, government, learning, megasites (sites allowing users to search many sites from one location), personality, organizations, academic departments, counseling, publications, and tests. Each topic site has links to relevant Web pages, support groups, personal pages, government institutes, associations, articles, and other resources.

Warren Bush's Psychology Cyber-Synapse ⊙ ⊙
http://www.umm.maine.edu/BEX/Lehman/HomePage.Stuff/text/PSYCHOCYBER.html

This site provides numerous links to Web sites and other online resources on psychology related organizations, university departments, databases, bibliographies, and other reference sources, mailing lists and newsgroups, online journals, self-help, and links to fact sheets and other resources on mental disorders and other related issues.

5.4 **Awards and Honors**

Introduction
Public recognition of important contributions in medicine is achieved through awards and honors from major educational, scientific, nonprofit, and corporate organizations. We have included many such awards in this section. Awards and honors are subject to change at any time, however, and some awards may not be granted every year. Organizations periodically discontinue awards, change their terms and qualifications, or add new awards and honors. For these reasons, the reader should visit these Web sites directly to obtain the latest information on current awards and honors.

Achievement

Administrative Psychiatry Award
http://www.psych.org/opps_man/appg.html

An honorarium of $500 and a plaque are presented to a clinical executive making significant improvements in the management of mental health delivery systems, and serves as a role model for other psychiatrists.

Agnes Purcell McGavin Award

http://www.psych.org/opps_man/appg.html

A $1,000 honorarium and certificate, presented at the American Psychiatric Association convocation will be granted to a psychiatrist working in the preventative aspects of childhood emotional disorders, through framing concepts, developing proofs, or creating applications.

APA Assembly Warren Williams Awards

http://www.psych.org/opps_man/appg.html

Annual awards of $1,000 are conferred, either in whole or in part to the winners for recognition of distinguished contribution or activity in psychiatry and mental health.

Arnold L. van Ameringen Award in Psychiatric Rehabilitation

http://www.psych.org/opps_man/appg.html

This award of approximately $5,000 and a plaque are awarded to the individual, institution, or organization providing significant contribution to the field of psychiatric rehabilitation.

Bruno Lima Award for Excellence in Disaster Psychiatry

http://www.psych.org/opps_man/appg.html

An award certificate, personal recognition in Psychiatric News, and in the annual program will serve as recognition for exemplary contributions in the care and understanding of disaster victims by district branch members.

Isaac Ray Award in Memory of Margaret Sutermeister

http://www.psych.org/opps_man/appg.html

The award of $1,500 will be presented in even-numbered years to a person who has made notable contributions in the field of forensic psychiatry or the psychiatric aspect of jurisprudence. The winner will present a lecture or series of lectures on the subject(s) and publish their manuscript.

Jack Weinberg Memorial Award for Geriatric Psychiatry

http://www.psych.org/opps_man/appg.html

A plaque and $500 will be presented to a psychiatrist for their leadership or significant contribution in clinical practice, training, or research in the field of geriatric psychiatry.

Jacob Javits Public Service Award

http://www.psych.org/opps_man/appg.html

Presented to a public servant in recognition of their contributions to the field of mental health, award recipients will receive an honorarium of $1,000.

Kun-Po Soo Award (previously the Asian American Award)

http://www.psych.org/opps_man/appg.html

The winner of this award, which is presented in recognition of their significant contributions on the subject of Asian culture heritage and psychiatry, will receive $1,000 and may be asked to present a lecture at the American Psychiatric Association (APA) annual meeting. Nominees need not be Asians, Americans, APA members, or psychiatrists.

Norbert and Charlotte Rieger Award for Scientific Achievement

http://www.aacap.org/Web/aacap/awards/awards.htm

A $5,000 award is given to a child and adolescent psychiatrist who has published in the past year the most important paper in the *Journal of the American Academy of Child and Adolescent Psychiatry*.

Oskar Pfister Award

http://www.psych.org/opps_man/appg.html

The recipient of this award will be recognized for their significant contribution in the area of psychiatry and religion, and will receive a $1,000 honorarium, plaque, and a chance to present their work at the American Psychiatric Association (APA) annual meeting.

Simon Wile Award

http://www.aacap.org/Web/aacap/awards/awards.htm

This $1,000 honorarium is presented to a psychiatrist who has demonstrated leadership and significant contributions in the field of liaison child and adolescent psychiatry.

Solomon Carter Fuller Award

http://www.psych.org/opps_man/appg.html

A $500 honorarium and plaque are presented to an African-American citizen having made great improvements in an area of psychiatry, resulting in an enhanced quality of life for African Americans.

Authorship

Elaine Schlosser Lewis Award for
Research on AttentionDeficit Disorder

http://www.aacap.org/Web/aacap/awards/awards.htm

This annual award of $5,000 acknowledges the Journal's best paper on AD/HD written by a child and adolescent psychiatrist.

Francis J. Braceland Award for Public Service

http://www.psych.org/opps_man/appg.html

This award of $500 and a plaque is presented every other year to a member of the American Psychiatric Association who has made significant contributions as an author, spokesperson, and publicist in the service of the mentally ill and disabled.

Manfred S. Guttmacher Award

http://www.psych.org/opps_man/appg.html

This award, co-sponsored by the American Psychiatric Association and the American Academy of Psychiatry and the Law, is presented annually for substantial contributions to the literature of forensic psychiatry, presented at any professional meeting or published in the previous year. An honorarium of $500, up to $500 travel expenses to non-member winners, and an additional $500 honorarium will be given upon presentation of the literature at the American Psychiatric Association annual meeting.

Robert T. Morse Writer's Award

http://www.psych.org/opps_man/appg.html

This annual award of $1,000 and a plaque presented at the American Psychiatric Association (APA) convocation is given to popular writer(s) who have promoted public understanding of psychiatry and mental illness.

Educational

Nancy C. A. Roeske Certificate of Recognition for Excellence in Medical Student Education

http://www.psych.org/opps_man/appg.html

A certificate is awarded in recognition of American Psychiatric Association members or fellows that have contributed significantly to medical student education.

Pfizer Pharmaceuticals— Visiting Professorship Program in Psychiatry

http://Web.ortge.ufl.edu/fyi/v24n06/fyi033.html

A $6,000 award will be given to promote interchange between visiting scientists, scholars, physicians, and academics associated with medical school psychiatry departments in the United States.

Fellowship

APA Lilly Psychiatric Research Fellowship

http://www.psych.org/res_res/lilly.html

This one-year fellowship of $35,000 will be awarded to a resident that has significant research potential in the fields of either general or child psychiatry.

Lectureships

Adolf Meyer Lectureship

http://www.psych.org/opps_man/appg.html

This lectureship serves to promote exchange of new research information between outstanding scientists and psychiatrists in order to improve psychiatric research. A $3,000 honorarium will be awarded, and the winner will present a lecture at the American Psychiatric Association annual meeting.

Award for Patient Advocacy

http://www.psych.org/opps_man/appg.html

This award of $2,000, a plaque, and an opportunity to present a lecture during the APA annual meeting will be given to a public figure for their personal achievements, their promotion of improving the services for people with mental disorders and those coping with substance abuse, and for speaking about mental illness and psychiatric treatment experiences.

Benjamin Rush Lectureship

http://www.psych.org/opps_man/appg.html

This lectureship is awarded to a person who has made significant contributions to the history of psychiatry, and may include professionals from that field, or other fields such as medical history or anthropology. The honorarium is $1,000 for member winners and $500 for nonmember winners.

Seymour D. Vestermark Award for Psychiatric Education

http://www.psych.org/opps_man/appg.html

A $1,000 honorarium and an opportunity to present a lecture at the American Psychiatric Association (APA) annual meeting will be given to an educator that has made great contributions to undergraduate, graduate or postgraduate education, and career development in psychiatry.

Simon Bolivar Lecture

http://www.psych.org/opps_man/appg.html

This award of $500 and a plaque honors a prominent Hispanic statesman or spokesperson, and is designed to educate the American Psychiatric Association (APA) membership about the problems and goals of Hispanics. The winner presents a lecture at the APA annual meeting.

Research and Investigation

A.E. Bennet Neuropsychiatric Research Foundation Awards

http://www.sobp.org

Annual awards of $1,500 are presented to young investigators in basic and clinical research in the field of biological psychiatry.

Alexander Gralnick, M.D. Award

http://www.psych.org/sched_events/ann_mtg_99/gralnick.html

This annual award of $4,000 acknowledges the research contributions of psychiatrists working in early diagnosis and treatment of schizophrenia.

American Psychiatric Institute for Research and Education/Janssen Scholars in Research on Severe Mental Illness

http://www.psych.org/res_res/janssen.html

This new fellowship program, co-sponsored by the American Psychiatric Institute for Research and Education and Janssen Pharmaceutica, awards promising PGY-1, PGY-2, and PGY-3 psychiatric residents $5,000 during the second year of a two-year fellowship, assisting in research career development. A research mentor, chosen from nationally recognized leaders in clinical and health services research, will be assigned to oversee the resident's fellowship. Funds for travel to the APA Annual Meeting are also provided during the two years of fellowship. This program specifically encourages awardees to pursue careers in clinical and health services research in areas related to schizophrenia, bipolar illness, and other severe mental diseases. Applications and other materials can be downloaded from this address.

APA Award for Research

http://www.psych.org/opps_man/appg.html

An honorarium of $5000 is given to recognize a body of work or lifetime contribution having major impact on the field of psychiatry.

APA Early Career and Senior
Scholar Health Services Research Awards

http://www.psych.org/libr_publ/hsrawrd.html

The American Psychiatric Association will give an honorarium of $1,000 each to both an early career psychiatrist who has published the best nominated paper, and to a senior scholar with significant research contributions in the mental health services field.

APA Kempf Fund Award

http://www.psych.org/res_res/kempf.html

This $1,500 award will be presented to a senior researcher who has made meaningful contribution to schizophrenia research. In addition, $20,000 will be awarded to a young research psychiatrist working with the senior researcher award winner in a mentor-trainee relationship.

APA SmithKline Beecham Young Faculty Award

http://www.psych.org/res_res/beecham.html

This stipend of $35,000 will be awarded to a junior faculty member in the field of Biology and Psychopharmacology of mood disorders in order to support their research.

Association for the Treatment of
Sexual Abusers (ATSA)—Graduate Student Research Grant

http://www.atsa.com/pages/grant.html

Grants for up to $15,000 will be awarded for Graduate Student Investigator projects that provide new and original research on the treatment and causes of sexual abuse.

Blanche F. Ittleson Award for Research in Child Psychiatry

http://www.psych.org/opps_man/appg.html

An award of $2,000 and a plaque are presented to a child psychiatrist or group for their published research on children's mental health.

Hofheimer Prize: Award for Research in Psychiatry

http://www.psych.org/sched_events/ann_mtg_99/psych_award.html

This award is given to acknowledge lifetime contribution in the field of psychiatry, or a significant contribution or body of work that has had a major impact in the psychiatric field. The Hofheimer Prize is the most significant award for research granted by the American Psychiatric Association.

Irving Phillips Award for Prevention

http://www.aacap.org/Web/aacap/awards/awards.htm

This $2,500 award is presented annually to the Academy member and child and adolescent psychiatrists who have made significant lifetime research contributions, a body of work, or a single book, paper, or project in the discipline of child and adolescent mental illness prevention.

Marie H. Eldredge Award

http://www.psych.org/opps_man/appg.html

This $1,000 award is presented to an American Psychiatric Association (APA) member or resident working in Hawaii, Pennsylvania, or New Jersey whose research focuses on the cause and treatment of neuroses and retarded persons.

William T. Grant Foundation

http://fdncenter.org/grantmaker/wtgrant/scholars.html

This award, given to early career research in social and behavioral sciences, focuses on resilience and vulnerability to stress, and on factors that shape child and youth development. Awards up to $50,000 per year for five years will be made to the applicant's institution.

Ziskind-Somerfeld Research Foundation

http://www.sobp.org

Senior investigators in the field of biological psychiatry and members in good standing of the Society of Biological Psychiatry are eligible for annual awards of $2,500 in either basic or clinical research, with the purpose of stimulating investigations in psychiatry.

5.5 Psychiatry Grant and Funding Sources

Introduction

For additional information on grants and funding, see the profile of the National Institute of Mental Health later in this section, and also see "Grant and Award Guides" under "Professional Medical Topics" in part two of this volume.

American Psychiatric Association (APA) Roster of Awards

http://www.psych.org/opps_man/appg.html

Forty different awards conferred through the American Psychiatric Association are profiled at this site, each with detailed information on the name of the award, the purpose of the award, the type of recognition, and monetary aspects. Most of these awards are included separately in "Awards and Honors" section of this volume. Those interested in awards should visit this APA site, since awards change, are added, and are eliminated from time to time.

Links to Funding Sources ⚙

http://www.behavior.org/links/links_fund.html

A compilation of 14 links to sites offering information on research grants and funding is provided at this section of the Cambridge Center for Behavioral Studies Web site. Connections include the National Science Foundation, *Center for Biomedical Research Newsletter,* the National Institute of Mental Health (NIMH) Guide for Grants and Contracts, and the National Institutes of Health (NIH).

Mental Health Net: Grants Online ⚙ ⚙ ⚙

http://mentalhelp.net/guide/pro28.htm

This address lists major Internet sites providing grants information, including foundations, associations, universities, and government institutes. Grants listed cover all areas of research and scholarship. Each site link is listed with a rating and detailed description of resources found at the site. Sources for articles, publications, and software related to grant writing are also found through this site.

Program for Minority Research Training in Psychiatry (PMRTP) ⚙ ⚙

http://www.psych.org/res_res/pmrtp.html

This program, designed to increase the number of underrepresented minority men and women in the field of psychiatric research, is fully described at the PMRTP Web site. Program goals, eligibility, training sites, and application information are summarized.

Programs Offering Research Fellowship Opportunities ⚙ ⚙ ⚙

http://www.psych.org/res_res/fellowship_opportunities.html

Organized by research field, over 30 links are provided to psychiatric fellowships at some of the finest research facilities in the nation. Neuroscience at Vanderbilt, Geriatric Psychiatry at Johns Hopkins, and Addictions Psychiatry at New York University are a few in this collection of opportunities.

Research Fellowship Directory for Psychiatry ⚙ ⚙ ⚙

http://www.psych.org/res_res/fellow.html

This online directory of research fellowship opportunities in psychiatry is organized alphabetically by state or Canadian province. As a preliminary screening tool, users may use their own judgment to evaluate the merits and drawbacks of specific programs and the research training they offer.

Van Ameringen Foundation/
APA Health Services Research Scholars ◉ ◉ ◉

http://www.psych.org/res_res/vanam.html

With support from this organization, the American Psychiatric Association (APA), utilizes several important data sets containing information on utilization, costs, and outcomes related to mental healthcare. The Web site describes the organization's mission to make these data sets more widely available to the mental health researcher through encouragement of research. Online information regarding application information is provided.

5.6 National Institute of Mental Health (NIMH) Profile

National Institute of Mental Health (NIMH) ◉ ◉ ◉

http://www.nimh.nih.gov/home.htm

The National Institute of Mental Health provides national leadership dedicated to understanding, treating, and preventing mental illnesses through basic research on the brain and behavior, and through clinical, epidemiological, and services research. Resources available at the site include staff directories, information for visitors to the campus, employment opportunities, NIMH history, and publications from activities of the National Advisory Mental Health Council and Peer Review Committees. News, a calendar of events, and information on clinical trials, funding opportunities, and intramural research are also provided. Pages tailored specifically for use by the public, health practitioners, or researchers contain mental disorder information, research fact sheets, statistics, science education materials, news, links to NIMH research sites, and patient education materials.

The National Institute of Mental Health (NIMH) specific site features and resources are summarized in the following descriptions.

NIMH Departments and Services

Anxiety Disorders Education Program

http://www.nimh.nih.gov/anxiety/anxiety/whatis/objectiv.htm

The Anxiety Disorders Education Program is a national education campaign developed by the NIMH to increase awareness among the public and healthcare professionals. The site provides a summary of the Program, a description of anxiety disorders, including panic disorder, obsessive-compulsive disorder, posttraumatic stress disorder, phobias, and generalized anxiety disorder. News, public service announcements, and contact details are also found at the site. Visitors can access library resources through the site, including full-text brochures and lists of books, pamphlets, videotapes, and other materials provided by other organizations. Professional resources include a list of meetings presenting NIMH exhibits, and order information for patient education materials.

Clinical Trials

http://www.nimh.nih.gov/studies/index.cfm

Clinical Trials information includes general resources for taking part in clinical research studies at NIMH, a Participant's Guide to Mental Health Clinical Research, links to details of current NIMH intramural and extramural research projects, and recent articles related to clinical research. Other clinical trials databases accessible from this site include the Alzheimer's Disease Clinical Trials Database, Center Watch Clinical Trials Listing Service, and the Rare Diseases Clinical Research Database.

Depression Education Program

http://www.nimh.nih.gov/depression/index.htm

The Depression Education Program offers visitors depression facts for adolescents/students, employers, older adults, and women by topic, including bipolar disorder and co-occurrence of depression with medical disorders. General depression facts, research, and suicide facts are discussed, and an NIMH publications order form is accessible from the site.

Does This Sound Like You?

http://www.nimh.nih.gov/soundlikeyou.htm

Does This Sound Like You? This question is asked of visitors as they proceed through a series of pages describing anxiety disorders. Contact information is provided for additional information on each disorder, and the text stresses the prevalence of these disorders in the American population.

NIMH Library ○ ○ ○

http://www.nimh.nih.gov/anxiety/library/brochure/anxbrch.htm

At this site, both professionals and consumers can obtain information on the most common types of anxiety disorders, including panic, obsessive-compulsive disorders, phobias, generalized anxiety, and posttraumatic stress disorders. Consumers can also access general information on the symptoms, treatment, and treatment center locations for these anxiety disorders. Useful professional resources at the site include the NIMH consensus statement on panic disorder, literature references on a variety of anxiety disorders, conference information, and links to current news pertaining to anxiety disorders.

NIMH Strategic Plan Development

http://www.nimh.nih.gov/strategic/strategicplan.htm

The Institute encourages public participation in the NIMH Strategic Plan Development. Visitors can review an initial of the Draft NIMH Strategic Plan, a list of current Program Announcements and Requests for Applications, and the NIMH Fiscal Year (FY) 2000 Professional Judgment Budget Summary. Contact information is provided for sending comments and suggestions.

Research Resources

http://www.nimh.nih.gov/research/index.cfm

Research Resources summarize NIMH funding opportunities, research training activities, and employment opportunities. News for researchers, research reports, statistics, and links to NIMH Research Consortiums and other NIMH research Web sites are available.

Resources for Practitioners

http://www.nimh.nih.gov/practitioners/index.cfm

Resources for Practitioners include links to clinical trials information, patient education materials available for download, anxiety disorders information, research reports and publications, research fact sheets, statistics, and Consensus Conference Reports, offering statements developed during NIH Consensus Development Conferences of relevance to the mental health field.

Resources for the Public

http://www.nimh.nih.gov/publicat/index.cfm

Resources for the Public include fact sheets on various mental illnesses, research fact sheets on current investigations, information on mental disorders and medications, statistics, questions and answers about psychotherapy research, and educational materials on mental disorders research. Materials are available in English and Spanish.

Science on Our Minds Series

http://www.nimh.nih.gov/publicat/soms.cfm

The Science on Our Minds Series presents online articles on specific mental health topics, including general mental illness and government policy, youth and adolescent mental health topics, depression, suicide, bipolar disorder, anxiety disorders, schizophrenia, women's mental health, genetics, brain imaging and emotions research, and stress and brain development.

Suicide Research Consortium

http://www.nimh.nih.gov/research/suicide.htm

The Suicide Research Consortium coordinates program development in suicide research across the Institute, identifies gaps in the scientific knowledge base on suicide across the life span, stimulates and monitors extramural research on suicide, keeps abreast of scientific developments in suicidology and public policy issues related to suicide surveillance, prevention and treatment, and disseminates science-based information on suicidology to the public, media, and policy makers. The site offers: a transcript of the Surgeon General's Call to Action to Prevent Suicide, 1999; a suicide fact sheet; a graph of suicide rates by age, gender, and race; a selected bibliography on research on suicidal behavior; and suicide statistics and regional variations in suicide rates from the Centers for Disease Control and Prevention (CDC). A special article outlining the current suicide problem in the United States is also available.

NIMH Research

Extramural Funding Opportunities

http://www.nimh.nih.gov/grants/grantinfo.cfm

This site offers an overview, description, and listing of NIMH extramural funding activities. Research is supported in molecular and cellular neuroscience; behavioral neuroscience; developmental neuroscience; the biological aspects of behavior; psychopharmacology and neuropharmacology; cognitive and language processes; personality, emotion, and psychosocial processes; and factors influencing neural, behavioral, psychological, and sociocultural development. Studies of the biological, psychological, and psychosocial aspects of stress, including posttraumatic stress, are supported, as is research in behavioral medicine, psycho- and neuro-immunology, neurovirology, and AIDS. The study of the epidemiology, etiology, pathophysiology, diagnosis, treatment, and prevention of distinct mental disorders is supported. Specific programs emphasize research in the psychopathology and mental and behavioral disorders of children, adolescents, and the aging as well as programs devoted to schizophrenia, mood, anxiety, and personality disorders. In addition, NIMH supports research on service delivery within the mental health system; the provision of mental health services in other types of healthcare settings; economic factors influencing supply, demand, and costs of mental health services; and mental health issues related to antisocial, violent, and abusive behavior, and law and mental health interactions.

Intramural Research

http://intramural.nimh.nih.gov

The NIMH Division of Intramural Research Programs (DIRP) encompasses a broad array of research activities that range from clinical investigation into the diagnosis, treatment, and prevention of mental illness to basic neuroscience studies conducted at the behavioral systems, cellular, and molecular levels. The Division is composed of more than 500 scientists working in 22 Clinical Branches and Basic Research Laboratories, as well as a freestanding Unit on Molecular Neurobiology, three specialized Research Sections and a program-wide Research Services Branch under the Office of the Scientific Director. The site offers details on the organization, training opportunities, and technology transfer activities, future planning and evaluations reports, and links to the specific branches and laboratories within DIRP.

Research Grants

http://www.nimh.nih.gov/grants/grantinfo.cfm

The NIMH supports research grants, research training, and career development programs to increase knowledge and improve research methods on mental and behavioral disorders; to generate information regarding basic biological and behavioral processes underlying these disorders and the maintenance of mental health; and to develop and improve mental health treatment and services. Research and research training supported by the Institute may employ theoretical, laboratory, clinical, methodological, and field studies, any of which may involve clinical, sub-clinical, and normal subjects and populations of all age ranges, as well as animal models appropriate to the system or disorder being investigated and to the state of the field.

5.7 Other Psychiatry Government Resources

Center for Mental Health Services (CMHS) Federal Resources ◎ ◎ ◎

http://www.mentalhealth.org/links/FEDLINKS.htm

Throughout this division of the comprehensive Center for Mental Health Resources, many of the more prominent federal resource Web sites can be accessed. Divisions within the Executive Branch include the Center for Mental Health Services (CMHS), Substance Abuse and Mental Health Services Administration (SAMHSA), Center for Substance Abuse Prevention (CSAP), the Center for Substance Abuse Treatment (CSAT), the National Clearinghouse for Alcohol and Drug Information (NCADI), National Institute on Alcohol Abuse and Alcoholism (NIAAA), National Institute on Drug Abuse (NIDA), National Institute of Mental Health (NIMH), National Institute on Aging (NIA), and the Office of National Drug Control Policy (ONDCP).

Center for Mental Health Services (CMHS) Grantee Database ◎ ◎ ◎

http://www.cdmgroup.com/Ken-cf/CMHSGran.cfm

Searchable by city and state, this Web site of the Center for Mental Health Services provides an organization search engine for the discovery of over 150 CMHS grantees. Included are Projects for Assistance in Transition from Homelessness (PATH) and the Statewide Family Network Support Project. Contact information for each grantee is included.

Center for Mental Health Services (CMHS) State Resources Guide ⊙ ⊙

http://www.mentalhealth.org/publications/stateresourceguides.cfm

Users can choose between a pull-down menu or a United States map to locate regional mental health agencies. Individual state mental health agencies and advocacy organizations are included. Listings provide brief mission statements and complete contact information.

National Association of State Mental Health Program Directors ⊙ ⊙ ⊙

http://www.nasmhpd.org/nri

Reflecting and advocating for the collective interests of State Mental Health Authorities, the National Association of State Mental Health Program Directors Research Institute, Inc. (NASMHPD) offers a specialized profiling system for descriptive organizational grant information. A listing of the NASMHPD's publications, its current projects, and performance measures can be viewed. To encourage communication and community participation in the delivery of mental health services, a performance indicator survey allows the user to research organizations by quality factors. The Research Institute receives research and training grants from the National Institute for Mental Health, which are outlined, and the National Technical Assistance Center brings news and information about the organization's technical assistance and training activities.

National Center for Posttraumatic Stress Disorder (NC-PTSD) ⊙ ⊙ ⊙

http://www.ncptsd.org/Index.html

The National Center for Posttraumatic Stress Disorder, a government agency under the U.S. Department of Veteran Affairs, carries out a broad range of multidisciplinary activities in research, education, and training in an effort to understand, diagnose, and treat PTSD in veterans who have developed psychiatric symptoms following exposure to traumatic stress. The site provides information about the organization and its activities, staff directories, employment and training opportunities, a searchable database of traumatic stress literature, reference literature, table of contents to PTSD Research Quarterly and NC-PTSD Clinical Quarterly, assessment instruments, and links to information about the disorder for the public.

National Council on Sexual Addiction and Compulsivity (NCSAC) ⊙ ⊙

http://www.ncsac.org/main.html

This national nonprofit organization is devoted to the promotion of public and professional awareness of sexual addiction and compulsivity. In addition to detailed member information, there are media contact resources, a suggested reading list, NCSAC position papers on sexual addictions, support groups, and general information about sexual addiction and compulsivity.

National Information Center for
Children and Youth (NICHCY) with Disabilities ◎ ◎

http://www.nichcy.org

This national referral center serves professionals and nonprofessionals by providing information on children and adolescents with disabilities. At this site, one can access the Center's publications, including fact sheets, summaries, news articles, parent and student guides, reference lists, and other information. There are links to state resource documents, an FAQ section, training information, a newsletter, related organizations and centers, conference information, and contact listings.

National Institute on Drug Abuse (NIDA) ◎ ◎ ◎

http://www.nida.nih.gov/NIDAHome1.html

A component of the National Institutes of Health, this organization supports international research, advocacy and education on drug abuse and related issues. The site provides information on the mission and goals of the organization, current news, descriptive fact sheets on commonly abused drugs and their treatment, links to publications, monographs, teaching materials and reports on various aspects of substance abuse and addiction. Information on conferences, including summaries of previous meetings, relevant news articles, links to sites on the subdivisions of NIDA, funding and training opportunities and information, advocacy items, a clinical trial network, and links to the National Institutes of Health site and other professional organizations and centers related to substance abuse. This site also includes a search engine and employment listings.

Substance Abuse and Mental Health Services Administration ◎ ◎ ◎

http://www.samhsa.gov

The Substance Abuse and Mental Health Services Administration is the federal agency charged with improving the quality and availability of prevention, treatment, and rehabilitation services in order to reduce illness, death, disability, and cost to society resulting from substance abuse and mental illnesses. Resources include professionals, programs and budget information databases, information on substance abuse and mental health issues, statistics, contracts, updated news releases, and a search form for relevant documents. Links to other related centers are provided, as well as links to general information on substance abuse and mental health problems.

6. NEUROLOGICAL, DIAGNOSTIC, AND THERAPEUTIC ASPECTS OF PSYCHIATRY

6.1 Neurological Aspects of Psychiatry

Neuroanatomy

A Brief Introduction to the Brain ⊙ ⊙ ⊙
http://ifcsun1.ifisiol.unam.mx/Brain/segunda.htm

This site from scientists in Mexico City offers an educational resource on neuroanatomy, designed for those with at least a high school education. Topics include Action Potential, Neuron, Anatomy of the Nervous System, Neurotransmitters, Behavior, Perception and Sensation, Cerebral Cortex, Reflexes, Cognitive Functions, Second Messengers, Development of the Nervous System, Sense of Balance, Ion Channels, Sense of Hearing, Learning, Sense of Vision, Membrane Potential, Sleep, Memory, Synapse, and Neural Networks. Visual aids and links to more detailed discussions of important terms accompany educational text.

Biological Basis of Human Behavior, Northwest Missouri State University ⊙ ⊙ ⊙
http://www.nwmissouri.edu/nwcourses/dunham/bioofhumanbehavior.htm

A comprehensive tutorial on the biological basis of human behavior is offered from Northwest Missouri at this site, covering the structures of the nervous system. There are valuable supplemental resources for related topics.

Fetal and Young Child Nervous System, University of Iowa College of Medicine ⊙ ⊙ ⊙
http://www.vh.org/Providers/Textbooks/FetalYoungCNS/FetalYoungCNS.html

Virtual Hospital offers this comprehensive presentation of the fetal nervous system and the brain, including both normal and abnormal brain development, presented by Dr. Adel Afifi and Dr. Ronald Bergman.

Moravian College Science Instrumentation Network: Neuroanatomy Review Information ⊙ ⊙ ⊙
http://www.cs.moravian.edu/~kussmaul/cns/neuro.html

Useful glossaries explaining terms related to neuroanatomy, neurochemistry, and non-anatomical neurology concepts are available at this address. Unfamiliar terms are linked to a definition within the glossaries.

Neuroanatomy Study Slides, Tulane University ⊙ ⊙ ⊙

http://www.mcl.tulane.edu/student/1997/kenb/neuroanatomy/readme_neuro.html

Professor Ken Bookstein of Tulane University's School of Medicine has prepared this slide presentation on neuroanatomy, in full color. It is a very effective teaching tool. Slides are both labeled and unlabeled.

Neuroscience Tutorial, Washington University School of Medicine ⊙ ⊙ ⊙

http://thalamus.wustl.edu/Course

The basics of clinical neuroscience, through a detailed analysis of the human brain and its functions, are explored through this illustrated online tutorial from the Washington University School of Medicine created by Diana Molavi, Ph.D.

North Carolina State University: Nervous System Gross Anatomy ⊙ ⊙ ⊙

http://courses.ncsu.edu:8020/classes/psy502001/psy502/l4nsgros/ns_pg1.htm

This site offers an excellent educational resource for those requiring general information on neuroanatomy. The anatomy of the brain, spinal cord, cranial nerves, peripheral nerves, the sympathetic nervous system, and the parasympathetic nervous system are described with text and useful images.

Online Dictionary of Mental Health: Neuroanatomy and Neuropathology ⊙ ⊙ ⊙

http://www.human-nature.com/odmh/neuroanatomy.html

Links to 21 sites are found at this address, offering access to anatomy images, interactive brain maps, educational resources, labeled slides and diagrams, neural tissues images, muscle and nerve images, and resources specific to neuropathology. One site presents information in Italian.

ScienceNet: Brain and Nervous System ⊙ ⊙

http://www.sciencenet.org.uk/database/Biology/Lists/braintable.html

ScienceNet, an information service based in the United Kingdom, specializes in explanations of complex topics in everyday language. Ninety common questions about brain and nervous system morphology and function, diagnostic procedures, and other topics are answered through links at this site.

Whole Brain Atlas, Harvard University ⊙ ⊙ ⊙

http://www.med.harvard.edu/AANLIB/home.html

Every aspect of the human brain and associated brain disorders are explored through this extraordinary atlas developed by Dr. Keith A. Johnson, M.D. and J. Alex Becker of Harvard University.

Neurotransmitters

World Wide Web Course Tools: Neurotransmitters ⊙ ⊙ ⊙
http://www4.gvsu.edu/~adrianb/hs428/section3.htm
Neurotransmitters are explained in detail at this site, including a definition and criteria
for neurotransmitter classification. In-depth discussions of neurotransmitter synthesis
and storage, release, and actions and deactivation are available with diagrams. The site
also offers a chart of specific types of neurotransmitters, including catecholamines,
other monoamine neurotransmitters, and peptide neurotransmitters, listing the
synthetic enzyme, receptors, inactivation process, and special notes.

Houston Community College System: Neurotransmitters ⊙ ⊙
http://nwc.hccs.cc.tx.us/psyc/neuron2/index.htm
Slide presentations on types and specific examples of neurotransmitters are found at
this site. Specific discussions of acetylcholine, dopamine, dopamine hypothesis for
schizophrenia, seratonin and norepinephrine, gamma-aminobutyric acid (GABA),
endorphins, and psychoactive drugs are available at the address.

Cerebral Institute of Discovery: Neurotransmitters ⊙ ⊙ ⊙
http://cerebral.org/neurotrans.html
The Cerebral Institute of Discovery, started by parents of a son with cerebral palsy,
disseminates information on neurology to the general public. This page devoted to
neurotransmitters offers links to many relevant Internet resources, including educational sites for children and adults, multimedia resources, and images. Sites presenting
current research from four investigators are also found through this address.

Neuroendocrinology

Society of Behavioral Neuroendocrinology ⊙ ⊙
http://www.sbne.org
This Society targets research professionals in the fields of behavior and neuroendocrinology. The site includes conference information, membership information, society
officers, goals and bylaws of the Society, a link to related meetings. Publications
resources include access to the official journal of the Society, *Hormones and Behavior*,
and related journals, namely the *Journal of Neuroscience and Neuropeptides*.

Neuroimaging and Pathology

Cognitive Neuroimaging Unit ◉ ◉ ◉
http://james.psych.umn.edu

A division within both the Veterans Affairs Medical Center and the University of Minnesota School of Medicine, this Unit in interested in brain mapping of cognitive functions in both healthy individuals and those with mental disorders. The history and mission of the Unit, available facilities and resources, a staff directory, a bibliography of recent publications, a bulletin board highlighting recent activities, information on associated clinics, and links to related sites are all found at this address. Visitors can also access links to resources related to the tools the Unit uses to process, analyze, and display Positron Emission Tomography (PET) images.

Johns Hopkins Medical Institutions: Division of Psychiatric Neuroimaging ◉ ◉ ◉
http://pni.med.jhu.edu

The Division of Psychiatric Neuroimaging increases the understanding of the brain, behavior, genetics, and connections among these subjects through neuroimaging research. This site offers a mission statement, a faculty and staff directory, descriptions of current projects with methods, jobs, and internship information (when available), contact details, and a bibliography of publications. Users can download some full-text articles from the site.

National Institute on Drug Abuse (NIDA) Notes: The Basics of Brain Imaging ◉ ◉
http://www.nida.nih.gov/NIDA_Notes/NNVol11N5/Basics.html

This site describes the main neuroimaging techniques used in drug abuse research, including Positron Emission Tomography (PET), Single Photon Emission Computed Tomography (SPECT), Magnetic Resonance Imaging (MRI), and Electro-Encephalography (EEG). Visitors will find explanations of information collected from these techniques and how each technique is performed.

Proceedings of the National Academy of Sciences (PNAS): Papers from an NAS Colloquium on Neuroimaging of Human Brain Function ◉ ◉ ◉
http://www.pnas.org/content/vol95/issue3/index.shtml#COLLOQUIUM

Twenty-three full-text articles related to neuroimaging are available through this site. Visitors can read the article online or download a copy. Other resources include a list of papers citing the article, links to similar articles found at PNAS Online and PubMed, a link to the article's PubMed citation, and the ability to search MEDLINE for articles with the same authors.

Whole Brain Atlas, Harvard University ⊙ ⊙ ⊙

http://www.med.harvard.edu/AANLIB/home.html

This comprehensive resource for images of normal and abnormal brain tissues offers an introduction to neuroimaging, an atlas of normal brain structure and blood flow, images of the "top 100 brain structures." vascular anatomy images, and images related to normal aging. Images related to specific cerebrovascular, neoplastic, degenerative, inflammatory, and infectious diseases are available at the site. Explanatory tours are available with some images.

Neuropsychiatry

American Academy of Clinical Neuropsychology (AACN) ⊙ ⊙

http://www.med.umich.edu/abcn/aacn.html

This site presented by the American Academy of Clinical Neuropsychology allows users to search the AACN directory of members, view the articles and bylaws of the Academy, view current AACN news, and access continuing education materials. Links to other neuropsychology sites are present.

American Board of Psychiatry and Neurology, Inc. ⊙ ⊙ ⊙

http://www.abpn.com

The mission of the American Board of Psychiatry and Neurology is to improve the quality of psychiatric and neurological care through a voluntary certification process for professionals. This site is designed to provide information on board certification, examinations, and policies of the board, and has an informative frequently asked questions (FAQ) section. The site also offers links to other related boards.

American Neuropsychiatric Association (ANPA) ⊙ ⊙

http://www.neuropsychiatry.com/ANPA/index.html

Resources offered by the ANPA at this site include program and registration information for the group's 2000 Annual Meeting, contact information, membership applications, an e-mail news subscription service, a directory of members, an online newsletter, journal information, and links to related sites of interest to neuroscientists. Internet access for this site is made available by Butler Hospital, and the site is supported by an unrestricted educational grant from Hoechst. A list of ANPA officers is also provided.

Association for Research in
Nervous and Mental Disease (ARNMD) ⊙

http://cpmcnet.columbia.edu/www/arnmd

The Association for Research in Nervous and Mental Disease is the oldest society of neurologists and psychiatrists. The site provides links to the history and mission of ARNMD, the board of trustees, ARNMD publications from 1920, an events calendar, 1998 meeting abstracts, and a list of program speakers and talks from the 1998 annual course.

Beth Israel Deaconess Medical Center and Harvard Medical
School Division of Behavioral Neurology-Neuropsychiatry ⊙ ⊙

http://www.bih.harvard.edu/behavneuro/Npsychiat.html

The Behavioral Neurology Unit presents an overview of psychiatry and neuropsychiatry services available, lists reasons for referral, and offers information on fellowships at this site. Clinical and laboratory research information is available by topic, and the site also offers a bibliography of recent publications and a faculty directory.

Centre for Clinical Research in Neuropsychiatry ⊙ ⊙

http://www.ccrn.uwa.edu.au

This center for psychiatric and neuroscience research, located in Western Australia, "focuses on the etiology, epidemiology, course, and outcome of major psychiatric disorders in adults and children," with special interest in genetics and family studies. Information about the Centre, a staff directory, research details, a bibliography of recent publications, and seminar details are found at this site.

Division of Intramural Research: NIMH—Neuropsychiatry Branch ⊙ ⊙

http://silk.nih.gov/silk/npb

The main focus of the Neuropsychiatry Branch (NPB) of the National Institute of Mental Health is to study the effects of early intervention on the course of psychotic disorders, particularly schizophrenia. The site contains a bibliography of recent publications, employment opportunities, notice of meetings, references relevant to the study, treatment, and prevention of various neuropsychiatric disorders, a list of early intervention research and treatment facilities, and links to related sites. Descriptions of the NPB PREVENT program, a forum for the discussion and exchange of information between groups studying various forms of prevention for neuropsychiatric disorders, and the National Collaborative Study of Early Psychosis and Suicide (NCSEPS) are also available.

Leicester University's Preclinical Sciences Neuroscience Page
http://www.le.ac.uk/pcs/links/anlineur.html

This concise yet useful list of links provides general neuroscience resources as well as Home Pages to premier online neuroscience centers, including the Yale Center for Neuroscience and the UCLA Laboratory of Neuro Imaging. Incorporated into the list are the neuroscience topics Parkinson's and Alzheimer's disease, neuroanesthesiology, neuroanatomy, and neuroimaging. Links to neuroanatomy study slides and the WWW Virtual Library on Neurobiology complete this neuroscience resource site.

Literature, Cognition, and the Brain ⊙ ⊙
http://www2.bc.edu/~richarad/lcb

In addition to a descriptive bibliography on the linkage of cognitive sciences and neurosciences with literature, there are links to conference information, abstracts, current research projects, reviews of relevant books, and a number of links to related Web sites, discussion groups, and other online resources.

Mental Health Net: Neurosciences and Neuropsychology ⊙ ⊙ ⊙
http://mentalhelp.net/guide/pro10.htm

This address contains links and reviews of sites providing resources related to neurosciences, neuropsychology, biofeedback, neurofeedback, neurophysiology, and brain images. Site descriptions are often detailed, and include suggested target audiences, resources found at the site, and site sponsors. General Web resources, newsgroups, mailing lists (with one-click subscription capabilities), journals, publications, research papers, professional organizations and centers, assessment tools, images and imaging resources, product suppliers, software, training programs, and tutorials are found at this valuable site. Other resources at the site includes an online bookstore with book reviews, a searchable calendar of conferences and workshops, disorder treatment information, chat forums on many subjects, employment listings, news, a search engine of professional psychology journals, and a directory of clinicians.

Neuropsychiatry.com ⊙ ⊙ ⊙
http://www.neuropsychiatry.com/NPcom/wwwlinks.html

This site contains a catalog of Internet resources by disorder category, and users can search the site to quickly locate links to relevant sites. Resources are provided in neurology, neuropsychiatry, neuropsychology, psychiatry, and psychology. Some links are listed with short descriptions. Drug information, associations, support groups, continuing education resources, government sites, and funding sources are typical of the resources found under each disorder category.

Neuropsychology Central ◎ ◎

http://www.neuropsychologycentral.com

This searchable site contains an online forum for interested professionals and consumers, informative resources for professionals, and links to sites on assessment, forensic, geriatric, organizations, pediatric publications, training, and other topics of interest.

Neuroscience and Mental Health on the World Wide Web ◎ ◎ ◎

http://www.neuropsychiatry.com/NPcom/wwwlinks.html

This address houses a valuable directory of Internet resources related to neuroscience and mental health. Sites are listed by disorder information or type of resource available at the address. Links are included to sites offering general resources, medication information, societies, academic departments, support groups, and government agencies. Some specific resources found at this site include conference listings, Continuing Medical Education resources, funding sources, journals and publishers, neuroanatomy and brain atlases, newsgroups and discussion forums, reference sources, and databases.

What's New in Neuropsychiatry ◎ ◎

http://www.cyberfax-med.com

This site offers links to news articles related to general psychiatric and neuropsychiatry issues. Summaries are available in French, but links lead to English language articles.

6.2 Diagnostics

Assessment and Testing

American Academy of Child and Adolescent Psychiatry (AACAP): Summary of the Practice Parameters for the Psychiatric Assessment of Infants and Toddlers ◎ ◎ ◎

http://www.aacap.org/clinical/infntsum.htm

This full-text article includes an abstract, considerations in the assessment of infants and toddlers, assessment techniques, diagnostic formulation, treatment planning, and detailed guidelines for a suggested infant and toddler mental status exam.

Australian Transcultural Mental Health Network: Research Literature on Multilingual Versions of Psychiatric Assessment Instruments ◎ ◎

http://www.atmhn.unimelb.edu.au/research/research_papers/mi/mi-faoct.html

Bibliographic information is available at this site for articles describing research evaluating or utilizing specific psychiatric assessment instruments. Articles are listed by psychiatric assessment instrument and subcategorized by language. The site provides a list of over 30 languages, and indicates if an article related to a specific assessment tool is available in each language.

ERIC/AE Test Locator ◎ ◎ ◎

http://ericae.net/testcol.htm

The Test Collection covers a broad array of tests, including educational and managerial fields of testing. The site allows users to search test databases from the site's sponsors: the ERIC Clearinghouse on Assessment and Evaluation, the Library and Reference Services Division of the Educational Testing Service, the Buros Institute of Mental Measurements at the University of Nebraska in Lincoln, the Region III Comprehensive Center at George Washington University, and Pro-Ed test publishers.

Mental Health Net: Assessment Resources ◎ ◎ ◎

http://mentalhelp.net/guide/pro01.htm

This address lists more than 50 sources and online locations of psychiatric assessment tests, providing descriptions and ratings with site links. Resources include tools for assessing depression, mania, emotional intelligence, childhood behavioral problems, and sexual disorders, as well as links to sites providing catalogs of assessment resources. Resources are available for both professionals and non-professionals searching for self-assessment tools. Links to newsgroups, journals, publications, and research papers, professional organizations and centers, additional assessment resources, product suppliers, and software companies are also available. Users can subscribe to mailing lists for e-mails of specific news and information at the site.

NYU Department of Psychiatry— Psychiatry Information for the General Public ◎ ◎ ◎

http://www.med.nyu.edu/Psych/public.html

This site provides links to general online psychiatry resources for the general public, including NIMH information, online screening tests for depression, anxiety, sexual disorders, attention-deficit/hyperactivity disorder, personality disorders, and resources for the diagnosis of psychiatric disorders and depression. Treatment resources are available, with topics including psychotherapy, medications, group psychotherapy, psychoanalysis, and cognitive behavioral therapy. Links are also included to self-help resources, advocacy groups, fact sheets, articles and other publications, and search engines.

Psychological Assessment Online ⊙ ⊙ ⊙ (free registration)
http://www.psych-assess.com/main.htm

This site is devoted to providing information on psychological testing or assessment. The site is divided into sections containing general or professional resources. Professional resources include technical information on assessment, such as test administration, interpretation, clinical interviewing, and forensic assessment. General resources include links to online essays, publishers, basic concepts in psychological assessment, meetings, a bookstore, and other related links.

Classifications

BehaveNet APA DSM-IV Diagnostic Classification ⊙ ⊙
http://www.behavenet.com/capsules/disorders/dsm4classification.htm

Diagnostic classifications and categories of psychiatric disorders and associated conditions are listed. Specific disorders are listed by category. Ordering information is available for the *American Psychiatric Association DSM-IV,* related publications, and books and other media through Amazon.com.

DSM-IV Complete Criteria for Mental Disorders ⊙ ⊙ ⊙
http://www.chesco.com/~snowbaby/DSM-IV.html

Divided into different sections, professionals and consumers can view the complete criteria for psychiatric illnesses such as childhood disorders, cognitive, substance-related, schizophrenia and other psychotic disorders, mood and anxiety disorders, somatoform, factitious and dissociative disorders, sexual and gender identity disorders, eating disorders, sleep disorders, impulse-control and adjustment disorders, and personality disorders. Complete criteria for each set of disorders is provided at the site.

International Classification of Diseases: Psychiatry ⊙ ⊙
http://www.informatik.fh-luebeck.de/icd/welcome.html

Primarily for clinicians and other professionals, this site offers an organized list of psychiatric disorders, according to the International Classification of Diseases, from the World Health Organization. This site for the reference manual features a hypertext document of Chapter V. This reference manual allows searches by disorder categories, alphabetical lists, and by keywords. A basic description of the disorder or group of related disorders is presented, as well as links to additional psychiatry sites.

Clinical Diagnosis

American Board of Mental Health Diagnostics ◎ ◎
http://www.diagnostics.org

This site contains a large listing of links to all aspects of mental health diagnoses, including assessment tools and diagnostic criteria outlines. Also included are links to statements and articles on family assessment and other psychiatry articles. Comprehensive information regarding certification by the board is available.

Clinical Disease Management for Psychiatric Disorders ◎ ◎ ◎
http://www.slis.ua.edu/cdlp/WebDLCore/clinical/psychiatry/index.htm

This site offers links to chapters in the Merck Manual and to other clinical sources for diagnosis and treatment of specific disorders, including libraries of pathology images, clinical practice guidelines, and clinical management resources. Links take the visitor to relevant sections of CHORUS (Collaborative Hypertext of Radiology), CliniWeb, Internet Mental Health, Family Practice Handbook, National Guideline Clearinghouse, and other Internet information sources.

Internet Mental Health: Diagnosis and Disorders ◎ ◎ ◎
http://www.mentalhealth.com/p71.html

An excellent site for concise diagnostic information regarding most of the more common mental health disorders, this Web site provides descriptive information for the physician or patient user. A life quality analysis is available through a 57 question Quality of Life Questionnaire that gives the patient or physician a summary of characteristics and an associated numerical measurement. American and European descriptions of 37 disorders and online diagnostic screenings for each are available. Additionally, research, treatment, and related Internet links are provided for each condition. Personality disorders, anxiety disorders, and substance-related disorders are included.

Merck Manual of Diagnosis and Therapy: Psychiatric Disorders ◎ ◎ ◎
http://merck.com/pubs/mmanual/section15/sec15.htm

Topics available through this portion of the Merck Manual include psychiatry in medicine, somatoform disorders, anxiety disorders, dissociative disorders, mood disorders, suicidal behavior, personality disorders, psychosexual disorders, schizophrenia and related disorders, psychiatric emergencies, drug use and dependence, and eating disorders. Specific disorders under these headings are described, and resources on each subject typically include etiology, symptoms and diagnosis, prognosis, and treatment.

University of Iowa Family Practice Handbook ☉ ☉ ☉

http://www.vh.org/Providers/ClinRef/FPHandbook/15.html

The Psychiatry Chapter of the University of Iowa's Family Practice Handbook explores mood disorders, anxiety disorders, substance-use disorders, acute psychosis, schizophrenia, and eating disorders. Each section has extensive clinical practice guideline and treatment information.

Using DSM-IV Primary Care Version:
A Guide to Psychiatric Diagnosis in Primary Care ☉ ☉ ☉

http://www.aafp.org/afp/981015ap/pingitor.html

As a courtesy of the American Family Physician, this article reviews the *Diagnostic and Statistical Manual of Mental Disorders,* 4th ed., primary care version (DSM-IVPC), examining the methods by which it accommodates the family physician in clinical practice. A comparison between the DSM-IV and DSM-IVPC is made in regard to the diagnostic features unique to DSM-IVPC as well as unresolved clinical issues regarding the primary care algorithms and other limitations to the family physician model with respect to hard to diagnose disorders.

Mental Status Examination

Mental Status Examination:
Lecture, Indiana University School of Medicine ☉ ☉ ☉

http://php.iupui.edu/~flip/g505mse.html

This Indiana University lecture on the mental status examination provides an excellent resource for this important diagnostic tool. There is significant detailed information on every aspect of the examination, such as utility, method, procedure and focal issues, and findings.

Psychiatry LectureLinks ☉ ☉ ☉

http://omie.med.jhmi.edu/LectureLinks/PsychiatryLinks.html

This online lecture and tutorial contains an introduction to psychiatry and behavioral sciences. There is a mental status exam and a cognitive exam. Disorders and illnesses that are discussed include dementia, mood disorders, schizophrenia, childhood autism, and substance abuse. Many other topics are discussed and introductions to the various sections are also provided.

Online Diagnosis

Internet Mental Health: Online Diagnosis ◎ ◎ ◎
http://www.mentalhealth.com/fr71.html

This site allows visitors to use interactive question and answer programs for provisional diagnoses of mental disorders, including anxiety disorders, childhood disorders, eating disorders, mood disorders, personality disorders, schizophrenia, and substance-related disorders. Descriptions, treatment, research, educational booklets, articles, and links to additional resources are available for each disorder.

6.3 **Therapies**

Alternative Therapies

Alternative Therapy:
Focus on Herbal Products ◎ ◎ (free registration)
http://www.med.virginia.edu/cmc/pedpharm/v4n5.htm

This article from *Pediatric Pharmacotherapy* offers a discussion of several popular herbal products. The National Institutes of Health alternative therapy criteria, FDA regulations, and current statistics on the use of alternative therapies are available, as well as discussions of Echinacea, St. John's wort, and ginseng. The article identifies active ingredients in each featured herbal product, contraindications, possible side effects, and history of use. Clinical studies of herbal products are referenced for additional information. A list of sources for information on herbal therapies is also found in the article.

Knowledge Exchange Network: Alternative Treatment ◎
http://www.mentalhealth.org/links/alternative.htm

Links at this site provide users with access to centers and other organizations offering information on music therapy, drama therapy, and other alternative approaches to mental wellness.

National Coalition of Arts Therapies Associations (NCATA) ◎ ◎
http://www.ncata.com/home.html

This alliance of professional associations dedicated to the advancement of art therapy represents six organizations. Art therapy, dance/movement therapy, drama therapy, music therapy, psychodrama, and poetry therapy are defined and discussed at this site. Information on upcoming conferences and contact details for professional organizations are available.

National Institute of Mental Health (NIMH): Questions and Answers about St. John's Wort ◎ ◎
http://www.nimh.nih.gov/publicat/stjohnqa.htm

Visitors to this site can read answers to questions about the use of St. John's wort in the treatment of depression. A large-scale clinical trial will be conducted by the National Institute of Mental Health (NIMH), in collaboration with the NIH National Center for Complementary and Alternative Medicine and the NIH Office of Dietary Supplements (ODS), on the therapeutic effect of St. John's wort in the treatment of clinical depression. The questions concern European studies of St. John's wort, possible dangers of the herb, contact information for clinical trial enrollment, and details of the upcoming clinical trial.

Behavior Therapy

Association for Behavior Analysis ◎ ◎
http://www.wmich.edu/aba/contents.html

The Association for Behavior Analysis, an international organization based at Western Michigan University, promotes experimental, theoretical, and applied analysis of behavior. Visitors to the site can access a job placement service, lists of affiliated chapters, student committees, special interest groups, annual convention details, membership details, a member directory, Association publications, and links to related Web sites.

Behavior Analysis ◎ ◎
http://www.coedu.usf.edu/behavior/behavior.html

Located within the University of South Florida, this site has a number of links to Web pages, associations, journals and other resources related to behavior analysis. In addition, educational training resources, graduate program information, and related Web sites are listed.

Behavior Online ◎ ◎ ◎
http://www.behavior.net

This is a professional site providing a structured discussion environment on over 25 behavioral therapies and topics such as anxiety disorders, evolutionary psychology, legal issues for therapists, online clinical work, and behavioral medicine, and primary care. Described as an online gathering place for mental health and behavioral science professionals, visitors can join in on the numerous discussion forums, use the links to obtain conference information, visit home pages for related organizations and institutes, and visit other related Web sites.

Behavior Therapy Links ⊙ ⊙ ⊙
http://home.wxs.nl/~tgth/links_en.htm

Behavior therapy resources at this site include links to general information sources, associations, newsgroups, journals, and sources for psychological tests and software information. Most resources found at the site are technical, and not for untrained audiences.

Cambridge Center for Behavioral Studies ⊙ ⊙ ⊙
http://www.behavior.org

The Cambridge Center for Behavioral Studies is a nonprofit organization aimed at using behavioral science for the resolution of challenges in the home, school, and workplace. The site offers a detailed discussion of behavior analysis, a bibliography of publications with ordering information, book reviews, behavior analysis articles, and news. Specific sections are devoted to information on animals/pets and behavior analysis, autism, education, parenting, behavioral safety, and performance management. Twenty-six links are available, providing access to academic sites, a bibliography of B. F. Skinner, classroom reference materials, information on educating disadvantaged children, a glossary of behavioral terms, additional Internet directories for behavioral information, and other resources. The home pages of 28 professional societies are also accessible through this site. International, American, Canadian, regional, and state organizations are listed.

Encylcopedia.com: Behavior Therapy ⊙ ⊙
http://encyclopedia.com/printable/01275.html

A concise definition of behavior therapy is offered at this site, including links to explanations of related terms. Links to additional suggested resources are provided with some related terms.

Journal of the Experimental Analysis of Behavior ⊙ ⊙ ⊙
http://www.envmed.rochester.edu/wwwrap/behavior/jeab/jeabhome.htm

This psychology journal primarily publishes findings relevant to the behavior of individual organisms. The site provides subscription information, instructions on preparation of manuscripts, a history of the journal, table of contents and abstracts of current and archived issues, selected electronic reprints of articles, commentaries, audio presentations, video clips, and links to related journals and organizations. Visitors can search abstracts for relevant material by keyword.

Bio- and Neurofeedback

Association for Applied Psychophysiology and Biofeedback (AAPB) ◉ ◉ ◉ (fee-based)
http://www.aapb.org

This nonprofit organization of clinicians, researchers, and educators is dedicated to advancing the "development, dissemination and utilization of knowledge about applied psychophysiology and biofeedback to improve health and the quality of life through research, education, and practice." General information at the site includes a description of biofeedback and psychophysiology, a list of common health problems helped by biofeedback, meetings and workshop information, membership information, a bibliography of recent research articles related to biofeedback and psychophysiology, links to related sites, an online bookstore, and content lists of AAPB publications. The site offers a directory of biofeedback practitioners and a forum for asking questions of biofeedback experts. Submission instructions are available for the AAPB 2000 Annual Meeting.

Biofeedback Network ◉ ◉ ◉
http://www.biofeedback.net

This online network of biofeedback/neurofeedback resources is a powerful, holistic tool. Association listings, equipment training and technology, treatment centers, practitioners, and employment and equipment-related classified ads are all available.

Biofeedback Therapies ◉ ◉
http://www.biofeedbacktherapies.com

This site describes biofeedback therapy and offers contact information for ordering associated tools and other services. These services, neurotherapy, and the use of biofeedback during treatment are described in detail.

EEG Spectrum Home Page ◉ ◉ ◉
http://www.eegspectrum.com

Neurofeedback research and clinical services are the subject of this encyclopedic site, which offers separate menus for the public and professional audiences. General resources pertaining to specific disorders for which neurofeedback may assist functioning are compiled and easily accessed. Articles on the origins of biofeedback and current applicable analysis are included. Training courses for professionals, the week's news in review, and a site-specific search engine make EEG Spectrum an excellent resource for the most current information on neurofeedback.

Freedom from Headaches ☉ ☉ ☉

http://lifematters.com/headache

The Freedom from Headaches site and Headache Reduction Training are the culmination of years of experience in the area of behavioral management for chronic pain disorders. The site and the online training focus on what the patient can do to better manage headaches, taking the user through the process step-by-step to ensure better headache management. A free newsletter, scientific literature, and information on an eight-week Headache Reduction Training Program that focuses on behavior identification and change are covered.

Frequently Asked Questions ☉ ☉ ☉

http://www.eegspectrum.com/articles/proffaq.htm

As a service of EEG Spectrum, Neurofeedback Research and Clinical Services, mental health professionals provide general information here to the most commonly asked questions about EEG neurofeedback training, its use, and history.

Neurofeedback Today ☉ ☉ ☉

http://www.eegspectrum.com/nftoday/current.htm

An online news and information source from the world of mental health, neuropsychology, neuropsychiatry, and neuroscience, Neurofeedback Today provides book listings, journal articles, announcements, and chats of the day for a wide range of topics relevant to the mind/body connection in disease. Addiction, EEG and cognitive neurosciences, pain, and fatigue are just a handful of subjects covered; all-inclusive.

Neurofeedback Yellow Pages Worldwide ☉ ☉ ☉

http://www.thegrid.net/dakaiser/nfyp

At Neurofeedback Yellow Pages Worldwide, the user may click anywhere inside a country's border to view a listing of neurofeedback practitioners in that region. Neurofeedback practitioners may add, modify, or remove information as necessary.

Self-Improvement Online-Biofeedback Sites ☉ ☉

http://www.selfgrowth.com/biofeedback.html

This site contains a listing of Web sites offering information on biofeedback and related therapies. Online articles, organizations, prevention and self-help resources, and institutes are included at the site.

Society for Neuronal Regulation (SNR) ☉ ☉

http://www.snr-jnt.org

This organization consists of professionals interested in neurofeedback training and research. Site resources include a glossary, a reference center, a listing of neurofeedback providers, conference information, and a neurofeedback archive of online abstracts and papers from selected SNR meetings. There is also free access to the *Journal of Neurotherapy*.

Brief Solution-Focused Therapy

Brief Solution-Focused Therapy ◎ ◎
http://inetarena.com/~bneben

This site offers information on a mailing list providing an ongoing therapy discussion, providing a resource to professionals interested in brief therapy, solution-focused therapy, strategic, structural, and related models. Visitors can subscribe to the list, find links to several related sites, access an online bookstore, read an article on brief therapy and managed care, and find a reference list of related articles.

Depth Oriented Brief Therapy (DOBT) ◎ ◎
http://www.dobt.com

Designed for professionals interested in brief solution focused therapy, the Depth Oriented Brief Therapy's methodology and concepts are available via literature, the DOBT video series, and training seminars for psychotherapists and other healthcare professionals. Professional references and links to the depth oriented brief therapy case studies can be accessed.

Cognitive-Behavior Therapy

American Institute for Cognitive Therapy ◎ ◎ ◎
http://www.cognitivetherapynyc.com

This site describes the process and concepts of cognitive therapy, lists psychiatric problems addressed at the Institute, and provides common questions, answers, and transcripts of recent news articles related to cognitive therapy and the Institute. Suggested readings, staff member biographies, fact sheets, an online newsletter, links to related sites, and fellowship details are also available.

Beck Institute for Cognitive Therapy and Research ◎ ◎ ◎
http://www.beckinstitute.org

The Beck Institute for Cognitive Therapy and Research, under the direction of the founder of Cognitive Therapy, Aaron T. Beck, M.D., Emeritus Professor of Psychiatry, University of Pennsylvania School of Medicine, and Director Judith S. Beck, Ph.D., Clinical Assistant Professor of Psychology in Psychiatry at the University of Pennsylvania, offers cognitive therapy training programs for mental health and medical professionals. Details of training programs, certification information, an online bookstore, an online newsletter, Dr. J. S. Beck's speaking schedule, and links to related sites are all available at this address. Visitors can also download an application for training programs at the site.

Center for Cognitive Therapy (Southern California) ◎ ◎
http://www.padesky.com

This Center was founded by request from the founder of Cognitive Therapy, and offers consultation, therapy for therapists, licensing preparation services for Ph.D. level psychologists in California, and training workshops. The site provides information on upcoming workshops, links to details of worldwide workshops, suggested readings with ordering links, conference news, and membership information.

Cognitive Therapy: The Basics of Cognitive Therapy ◎
http://mindstreet.com/cbt.html

Cognitive therapy is discussed at this site, including a definition, research background details, descriptions of cognitive therapy sessions, and suggestions for locating additional resources. Suggested readings are listed at the site.

MindStreet Cognitive Therapy: A Multimedia Learning Program ◎ ◎
http://mindstreet.com/mindstreet

This site describes the first computer program to combine interactive multimedia with psychiatric techniques of cognitive therapy. The program consists of full-screen, full-motion video, and a take-home manual with customized patient homework assignments. The program is designed to help patients cope with emotional problems, assist therapists in reaching treatment goals, and reduce healthcare costs. The site includes a program synopsis, an introduction to cognitive therapy, and a description of the learning environment and training applications. Additional features include ordering information, comments and reviews, author information, credits, system requirements, and general information about MindStreet.

National Association of Cognitive Behavioral Therapists ◎ ◎ ◎
http://www.nacbt.org

Up-to-date information and news is provided at the official site of the National Association of Cognitive-Behavioral Therapists, including back issues of the *Rational News* newsletter. A referral database sends you to the organization's national database of certified cognitive-behavioral therapists. Professional certifications offered by the organization are outlined, and a professional and self-help resources store is provided online. Products for professionals include home study courses, books, and audiovisual materials. Likewise, self-improvement courses, and multimedia materials are available to the lay community.

Social Cognition Paper Archive and Information Center ◎ ◎
http://www.psych.purdue.edu/~esmith/scarch.html

In addition to fact sheets, presentations, articles, and abstracts about social cognition and related subjects, professionals and consumers can access one of the many related links as well. Information on various researchers working in the field of social cognition is also available.

University of Pennsylvania Health System (UPHS): Department of Psychiatry—Center for Cognitive Therapy ◎ ◎
http://www.med.upenn.edu/~psycct

The Center for Cognitive Therapy offers tertiary care, therapy, education, clinical training, and research programs. The site provides a staff listing, information on educational programs, answers to frequently asked questions, links to related sites, information on the Center's case consultation service, employment listings, a referral list of cognitive therapists, consulting, and lecture series.

Community-Based Psychiatric Treatment

American Association of Community Psychiatrists ◎ ◎
http://www.comm.psych.pitt.edu/find.html

The American Association of Community Psychiatrists promotes excellence in inpatient mental healthcare, solves common problems encountered by psychiatrists in a community setting, establishes liaisons with related professional groups for advocacy purposes, encourages psychiatrist training, improves relationships within community settings between psychiatrists and other clinicians and administrators, and educates the public about the role of the community mental health system in the care of the mentally ill. This site provides information on the mission of the Association, board members, and membership information. The present and previous newsletters and issues of *Community Psychiatrist* are available, as well as links to relevant training and research programs in the discipline.

Assertive Community Treatment (ACT) ◎ ◎
http://actassociation.com/main_1.htm

Assertive Community Treatment, a specific approach providing community-based psychiatric treatment, rehabilitation, and support, is described in detail at this site. Topics include a description of people served by ACT and minimum characteristics a service must meet to be considered an ACT provider.

Knowledge Exchange Network: Community Support Programs
http://www.mentalhealth.org/cmhs/communitysupport/index.htm

Community Support Programs of the Center for Mental Health Services facilitate the effective delivery and implementation of mental health services in local communities. The site offers state resource guides, publications, Program of Assertive Community Treatment standards, archived activity updates, a program fact sheet, and specific community support program summaries. Links are available to sites offering resources related to accessibility issues, employment, self-help/support groups, and patients' rights.

National Council for Community
Behavioral Healthcare ⊙ ⊙ ⊙ (some features fee-based)
http://www.nccbh.org

The National Council for Community Behavioral Healthcare conducts advocacy and educational activities for community behavioral healthcare organizations. Resources at the site include a description of membership benefits, current advocacy issues and initiatives, recent letters to Congress, news, and conference details. Educational materials include books available to order, an online newsletter highlighting recent legislation, an online journal of educational articles, and a detailed discussion of behavioral health statistics and the impact of behavioral disorders on society. Services and employment opportunities are listed at the site. Paid membership allows access to current public policy reports, news, online communications, and a networking directory.

Electroconvulsive Therapy (ECT)

American Academy of Family Physicians:
Electroconvulsive Therapy (ECT) for Severe Depression ⊙ ⊙
http://home.aafp.org/patientinfo/depress.html

This site answers important questions about electroconvulsive therapy (ECT). Visitors will find a list of conditions treated with ECT, a description of the procedure, common precautions and preparations for the procedure, a description of the ECT session, and a discussion of possible side effects and outcome.

Electroconvulsive Therapy Internet Resources ⊙ ⊙
http://www.epub.org.br/cm/n04/historia/ectrec_i.htm

This site lists links to resources providing patient information, articles, and position statements concerning Electroconvulsive Therapy (ECT). Sites advocating and discrediting this form of therapy are listed.

Electroconvulsive Therapy—National Institutes of Health Consensus Development Conference Statement ◉ ◉
http://stripe.colorado.edu/~judy/depression/ect.html

This site contains a full transcript of the National Institutes of Health Consensus Development Conference Statement related to Electroconvulsive Therapy (ECT), developed in 1985. The document describes evidence that ECT is effective for specific mental disorders, risks and adverse effects, factors to consider when determining if ECT treatment is appropriate, guidelines for administering ECT, and directions for further research.

University of Pennsylvania Health System (UPHS): Commonly Asked Questions Concerning Electroconvulsive Therapy (ECT) ◉ ◉
http://www.med.upenn.edu/ect/ectfaq.htm

The site answers common questions on ECT, discussing the process of ECT, common patients, ECT safety, common side-effects, risks and benefits, number of treatments, when to stop ECT, testing prior to ECT treatment, the ECT treatment plan, therapeutic strategies after the initial course of treatments, and maintenance ECT.

What You Should Know about Electroconvulsive Therapy (ECT) ◉ ◉
http://www.harborside.com/~equinox/ect.htm

This site, presented by the Committee for Truth in Psychiatry, attempts to warn visitors of possible dangers associated with ECT. A prototype informed consent statement, a description of shock therapy, and articles discouraging this form of therapy are available at the site.

Eye Movement Desensitization and Reprocessing (EMDR)

Eye Movement Desensitization and Reprocessing (EMDR) Institute ◉ ◉
http://www.emdr.com

EMDR, an innovative treatment for depression, addictions, phobias, trauma, and other disorders, is described at this site for both consumers and professionals. The site also describes training at the Institute and offers faculty profiles, publications and controlled studies, information on humanitarian assistance by the Institute, discussion groups, study groups, and a system for ordering books and other products. Contact information for clinician referrals is also available.

Gene Therapy

Access Excellence Activities Exchange—Genetic Counseling: Coping With The Human Impact Of Genetic Disease ◎ ◎ ◎
http://science.peoriaud.k12.az.us/ScienceWebs/Genetech/counsel3.htm

This site provides visitors with links to information related to genetic counseling, including Internet resources, organizations, and suggested printed articles, books, and video. Descriptive information is given with each Internet link. A glossary of terms related to genetic counseling is available at this site, targeting a general, nontechnical audience.

University of Wisconsin Biotechnology Center: Genetic Counseling and Gene Therapy ◎ ◎
http://www.biotech.wisc.edu/Education/Poster/counseling.html

This site, designed for a non-technical audience, describes genetic and DNA analysis techniques and their use in genetic counseling and gene therapy research. Discussions of the tools of biotechnology, industries utilizing biotechnology advances, and genetic engineering are also available.

Group Therapy

American Psychological Association (APA): Group Psychology and Group Psychotherapy (Division 20) ◎ ◎
http://www.pitt.edu/~cslewis/GP2/Hello.html

The Group Psychology and Group Psychotherapy Division offers a history of the division, committee lists, general awards information, a directory of officers, details of publications, membership details, news, and an e-mail mailing list. Links are available to related sites, including research centers, online journals, and other professional associations.

Association for Specialists in Group Work ◎ ◎ ◎
http://www.psyctc.org/mirrors/asgw

The Association for Specialists in Group Work (ASGW) presents a resource starting point for practitioners of group therapy. The ASGW Web site describes the organization's primary mission of establishing standards for professional practice and for the support and dissemination of research knowledge in the field. Descriptions of core group work skills are illustrated in the Group Work Rainbow and core group work training standards are established and prepared for counselors and other professionals. The ASGW products including publications, audiovisual materials, and software are all available to facilitate training, practice, and research. A calendar of events and links to further resources exist at the site for the enhancement of the research and practice of group work.

Interactive Group Therapy ◎ ◎ ◎
http://www.earley.org/Group%20Therapy/group_therapy_frame.htm

This Web address includes listing of articles, books, and training opportunities for the professional psychotherapist involved in group therapy work in addition to information for the general public on interactive group therapy. Annotated transcripts of group therapy sessions, articles for therapists, and handouts for group members that encourage interactive work are all available. A professional publication on the pattern system as it applies to group therapy may be accessed online, and a host of professional group therapy organizations and e-mail lists can be found.

International Association of Group Psychotherapy ◎ ◎
http://www.psych.mcgill.ca/labs/iagp/IAGP.html

The Association is dedicated to the development of group psychotherapy; as a field of practice, training, and scientific study; by means of international conferences, publications, and other forms of communication. The Web page consists of membership information and a directory of the executive and board of directors. The site also offers links to conference information, an electronic forum, and links to other sites of interest. Upcoming links include abstracts of scientific articles relating to group psychotherapy.

Shame and Group Psychotherapy ◎ ◎
http://members.tripod.com/~birchmore/index.html

This site offers a discussion of shame and group psychotherapy, as well as patient education booklets, links to related sites, references on shame, and references on scapegoating, bullying, cruelty, and persecution.

Hypnotherapy

American Board of Hypnotherapy ◎ ◎
http://www.hypnosis.com/abh/abh.html

The American Board of Hypnotherapy supports over 4,000 members, located in the United States and throughout the world. The site offers a detailed explanation of the organization's purpose, membership information, registration and certification activities, and contact details for additional information.

American Psychotherapy and
Medical Hypnosis Association (APMHA) ◎ ◎ ◎

http://fourohfour.xoom.com/Members404Error.xihtml

The APMHA was founded in 1992 for state board licensed and certified professionals in multi-disciplines of Medicine, Psychology, Social Work, Family Therapy, Alcohol and Chemical Dependency, Professional Counseling, Dentistry, and Forensic and Investigative Hypnosis. The site provides a description of hypnosis, membership information and application, professional referrals, training and certification program information, links to related sites, ordering information for professional video training tapes, and contact details.

Hypnodirect.com:
Official Hypnotists Directory of the United States ◎ ◎ ◎

http://www.hypnodirect.com

Links to directory usage, a search engine, and referral services are available at this site. International services chat room, bulletin board, training information, hypnosis schools, products, related organizations, access to the newsletter, and information about hypnosis itself can be found at this site. Links to related sites are also available.

Hypnosis, Brief Therapy,
and Altered States of Consciousness Web Site Links ◎ ◎

http://www.inmet.com/~dlb/hypnosis/hypnosis.html

This personal Web page provides links to sites providing resources on hypnosis and related topics, altered states of consciousness, parapsychology, brief therapy, and lucid dreaming. Personal notes from recent hypnosis conferences are available.

Hypnotherapy & Clinical Hypnosis Links ◎ ◎ ◎

http://easyweb.easynet.co.uk/~dylanwad/morganic/links.htm

Links to professional journals, United Kingdom based organizations and hypnotherapy providers, discussion sites, and personal sites related to hypnotherapy are found at this address.

Marriage and Family Therapy

American Association of Marriage
and Family Therapists (AAMFT) ◎ ◎ ◎ (fee-based)

http://www.aamft.org

The American Association for Marriage and Family Therapy is the professional association for the field of marriage and family therapy, representing the professional interests of more than 23,000 marriage and family therapists throughout the United

States, Canada, and abroad. This site allows professionals and other interested parties to search directories for therapist listing and provides information on the Association. General information includes clinical updates on various marriage and family mental health issues; the link for practitioners lists information on conferences and conference highlights, resources, a referral section, publications, education, training, licensing links, and membership information.

American Family Therapy Academy ⚙

http://www.afta.org

This nonprofit professional organization fosters an exchange of ideas among family therapy teachers, researchers, and practitioners. The site presents the organization's objectives, policy and press releases, membership details, a membership directory, excerpts of the organization's newsletter, and lists of recent awards with recipients. The site will soon offer links to related professional organizations.

Family Therapy Net: Online Counseling ⚙ ⚙ ⚙

http://www.familytherapynet.com/index.htm

Visitors to this site can e-mail a professional with advice concerning marriage, relationships, family, and stepfamilies, and access facts about parenting, divorce, abuse, and children. Personal online counseling sessions are available, and visitors can also read recent mailings with professional responses. Links are provided to Internet resources related to family therapy, mental health, addiction and recovery, co-dependency, and stepfamilies.

Family Therapy Web Sites ⚙ ⚙

http://www.abacon.com/famtherapy/links.html

This site contains links to family therapy resources on the Internet, including associations, journals, home pages of practitioners and groups, and sites offering general resources. Short site descriptions are provided with most links.

Marital and Family
Therapy Pathfinder Directory ⚙ ⚙ ⚙ (some features fee-based)

http://clunet.edu/iss/path/therapy/thleft.html

California Lutheran University (CLU) offers this helpful directory of marital and family therapy Internet resources. Categories of resources include periodicals, databases, electronic journals, CLU journals, reference sources, encyclopedias, assessment tools, statistical information, Web directories, newsgroups, associations and organizations, and universities and institutes. Resources are also listed alphabetically. Some material is available only to CLU students, faculty, and staff.

Marriage and Family Therapy (MFT) Info Link ⊚ ⊚ ⊚

http://www.enol.com/~sherman/MFT/MFT.html

Sites listed at this Internet directory of marriage and family therapy resources include those related to specific theoretical foundations and therapies, consumer resources, a bibliography of professional articles, graduate programs, professional organizations, e-mail discussion lists, institutes, professional liability insurance resources, regulatory bodies, and business resources. The site also answers students' frequently asked questions and offers a marriage and family therapy Graduate Student/Therapist Survival Guide.

National Association of Social Workers (NASW) ⊚ ⊚

http://www.naswdc.org

This international organization of professional social workers is devoted to the professional growth of its members, the creation and maintenance of professional standards, and the advancement of social policies. Membership details, chapter listings, publications information, a directory of social workers, continuing education resources, employment notices, an online store, news, and advocacy activities are listed at the site. Links are available to state chapters, professional organizations, government and advocacy resources, child abuse prevention and child welfare resources, health, mental health, substance abuse resources, and commercial partners.

National Council on Family Relations (NCFR) ⊚

http://www.ncfr.org/body.html

The NCFR is comprised of family researchers, educators, policy makers, and practicing professionals, sharing knowledge and information resources. Site visitors can access membership details, register for monthly teleconferences, and peruse job listings.

Occupational Therapy

American Occupational Therapy Association, Inc. ⊚ ⊚ ⊚

http://www.aota.org

This organization offers information on occupational therapy, news, membership details, details of events, products and services, academic accreditation resources, continuing education resources, publications, and information on academic and fieldwork education. Student resources include journals and information on educational programs, fieldwork, and careers. Consumers can access information on occupational therapy, fact sheets, case studies, a directory of practitioners, and links to related sites. Conference details and links to related sites are also found at this address.

Occupational Therapy: Movers & Shakers in Mental Health ◎ ◎

http://web2.airmail.net/cybervyl/list.htm

An informative question and answer session introducing the topic of occupational health in treating mental illness is located at this site. In addition, there is related meeting information, documents that advocate this type of therapy, a discussion list, articles, research information, treatment suggestions, a reading list, and a number of links to related Web sties. In addition, there are personal accounts from patients who have benefited from occupational therapy.

Occupational Therapy Resources ◎ ◎

http://www.qldnet.com.au/tvhs/occ-ther.htm

This site catalogs links to Internet resources in occupational therapy and rehabilitation by topic. Associations, organizations, general information sites, and online forums are included in the list. Some of the topics covered include disability, schizophrenia, attention-deficit/hyperactivity disorder, arthritis, AIDS, and carpal tunnel syndrome.

Primal Psychotherapy

Daniel's Primal Psychotherapy Web Site ◎ ◎

http://planet.nana.co.il/temichev

For those interested in regressive deep feeling psychotherapies, this Web site contains important information regarding the theory of primal therapy, links to other primal therapy Web sites, and related reference material. Included topical material such as Reiki techniques and primal parenting can be found. Lists to primal centers worldwide and sites connecting the user with primal discussion groups and book reviews are offered.

Primal Psychotherapy Page ◎ ◎

http://home.att.net/~jspeyrer

This useful site offers a site search engine, news, book reviews, a list of centers specializing in primal psychotherapy, questions and professional answers, links to related sites, articles, a newsletter, chat forums, articles on birth trauma, and special program information. Primal psychotherapy is discussed, including a description of conditions benefiting from this form of therapy.

Psychiatric Emergencies

Crisis Intervention Resource Manual ◎ ◎ ◎
http://www.bartow.k12.ga.us/psych/crisis/crisis.htm

This manual, developed for the Bartow County School System (Georgia), offers counselors, principals, and other school staff a resource for dealing with a variety of crisis situations, including suicide, death/grief, and natural disasters. Crisis team handouts, parent/teacher handouts, and sample letters and memoranda are available at the site. A list of suggested reading resources, emergency telephone numbers (for Bartow County), reference citations, and links to sites offering resources on crisis intervention are also found at this address.

Emergency Psychiatry, University of Iowa Hospitals and Clinics ◎ ◎ ◎
http://www.vh.org/Providers/Lectures/EmergencyMed/Psychiatry/TOC.html

Psychiatric emergencies, such as suicide, extreme agitation and violence, intoxication, and other conditions are explored in this Emergency Psychiatry Service Handbook by Gerard Clancy, M.D., offered through Virtual Hospital.

Federal Emergency
Management Agency: Response and Recovery ◎
http://www.fema.gov/r-n-r/counsel.htm

The Federal Emergency Management Agency describes crisis counseling services available to survivors of Presidentially-declared major disasters at this address. Hotline numbers and a link to additional resources are also available.

Merck Manual: Psychiatric Emergencies ◎ ◎ ◎
http://www.merck.com/pubs/mmanual/section15/chapter194/194a.htm

Information is available at this site for physicians treating patients with psychiatric symptoms in an emergency situation. The general nature of this situation is discussed, followed by a list of emergencies requiring a general medical evaluation, hospitalization or other institutional support, minimal pharmacologic intervention, and more comprehensive intervention. For each condition, a list of medical conditions presenting the mental condition, possible causes (when known), and suggested therapies are included.

Psychoanalysis

Academy for the Study of the Psychoanalytic Arts ⊙

http://www.academyanalyticarts.org

This site provides professionals with free online access to program papers, articles, and other reference materials on the topics of psychoanalysis and related fields. The organization's background, meeting, and membership information is also provided.

American Academy of Psychoanalysis ⊙ ⊙

http://aapsa.org

The American Academy of Psychoanalysis represents the National Academy of Professional Medical Psychoanalysists. Informative links to the *Journal of the American Academy of Psychoanalysis*, selected articles from the *Academy Forum*, related meetings, member roster, organization information, publications, and research details are available at the site.

American Psychoanalytic Association ⊙ ⊙ ⊙

http://apsa.org

The American Psychoanalytic Association is a professional organization of psychoanalysts throughout the United States. Press releases, a calendar of events and meetings, general information about psychoanalysis, fellowship details, an online book store, a directory of psychoanalysts, *Journal of the American Psychoanalytic Association* abstracts, and an online newsletter are all available at the site. An extensive catalog of links to related online journals, institutes, societies, organizations, libraries, museums, and general sites are offered through the site. The Jourlit and Bookrev databases are also available, together constituting a formidable bibliography of psychoanalytic journal articles, books, and book reviews. Information on obtaining journal reprints is supplied.

American Society of Psychoanalytic Physicians ⊙

http://pubweb.acns.nwu.edu/~chessick/aspp.htm

This Society and Web site were created to provide a forum for psychoanalytically-oriented psychiatrists and physicians. The purpose of the Society, as well as a list of the officers and editorial board is available.

Association for Psychoanalytic Medicine ⊙ ⊙

http://cpmcnet.columbia.edu/dept/pi/psychoanalytic/APM

The Association for Psychoanalytic Medicine (APM) is a nonprofit organization, and is an affiliate society of both the American Psychoanalytic Association and the International Psychoanalytic Association. Most members are graduates of the Columbia University Center for Psychoanalytic Training and Research, participating in professional development and community outreach activities. An extensive list of the association-sponsored lectures, held at the New York Academy of Medicine, as well as online access to publications, such as *The Bulletin—the Journal of the APM,* and *The Shrink.* There is information on awards, and a membership roster. Other links include postgraduate education information, and mental health resources.

Center for Modern Psychoanalytic Studies ☺ ☺

http://www.cmps.edu

The Center for Modern Psychoanalytic Studies is dedicated to training and research in psychoanalysis. Within this Web site, professionals will find reference materials, including online access to the table of contents to the journal, *Modern Psychoanalysis,* workshop bulletins, a book list, as well as membership information and conference listings.

Cyberpsych.org ☺ ☺

http://www.cyberpsych.org

This site offers descriptions and links to professional psychoanalytical societies and psychoanalytical forum discussions.

International Psychoanalytical Association (IPA) ☺ ☺ ☺

http://www.ipa.org.uk

Described as the world's primary psychoanalytic accrediting and regulatory body, the Association's Web site has numerous links to the various conferences and congresses organized by the Association, as well as links to special committees' synopses, a message forum, access to IPA newsletters, and other related links.

NYU Psychoanalytic Institute— New York University Medical Center ☺ ☺ ☺

http://www.westnet.com/~pbrand

NYU Psychoanalytic Institute educates qualified individuals from a variety of professional backgrounds in the theory and practice of psychoanalysis. The site describes psychoanalysis, educational programs provided by the Institute, consultation and treatment services at the Institute, and provides links to related sites.

Psychoanalytic Therapy FAQ ☺ ☺ ☺

http://users.erols.com/henrywb/Psyan.html

This Web site contains brief answers to over 30 questions about psychoanalytic therapy, with topics including benefits, role of the therapist and patient, dreams, the unconscious, different schools, length of treatment, cost, choosing a therapist, and more.

Psychotherapy

American Association of Psychotherapists   ☢ (fee-based)

http://www.angelfire.com/tx/Membership/index.html

The American Association of Psychotherapists is a national nonprofit, multidisciplinary professional organization of certified clinicians dedicated to the support and development of psychotherapy. This Web site was created to provide networking opportunities for professionals. The site provides a message board, chat room, and online membership application.

American Group Psychotherapy Association   ☢ ☢ ☢

http://www.groupsinc.org

The American Group Psychotherapy Association works to enhance the practice, theory, and research of group therapy. The Association offers information about group therapy, a directory of group therapists for interested patients, news, contact information, a meetings and events calendar, and publications details at this site. Specific resources for group therapists and students include ethical guidelines for group therapists, training opportunities information, certification details, government reports, advanced principles of psychotherapy, and links to affiliated societies.

Carol Matseoane's Public Service
Communications Network: Psychotherapy Links   ☢ ☢

http://members.tripod.com/CarolM_1/psychotherapy/psychotherapy_links.htm

This address contains links to various sites offering information on psychotherapy, and includes associations, institutes, news groups, and scientific resources. Comments are provided with some links.

Group-Psychotherapy   ☢ ☢ ☢

http://www.diac.com/~haimw/group2.html

Resources for professional group psychotherapists at this site include a discussion forum, a basic bibliography of group psychotherapy publications organized by specific subjects, and suggested video resources. Links are available to important journals and MEDLINE, conference details, grants and awards information, material on courses and studies, and other resources related to group psychotherapy.

Health Center.com: Therapy   ☢ ☢

http://site.health-center.com/brain/therapy

Devoted to providing information on all aspects of psychological therapy, consumers and professionals can use links to find resources on therapy, assistance in obtaining therapy, the different types of therapy, and links to specific mental disorders and an overview of symptoms and available treatments.

Psyche Matters: Group Therapy, Group Dynamics, and Analysis Links ◎ ◎ ◎

http://psychematters.com/group.htm

This site lists links to institutes, organizations, publications, conference details, and general resources related to group therapy. Short descriptions are available with some site links.

Psychotherapy Central ◎ ◎

http://www.gn.apc.org/noharm/crp/crpaltri.htm

This site catalogs Internet resources in psychotherapy, psychopathology, psychiatry, and health psychology. General sites, associations, journals, newsletters, and sites offering services are included in the list, organized by topic.

Psychotherapy Innovations ◎ ◎

http://www.psychinnovations.com

This site offers information on new advances, techniques, and tools in psychotherapy for the general public and professionals. Journals and other online information resources, books, information on visualization and awareness processes, rapid acting or power therapy resources, discussion lists, an online newsletter, an online ordering service, and contact details are listed at the site.

Psyweb.com: Psychotherapy ◎ ◎

http://www.psyweb.com/psywebsub/MentalDis/AdvPsych.html

Visitors to this site will find short descriptions of many psychotherapy schools, including Adlerian, behavior, existential, gestalt, person-centered, psychoanalytic, rational-emotive, reality, and transactional analysis therapies. These short overviews may be useful to both consumers and professionals.

Silvan S. Tomkins Institute ◎ ◎

http://www.behavior.net/orgs/ssti

Devoted to understanding human emotion, this Institute provides support for research on affect and script theory and related psychotherapy systems. Information about the different theories, online articles from the Institute's bulletin, continuing education, and other related information is available.

Society for the Exploration of Psychotherapy Integration (SEPI) ◎ ◎

http://www.cyberpsych.org/sepi.htm

"The primary objectives of SEPI are to encourage communication and to serve as a reference group for individuals interested in exploring the interface between differing approaches to psychotherapy." This site provides information on the society's mission, conference information, a list of influential books, training opportunities in psycho-therapy integration, an online article, and links of interest.

Transactional Analysis

United States of America Transactional Analysis Association ◎ ◎

http://usataa.org

This organization is a community of professionals utilizing transactional analysis in "organizational, educational, and clinical settings, and for personal growth." A history of the organization, membership details, events notices, and articles are available at the site. Links are provided to transactional analysis associations, online publications, and educational sites.

Transcranial Magnetic Stimulation (TMS)

Transcranial Magnetic Stimulation in Psychiatry ◎ ◎ ◎

http://www.musc.edu/tmsmirror/intro/layintro.html

Based on the use of pulsed magnetic fields, this new, near-painless treatment shows promise in terms of its potential in the treatment of mental illness. The principles of transcranial magnetic stimulation are described and the safety and efficacy of extracranial techniques are examined.

Transcranial Magnetic Stimulation (TMS) ◎ ◎ ◎

http://www.biomag.helsinki.fi/tms

An online movie demonstrating the spread of cortical electrical brain activity following transcranial magnetic stimulation is shown, and numerous links to detailed informa-tion regarding the principles and safety of this new technique are found. Terminology, journal articles, current research, and further Internet connections are provided.

Transcranial Magnetic Stimulation (TMS): Its Potential in Treating Neuropsychiatric Disorders ◎ ◎ ◎

http://www.mcleanhospital.org/psychupdate/psyup-I-4.htm

A detailed description of this novel, noninvasive technique is explored at the Web site, and recent clinical studies are outlined, including the results of patients found to be refractory to other treatments. Published reports of the use of transcranial magnetic stimulation in posttraumatic stress disorder (PTSD) patients, and the limited research on the therapy as applied to TMS and Parkinson's disease are mentioned. Side effects and the future of TMS are discussed, and references to additional reading for clinicians are also included.

6.4 **Psychopharmacology/Drug Therapy**

Anticholinergics

How Anticholinergics Work ⊙ ⊙ ⊙
http://www.nmhc.co.uk/moa-proc.htm

A hypothesis regarding anticholinergic activity of antipsychotics is presented at this Web site. Also outlined is the normal anatomy and physiology of chemical brain cell communication and excess dopamine activity that produces the symptoms of psychosis. Synapses, neurotransmitter functions, and symptoms of malfunction are reviewed. Examples of drugs that increase dopamine activity and possibly produce symptoms of anxiety or psychosis are discussed, as are the Parkinsonian or extra-pyramidal side effects common in those treated with dopamine receptor blockade. A summary of adjunct therapy with anticholinergics to prevent muscular rigidity and tremor is presented.

Anticonvulsants

Advancing the Art and Science of
Pain Management: Anti-Convulsant Medications ⊙ ⊙
http://www.paincareplus.com/anti-convulsant_meds_main.html

Indications of anticonvulsants in seizure disorders and special instructions and precautions for the most commonly prescribed anticonvulsant therapies are described at the Web address. For further physician knowledge and patient information, an adverse event list is included.

Anticonvulsants ⊙ ⊙ ⊙
http://www.puritan.com/healthnotes/Drug/Anticonvulsants.htm

This site provides information about anticonvulsants, a class of drugs used to prevent seizures in people with epilepsy. The site provides drug and brand names and details possible interactions with dietary supplements. Supplements discussed include biotin, carnitine, folic acid, melatonin, vitamin D, and vitamin K.

Anticonvulsants ⊙ ⊙
http://www.toxicology.lsumc.edu/ahpharm/anticonv.htm

This site contains a lecture on anticonvulsants that may be downloaded.

Anticonvulsants ⊙ ⊙ ⊙

http://www.ebando.com/band51/b51-3.html

From the Bandolier, this article provides information about the use of anticonvulsants in the treatment of head injury patients. The site describes studies and results. Graphics and references are included.

Antiepileptic Drugs ⊙ ⊙ ⊙

http://www.hsc.unt.edu/departments/pharm/99antic/index.htm

A 41-slide presentation on antiepileptic drugs is offered at this subsite of a medical pharmacology course at the University of North Texas Health Science Center. Outlined are the general principles of therapy, mechanisms of action of various antiepileptic classifications, their pharmacokinetics, indications for use, and drug interactions. Epilepsy classifications, facts on seizure incidence, and charts depicting the major characteristics of generalized and partial seizures are found.

Antiepileptics ⊙ ⊙

http://www.nmh.org/netreach/html/anticon1.html

Northwestern Memorial Hospital presents this online fact sheet regarding antiepileptic medications for the control and prevention of seizures. Administration, adverse events, and special patient instructions provide convenient, consumer advice. A list of generic and name brand antiepileptics is provided.

Antidepressants

Major Depression and the Neurotransmitter Serotonin ⊙ ⊙ ⊙

http://www.lafayette.edu/~loerc/ander.html

The biological role of serotonin in subgroups of depressed patients is explored at this online article. The hypothesis that depression may result from a deficiency of available serotonin is supported by the effectiveness of selective serotonin reuptake inhibitors (SSRIs) in treatment. Additional genetic studies, reduced levels of serotonin metabolites in depressed patients, and decreased levels of platelet serotonin are also discussed in support of the correlation between an abnormal serotonergic system and depression.

Selective Serotonin Reuptake Inhibitors (SSRIs) ⊙ ⊙

http://www.biopsychiatry.com/ssrispec.htm

This site contains several interrelated abstracts. An update on SSRIs is provided which summarizes the safety, efficacy, and common side effects. In addition, the selection of SSRIs as the treatment of choice in instances of eating disorders, premenstrual dysphoria, panic disorder, depression, and obsessive-compulsive disorder, is discussed. Links to additional article abstracts highlighting the progress made with specific SSRIs, further information on SSRIs mechanisms of action, and SSRI selection suggestions are found.

Serotonin and Judgment ⊙ ⊙ ⊙

http://www.sfn.org/briefings/serotonin.html

By selectively restoring serotonin's activity level in patients with depression, researchers hope to prevent impulsive and destructive behaviors that often lead to suicide. This online Brain Briefing from the Society for Neuroscience outlines current study that may lead to the use of brain imaging techniques for identification of those at greatest risk for destructive behavior. An explanation of possible new insights into the mechanisms of serotonin and the identification of components that play a role in defective serotonin processing are presented.

Antipsychotics/Neuroleptics

Antipsychotic Drugs ⊙ ⊙ ⊙

http://www.gvsu.edu/adrianb/HS311Web/antipsyc.htm

Visitors will find the signs and symptoms of schizophrenia, possible pathology, and a listing of typical antipsychotic agents at the Web site. Additional indications for antipsychotics, a review of their anticholinergic effects, and the adverse events associated with their administrations are summarized. A convenient chart is provided, outlining drug class, usage, pharmacodynamics, side effects, routes of administration, and pertinent comments.

Common Neuroleptics ⊙ ⊙ ⊙

http://biochem2.kenyon.edu/neurochem/common_neuroleptics.htm

This site describes common neuroleptics. Drugs discussed include chlorpromazine and reserpine.

Dopamine Receptor Blockade: Antipsychotic Drugs ⊙ ⊙ ⊙

http://www.williams.edu:803/imput/IIIB4.html

The chemical structure of various typical and atypical antipsychotics and their properties allowing them to block dopamine receptors are discussed at the Web site. Features of typical antipsychotics, helpful in alleviating the positive symptoms of schizophrenia, are discussed, as well as the atypical antipsychotics, which lack the undesirable side effects present with the traditional antipsychotics. A page summarizing the clinical application of dopamine discusses the splitting of cognitive function in schizophrenia, symptoms hypothesized to be from dopaminergic dysfunction, and the *DSM-IV* categories of schizophrenia.

Neuroleptics ◎ ◎ ◎

http://neuroland.com/psy/neuroleptics.htm

Information regarding formulations, dosage, and pharmacologic considerations of administration of neuroleptics are outlined at this Neuroland Web site. Phenothiazines, thioxanthenenes, butyrophenones, and heterocyclics are all included categories.

Newer Generation Antipsychotic Drugs ◎ ◎ ◎

http://www.nlpra.org.hk/1stSymposium/NGAD.html

Limitations to traditional antipsychotics and an introduction to the more novel drug treatments in schizophrenia are reviewed, with a focus on effectively treating both the positive and negative symptoms of the illness. Extrapyramidal, anticholinergic, anti-adrenergic, and other side effects of traditional neuroleptics are summarized, in addition to the recent advances in the improvement of adverse event profiles.

Anxiolytics

Anti-Anxiety Drugs ◎ ◎

http://www.chre.vt.edu/f-s/kredican/EDHL3534MM/ANTI.html

The major uses, principal types, and clinical applications and mechanisms of action for antianxiety agents are briefly outlined at the Web site.

Benzodiazepines ◎ ◎

http://www.adhl.org/benzodi.html

A listing of the most commonly prescribed benzodiazepines is offered, with additional information regarding duration of action, detection in urine, psychological and physical effects, and symptoms of withdrawal.

Common Benzodiazepines ◎ ◎

http://biochem2.kenyon.edu/neurochem/benzodiazepines.htm

A concise description regarding two of the most common benzodiazepines, Librium and Valium, includes their addictive qualities, sedating effects, and potential depressive potentials when combined with alcohol or barbiturates.

Drug Review: Anxiety Drugs ◎ ◎

http://pathcuric1.swmed.edu/ScribeService/
Resources/pharm/quickreview/Drug_Review-Anxiety.html

This quick review of antianxiety agents offers visitors a listing of general features, therapeutic uses, side effects, and information on the toxicity potentials for benzodiazepines, barbiturates, and alcohol.

Medication Profiles: Benzodiazepines (BZs)   ⊙ ⊙ ⊙
http://anxieties.com/8Meds/BZs.htm

This Web page, courtesy of Anxieties.com, provides information on the benefits, side effects, and disadvantages of benzodiazepine usage. A chart outlining the possible symptoms associated with drug withdrawal, suggestions for dosage tapering, and individual profiles of the more commonly prescribed benzodiazepines are provided.

New Ways To Stop Worrying: Future Anxiolytics   ⊙ ⊙ ⊙
http://www.biopsychiatry.com/anxfut.html

This article abstract, an excerpt from a major psychiatric medical journal, offers summary format information on the current state of development regarding new, anxiolytic alternatives to benzodiazepines in the treatment of anxiety. Mention of their beneficial targeting of neurotransmitter receptors and citing of partial antagonists with beneficial clinical profiles are found. Serotonin receptor subtype targeting and simultaneous targeting of multiple receptor sites in future treatment are discussed. Additional therapies and the future of the neurobiological regulation of anxiety are summarized.

Clinical Pharmacology

American College of Neuropsychopharmacology (ACNP)   ⊙ ⊙ ⊙
http://www.acnp.org

To further education and research in the field, the American College of Neuropsycho-pharmacology provides information on panel, poster, and study-group abstract submissions, the Archives in Psychopharmacology at Vanderbilt University, and the organization's annual meeting. Current and archived issues of the online *ACNP Bulletin* are available in Adobe Acrobat format, and the site's scientific link direct visitors to a searchable, online version of the ACNP professional publication, *Neuropsychopharmacology*. Related advocacy affiliates and scientific links are provided.

Clinical Psychopharmacology Seminar, University of Iowa College of Pharmacy   ⊙ ⊙ ⊙
http://www.vh.org/Providers/Conferences/CPS/contents.html

Forty-five major topics related to clinical psychopharmacology are explored through this menu provided by the University of Iowa College of Pharmacy, such as specific disorder treatments, dosing, primary therapeutic action, and side effects.

Harvard Psychopharmacology Algorithms Project ◎ ◎ ◎
http://www.mhc.com/Algorithms

This site allows professionals to view and download the computerized algorithms created by this project. The depression and schizophrenia algorithms are complete, and these programs provide advice and guidance on drug therapy in various psychoses. Confidence ratings inform as to the quality of research evidence to fortify each step of the algorithm. A publications bibliography is also included.

MedWebPlus: Psychopharmacology ◎ ◎ ◎
http://www.medwebplus.com/subject/Psychopharmacology.html

MedWebPlus supplies links to journal titles, abstracts, and sometimes full-text articles, listing articles by subject. Full journal information is also provided. Psychopharmacology topics include bibliographies, consumer health, history of medicine, internship and residency resources, neurology, neuropharmacology, patient education, periodicals, pharmacology, psychiatry, psychophysiology, religion and medicine, societies, scientific societies, and substance-related disorders.

Neurology Pharmacotherapeutics ◎ ◎ ◎
http://wizard.pharm.wayne.edu/medchem/pha422.html

This online medicinal chemistry tutorial provides information on general and local anesthetic agents, opioid analgesics, and antiseizure agents. Stages of general anesthesia, specific agents, and chemical structural components are examined.

Pharmacological Management of Acute Delirium ◎ ◎ ◎
http://www.vh.org/Providers/Conferences/CPS/02.html

This peer-reviewed, clinical psychopharmacology seminar reviews the pharmacologic management of behavioral disturbances secondary to delirium. Antipsychotics, treatment of acute and chronic delirium, studies comparing benzodiazepines to antipsychotics, and summaries on lithium and anticonvulsants are all included. An outcome table for measurement of efficacy of treatment with non-neuroleptics is provided.

Psychopharmacology Links ◎ ◎
http://www.links.co.nz/culture/drugs/psycho.htm

Resources provided at this site include links to psychopharmacology forums, search tools, substance abuse resources, basic pharmacology information related to antidepressants, publications, journals, articles, associations, and pediatric psychopharmacology information.

Psychopharmacology Tips ◎ ◎ ◎

http://uhs.bsd.uchicago.edu/~bhsiung/tips/intro.html

Visitors to this site will find general information on the psychopharmacological treatment of psychiatric disorders based on a chat forum of therapists at the site. Specific drugs and psychiatric disorders can be chosen to include in a site search, and users can also search by keyword. Links are available to another chat forum, Internet resources in psychiatry and psychopharmacology, and a list of answers to questions posted by patients and caregivers.

Drug Databases

Clinical Pharmacology ◎ ◎ (fee-based)

http://www.cponline.gsm.com

As an electronic drug reference site, professionals and laypersons can use the searchable database for drug information, available as a brief summary or mini-monograph. Full monograph access requires subscription to the online service.

Internet Mental Health: Medications ◎ ◎ ◎

http://www.mentalhealth.com/fr30.html

Resources on more than 150 psychiatric medications are available at this site. Information on each drug, taken from Canadian monographs, includes pharmacology, indications, contraindications, warnings, precautions, adverse effects, overdose, dosage, supplied dose, and any details on current research related to the drug. The site also offers links to sites containing additional drug information and an online medical dictionary.

Medical Science Bulletin:
Psychopharmacologic and Neurologic (CNS) Drug Reviews ◎ ◎

http://pharminfo.com/pubs/msb/msbpsyc.html

Supported by Pharmaceutical Information Associates, Ltd., this site contains a broad list of drug reviews for various central nervous system (CNS) mental health issues, including Alzheimer's disease, antipsychotics, drug addiction, depression, eating disorders, Parkinson's disease, and general topics in mental illness.

National Institute of Mental Health (NIMH): Medications ◎ ◎ ◎

http://www.nimh.nih.gov/publicat/medicate.htm

This address offers an online Medications booklet from the National Institute of Mental Health, designed to help patients understand how and why drugs can be used as part of the treatment for mental health problems. An introduction to drugs and their use in the treatment of mental illnesses, important considerations about drug therapy, and important questions for a patient's doctor are found at the site. Detailed information is available on antipsychotic medications, anti-manic medications, antidepressant medications, and anti-anxiety medications. A discussion of medications in children, the elderly, and pregnant or nursing women is available, as well as an index of medications listing generic and trade names, and a bibliography of reference articles.

Neuro Med Pharmacology Page ⊙ ⊙ ⊙

http://www.neuroland.com/neuro_med.htm

Dosage information on neuropharmacotherapies is provided at this Neuroland Web site. With 30 medication categories including antidepressants, anticonvulsants, muscle relaxants, and spasticity treatments, practitioners can quickly scan administration and adverse event information. For each pharmaceutical choice, alternative treatments and related readings may be obtained.

PharmInfo Net: Medical Sciences Bulletin:
Psychopharmacologic and Neurologic (CNS) Drug Reviews ⊙ ⊙

http://pharminfo.com/pubs/msb/msbpsyc.html

This site contains news articles related to new drugs used in the treatment of Alzheimer's disease, depression, migraine, stroke, epilepsy, schizophrenia, and other central nervous system (CNS) or psychiatric conditions. General topics are also discussed, and visitors can access drug reviews in other medical subjects.

Project Inform: Psychoactive Drugs ⊙ ⊙

http://www.thebody.com/pinf/drugbkix.html

Taken from the *HIV Drug Book,* this site contains concise explanations of drugs used to treat more common psychiatric disorders, such as anxiety, depression, insomnia, psychoses, and mania. Drug categories and specific drugs are listed, and links to fact sheets describing the type of drug, treatment information, and side effects are provided.

Psychiatric Medications ⊙ ⊙

http://www.mentalhealth.nu

This online book gives professionals and consumers a good overview of psychiatric drug therapy, and includes chapters devoted to antidepressants, antianxiety drugs, neuroleptics, and mood stabilizers. Each chapter considers drug treatments for different disorders, contraindicators, and general effects of the drugs.

Psychopharmacology and Drug References ⊙ ⊙ ⊙

http://mentalhelp.net/guide/pro22.htm

This site offers users the opportunity to ask specific drug questions of pharmacists and locate drug information by generic name, including pharmacology, indications, contraindications, warnings, precautions, adverse effects, overdose information, typical dosages, supplied dosages in typical pill forms, and research information. Visitors can also access links to newsgroups, mailing lists, journals, publications, research papers, professional organizations and centers, and other Internet resources.

Mood Stabilizers

Pharmacology ☺ ☺ ☺
http://www.walkers.org/noframes/stabilizers.htm

Links to six mood stabilizing drugs are offered at this site of the HealthCentral Rx Online Pharmacy. Visitors will find complete warnings and prescribing information, with access to clinical pharmacology, inactive ingredients, mechanisms of action, indications, precautions, patient information, and pregnancy risk category. The links also feature drug interactions, a system-by-system guide to side effects, and dosage and administration tables for all included drugs.

6.5 Clinical Practice

Clinical Guidelines and Practice

American Academy of Child and Adolescent Psychiatry (AACAP): Clinical Practice ☺ ☺
http://www.aacap.org/clinical

This site describes activities of the American Academy of Child and Adolescent Psychiatry organization aimed at improving clinical practice for both professionals and patients. Practice parameters and systems of care developed by the Academy, information on managed care issues, resources on current procedural terminology (CPT) codes, and efforts to preserve psychotherapy as the core of child and adolescent psychiatry are described at the site.

American Psychiatric Association (APA) Clinical Practice ☺ ☺ ☺
http://www.psych.org/pract_of_psych/index.html

This site links users to APA resources, including those for early-career psychiatrists. Other sections of the site include links to professional development resources, a final report from the APA Task Force on Quality Indicators, resources from the APA Commission on Psychotherapy by Psychiatrists, and a career-oriented mailing list. Resources are provided on mental retardation and developmental disabilities, the APA Practice Research Network, APA delivery systems and special-interest caucuses, cross-cultural APA resources, iAPA international practice and education activities, and the APA 1998 National Survey of Psychiatric Practice. Many resources for practice management, the Federation of State Medical Boards, and a worldwide directory of psychiatric organizations are also available from the site.

American Psychiatric Association (APA) Practice Guidelines ○ ○ ○

http://www.psych.org/clin_res/prac_guide.html

Practice guidelines from the American Psychiatric Association are available at this site including those for the treatment of patients with delirium, panic disorder, bipolar disorder, eating disorders, substance abuse disorders, Alzheimer's disease and other dementias, schizophrenia, nicotine dependence, and major depressive disorder. Guidelines also cover psychiatric evaluation of adults. Users can also access quick reference guides on treating delirium and schizophrenia, patient and family guides related to delirium and smoking cessation, and ordering information for print guidelines.

American Psychiatric Association (APA) Practice Research Network (PRN) ○ ○ ○

http://www.psych.org/res_res/background.html

The Practice Research Initiative is a network of psychiatrists cooperating in the collection of data and conduct of research studies on issues relating to clinical and health services delivery issues. The site offers a mission statement, research objectives, details of study collaborations, confidentiality, and convenience, PRN membership eligibility requirements, information on joining the PRN, current and upcoming PRN activities, and contact details for additional information.

Clinical Practice Guidelines for Mental Disorders ○ ○ ○

http://www.guideline.gov/BROWSE/browse_disease_body.asp?type=&view=disease

Over 50 guidelines are available for a variety of mental disorders, courtesy of the National Guideline Clearinghouse. Categories include sleep disorders, eating disorders, mood disorders, anxiety disorders, substance-related disorders, delirium, dementia, amnestic, and cognitive disorders, sexual and gender disorders, mental disorders diagnosed in childhood, and schizophrenia and other disorders with psychotic features. Users may opt to view brief summaries, complete summaries, or the complete text of the chosen guidelines and practice parameters.

Clinical Practice Guidelines for Mental Health Treatment and Intervention ○ ○ ○

http://www.guideline.gov/BROWSE/browse_treatment.asp?type=&view=treatment

With over 20 clinical practice guidelines individually accessible, this page of the National Guideline Clearinghouse offers guidelines regarding behavioral health treatment and interventions. Parameters specific to mental health services, personality assessment, psychological techniques, psychiatric somatic therapies, behavioral sciences, psychotherapy, and psychological tests may be accessed. Users may opt to view brief summaries, complete summaries, or the complete text of the chosen guidelines and practice parameters.

Clinical Practice Guidelines in Psychiatry ⊙ ⊙ ⊙
http://www.guideline.gov/index.asp

Over 90 clinical guidelines related to the practice of psychiatry are listed at this page of the National Guidelines Clearinghouse, which is updated weekly with new and revised information, allowing physicians and allied healthcare professionals access to current treatment protocols. To obtain a list of psychiatry guidelines, type "psychiatry" into the search tool at the main site. The browse function of the National Guideline Clearinghouse allows viewers to select other organization names from an alphabetically arranged list, or, alternatively, visitors may cross-reference using initials, acronyms, and abbreviations for better guideline browsing. Users may opt to view brief summaries, complete summaries, or the complete text of the chosen guidelines and practice parameters.

Expert Consensus Guidelines ⊙ ⊙ ⊙
http://www.psychguides.com

Visitors to this site can download expert consensus guidelines for the treatment of posttraumatic stress disorder, schizophrenia, agitation in older persons with dementia, obsessive-compulsive disorder, and bipolar disorder. Guidelines for psychiatric and behavioral problems in mental retardation, attention-deficit/hyperactivity disorder, and the treatment of depression in women are available. A description of methodology used in developing the guidelines, patient and family guides, conference details, and links to related sites are also available at this address. These guidelines have been supported by unrestricted educational grants from Abbott Laboratories, Bristol-Myers Squibb, Eli Lilly and Co., Janssen Pharmaceutica, Inc., Novartis Pharmaceuticals Corporation, Ortho-McNeil Pharmaceutical, Pfizer, Inc., Solvay Pharmaceuticals, and Zeneca Pharmaceuticals.

National Guideline
Clearinghouse (NGC): Nervous System Diseases ⊙ ⊙ ⊙
http://www.guideline.gov/BROWSE/browse_disease_body.asp?type=&view=disease

Eighty clinical guidelines relating to nervous system diseases are available at this site. Visitors can also access guidelines on related subconcepts of nervous system diseases, including neuromuscular diseases, neurological manifestations, nervous system neoplasms, mental retardation, nervous system abnormalities, central nervous system diseases, and peripheral nervous system diseases.

University of Groningen Department of Social Psychiatry: Schedules for Clinical Assessment in Neuropsychiatry (SCAN) ⊘ ⊘ ⊘

http://www.psy.med.rug.nl/0018

Schedules for Clinical Assessment in Neuropsychiatry (SCAN), developed within the World Health Organization, offers tools and manuals for "assessing, measuring, and classifying psychopathology and behavior associated with the major psychiatric disorders in adult life." This site offers a list of SCAN training centers worldwide, a bibliography of SCAN publications, answers to frequently asked questions, and a link to the World Health Organization SCAN home page. A discussion of SCAN includes a detailed description of methods used in assessment, SCAN software, suggested reference materials, a list of advisory committee members, and a short description of SCAN training courses.

Managed Care

American Psychiatric Association (APA) Managed Care Practice Management ⊘ ⊘ ⊘

http://www.psych.org/pract_of_psych/managed_care.html

The American Psychiatric Association site offers resources on practice management from the Office of Healthcare Systems and Financing at this address. Visitors can access the APA Handbook for the Development of Public Managed Care Systems, download an outpatient treatment report form, and find links to many valuable practice management resources. Additional resources include: access to the State Boards of Medical Licensure—Federation of State Medical Boards of the U.S., Inc., a directory of state Medicare carriers, a list of suggested readings related to managed care, information on capitation and deselection from managed care networks, information on the Employment Retirement Income Security Act, answers to frequently asked managed care questions, details on how to appeal managed care reimbursement denials, contacts for the APA managed care help line, recommendations for patients during changes in healthcare provider networks, CPT coding resources, information on practice management software, suggestions for what to do about unpaid claims, and information on managed care and Medicare private contracting. A thorough description and link to the National Practitioner Data Bank and a managed care newsletter are also available at the site.

Knowledge Exchange Network: Managed Care ⊘ ⊘

http://www.mentalhealth.org/links/managedcare.htm

Twenty-one links are available at this address, offering access to federal agencies, associations, education resources, institutes, organizations, and other information sources related specifically to mental health and/or managed care. The site serves as a valuable beginning to Internet searches for information on managed care.

Psychotherapy Finances and Managed Care Strategies ◎ ◎ ◎
http://www.psyfin.com

This Web site was created to aid behavioral health providers with the financial issues in practice and managed care. Updated news items relating to managed care, social work, and other mental health related topics are provided. Articles from the *Psychotherapy Finances* newsletters are available online. There is an online store, conference information, other therapists Web sites, a providers directory, and a link to a fact sheet on strategies related to mental health provision and finances. The Web site's database is searchable by keyword.

7. OTHER TOPICAL RESOURCES FOR PSYCHIATRY

7.1 Abuse, Neglect, and Domestic Violence

About.com: Abuse/Incest Support
http://incestabuse.about.com/health/incestabuse/?once=true&

About.com offers current news and policy information related to domestic abuse, as well as a guide to Internet resources related to domestic abuse and violence. Articles, therapy and professional resources, information and support for survivors of domestic abuse, hotline numbers, prevention resources, statistics, and general information on different forms of abuse are cataloged at this site.

Abuse Resources from the Center for Mental Health Resources
http://www.mentalhealth.org/links/abuse.htm

As a service of the Center for Mental Health Resources (CMHR), this site provides a variety of links related to abuse-specific topics. Comprehensive site connections include the National Clearinghouse on Child Abuse and Neglect Information, Abused Children With Disabilities, and the Borderline Personality Disorder Sanctuary. Links at this site offer plenty of information from forming one's own self-help group to communicating via real-time with other victims of abuse. This is a notable site for abuse survivors.

American Bar Association (ABA)—
Commission on Domestic Violence
http://www.abanet.org/domviol/home.html

The Commission on Domestic Violence is committed to developing a national response to domestic violence, and aims to improve and enhance existing policies and solutions in the constantly changing field of state and federal domestic violence law. The site offers suggestions on teaching law students about domestic violence, resources for research inquiries into domestic violence, selected domestic violence publications, a bibliography of materials on domestic violence published by ABA and other organizations, and more information about legal research and analysis of domestic violence. The site offers a guide identifying individuals and organizations able to take steps to help end domestic violence and details of a video series explaining the use of federal laws to stop violence against women. General information for victims of domestic violence, including contact details, finding legal aid, and safety planning is also available, as well as statistics, myths, and facts related to domestic violence. News, conference details, and internship resources are found at the site.

American College of Obstetricians and Gynecologists (ACOG) Violence Against Women Homepage ◎ ◎ ◎

http://www.acog.org/from_home/departments/dept_web.cfm?recno=17

This support site offers a directory of nationwide coalitions against domestic violence, abuse screening information, a link to publications on news and educational materials for affected persons, information on events, national support groups, and a fact sheet presenting statistics on violence against women. Also included is a bibliography on various aspects of sexual assault, and discussions of men and women's issues, psychosocial, elderly and medicolegal topics, a list of related sites, and general information about the ACOG.

American Professional Society on the Abuse of Children (APSAC) ◎ ◎

http://www.apsac.org

The mission of APSAC is to ensure that everyone affected by child maltreatment receives the best possible professional response. This professional society's site provides information on the society itself, membership information, legislative activities, professional education, state chapters, and public affairs, and current news. Information on the society's publications, such as the APSAC Advisor, the APSAC Guidelines for Practice, the APSAC Handbook on Child Maltreatment and Child Maltreatment are available online. There is also information for those interested in donating to the society.

Association for the Treatment of Sexual Abusers (ATSA) ◎ ◎

http://www.atsa.com

The Association for the Treatment of Sexual Abusers is an international organization focused specifically on the prevention of sexual abuse through effective management of sex offenders. The site provides membership information, Sexual Abuse journal table of contents, 1999 graduate research awards and ATSA research grants, position statements, conference information, internship and fellowship opportunities, employment opportunities, and book lists.

Child Abuse Prevention Network ◎ ◎ ◎

http://child.cornell.edu/capn.html

This site offers resources for reporting child abuse, and links to sites offering discussions of survivors' issues and childhood violence, newsgroups, federal resources, and organizations engaged in prevention activities. Parenting resources, the National Data Archive on Child Abuse and Neglect, and general child abuse Web sites are accessible from this site.

Family Violence and Sexual Assault Institute (FVSAI) ◎ ◎
http://www.fvsai.org

FVSAI is a nonprofit resource center offering a clearinghouse of categorized references and unpublished papers related to all aspects of family violence and sexual assault. Information is available on conferences, training, publications, and membership. Services listed at the site include resource of materials, a categorized reference database, program evaluation and research; program development, consultation, and assistance; speaker database; international and local conferences; professional workshops and certified training; and program prevention and intervention. Some resources are only available to those with a current membership, which requires an annual fee.

Feminist Majority Foundation—
Violence Against Women Internet Resources ◎ ◎ ◎
http://www.feminist.org/gateway/vs_exec2.html

This list of Internet resources offers links to sites presenting general information, emotional abuse resources, research, organizations, shelters, services, and similar resources, stalking, and self-defense. Each link is accompanied by a short paragraph providing helpful information about the site.

Men and Domestic Violence Index ◎ ◎
http://www.vix.com/pub/men/domestic-index.html

Chat transcripts, quotes, and other information sources on issues relating to men and domestic violence are available at this site. Topics include husband battering, child abuse, other domestic violence, other male abuse, and links to related references.

National Center for Missing and Exploited Children (NCMEC) ◎ ◎ ◎
http://www.missingkids.org

The National Center for Missing and Exploited Children, a nonprofit organization, is the nation's resources center for child protection. Organizational resources include program and activity details, new technology descriptions, and contact information. Visitors can search for child photos, report a possible sighting of a missing child, find donating and volunteering information, read success stories, and access news and events details. Information at the site is available in both English and Spanish.

National Clearinghouse on Child Abuse and Neglect ◎ ◎ ◎
http://www.calib.com/nccanch

A service of the Children's Bureau, Administration for Children and Families—Department of Health and Human Services, this national clearinghouse is provided to professionals seeking information on the prevention, identification, and treatment of child abuse and neglect, and related child welfare issues. The site broadcasts new initiatives, reports, and Internet resources, and provides access to a wide range of publications, including fact sheets, the "User Manual Series," statistical information, bibliographies, prevention resources, resource and support listings, and other documents. The site also offers a list of upcoming conferences, contact information, a catalog of publications, funding sources, databases containing documents, national organizations information, prevention programs, and links to related sites. Additional services provided by the clearinghouse to professionals are described at the site, including help with statistics, child welfare issues, child abuse and neglect prevention, and state statutes.

National Coalition Against Sexual Assault ◎

http://www.ncasa.org

This organization provides information, advocacy, and support for sexual assault. Within this site are links to conference and advocacy news, membership information, legal advice and court case summaries, and articles on sexual assault and violence. There is also a section on sexual assault myths and facts, as well as a list of related Web sites.

National Institute of Mental Health (NIMH): Helping Children and Adolescents Cope with Violence and Disasters ◎ ◎ ◎

http://www.nimh.nih.gov/publicat/violence.htm

This site offers a definition of trauma, a discussion of how children and adolescents react to trauma, suggestions on helping a victim, information on posttraumatic stress disorder, and treatment of this disorder. A discussion of current research, and a resource list for support and additional information sources are also offered.

Rape, Abuse, and Incest National Network (RAINN) ◎ ◎

http://www.rainn.org

This support site offers a searchable directory of rape crisis centers and hotline numbers, facts about the network, including contact information, and basic information on rape and related abuse statistics. Fact sheets on what to do if sexually assaulted, current news, and access to the RAINN newsletter and its archive are also available to visitors.

Recovered Memories of Sexual Abuse: Scientific Research and Scholarly Resources ◎ ◎ ◎

http://www.jimhopper.com/memory

This comprehensive Web site contains information about the author, research data, controversy and theories, a great number of research articles on recovered memories, related reference materials and legal information. The articles address various topics including false memory syndrome, the psychiatry of dissociation and memory, and other related topics. In addition, there are links to the psychiatric diagnosis of dissociative amnesia, support information, and related Web sites.

Safer Society Foundation ◎ ◎

http://www.safersociety.org

This national nonprofit organization provides advocacy, referrals, and research for the prevention and treatment of sexual abuse. At this site, professionals and consumers can find news updates, learn about the Foundation's information and referral services, training and consulting information, research resources, and order books, and other reference materials provided by the Safer Society Press. Contact information and links to related organizations are also provided.

Sexual Assault Information Page ◎ ◎ ◎

http://www.cs.utk.edu/~bartley/saInfoPage.html

This site serves as a clearinghouse for fact sheets, articles, links to Web sites, organizations, and other types of resources related to sexual assault, rape, sexual abuse, sexual harassment and other related topics. There is a section answering frequently asked questions, online access to previous issues of the newsletter, and a search engine for keyword searches of the site. In addition, the resources contained herein are divided into sections based on the type of sexual abuse or assault, domestic violence, legal issues, men's issues, professional and university resources, trauma-related issues, rape and rape crisis centers, newsgroups, and other related topics. The variety of topics covered and the amount of information present make this site valuable for consumers and professionals.

Substance Abuse and Mental Health Services Administration (SAMHSA): Women, Co-occurring Disorders and Violence Study ◎ ◎ (some features fee-based)

http://www.prainc.com/wcdvs/index.html

Program structure, principal investigators, and study sites are described at this address. Links are available to Web addresses associated with study sites and principal investigators.

Useful Victimology Links ◎ ◎ ◎

http://www.nursing.upenn.edu/Victimology

Supported by the School of Nursing at University of Pennsylvania, this site contains resources related to the study of victims and victims issues, including numerous links to organizations, articles, Web sites, documents, and support groups. The resources are divided into one of four categories—forensic resources, rape and child abuse, government and Pennsylvania resources, and domestic violence issues.

7.2 Academic Psychiatry

Association for Academic Psychiatry ○ ○

http://www.aapsych.org

The Association for Academic Psychiatry is devoted to psychiatry education issues, and provides a forum for members to discuss teaching techniques, curriculum, and other related topics. Visitors to the site can contact officers and committee chairs through e-mail and access online newsletters, membership details, teaching resources, and annual meeting information. Table of contents, abstracts, full-text articles, and archives of the Association's journal, *Academic Psychiatry*, are also available through this site.

Association for the Advancement of Philosophy and Psychiatry ○ ○

http://www.swmed.edu/home_pages/aapp

The mission of the Association for the Advancement of Philosophy and Psychiatry is to encourage interdisciplinary activity in philosophy and psychiatry and to advance knowledge, promote research, and facilitate understanding in both fields. The Association's mission statement is provided at the site, as well as links to the officers and executive council members, meetings and conferences, local and special interest groups, and free access to the official journal of the Association, *Philosophy, Psychiatry, and Psychology*.

7.3 Adoption

Adoption Network ○ ○ ○

http://www.adoption.org

The Adoption Network is a volunteer-operated general information resource for the adoption community. Links to live chat rooms, an Internet-based classified ad service, information and support for birth parents and adoptees, and a list of FAQs round out this informative, well-organized site.

American Surrogacy Center, Inc. ○ ○ ○

http://www.adopting.org/ar.html

Organization departments include current news about adoption, online support forums, a state-by-state adoption resource directory, and 24-hour chats for adoptive parents and adoptees. Complete adoption resources include listing of licensed agencies, assistance in finding children, as well as international adoption information. Novel features of this site include photolistings of available children, and birth family search information.

Support-Group.com Adoption ◎ ◎

http://www.support-group.com/cgi-bin/sg/get_links?adoption

At Support-Group.com Adoption, local listings of support groups and organizations may be accessed by state/country. An adoption bulletin board is available and a usenet group, alt.adoption, may be accessed with proper Web browser configuration.

7.4 Advocacy, Public Policy, and Law

Advocacy and Protection ◎ ◎ ◎

http://www.mentalhealth.org/links/advocacy.htm

The Center for Mental Health Services, a division of the Federal Substance Abuse and Mental Health Services Administration, has drawn together 25 organizations and programs covering advocacy for patients, consumers, and survivors. Each of these entries is a hot link to the primary organization, and will be helpful to any individuals who are concerned about the problems of mental illness and the individuals and families who are affected.

Advocacy Unlimited, Inc. ◎ ◎

http://mindlink.org.cnchost.com/links.htm

This Connecticut-based group promotes self-determination for individuals suffering or recovering from psychiatric disabilities. The site describes the organization's philosophies and goals, provides information on advocacy education, offers online application to education programs, lists special events and announcements, and contains employment opportunities, featured articles, a resource center for other publications, and an online bookstore. Links to related sites include other advocacy groups, associations, legal sites, and other consumer resources.

Advocacy/Consumers/Survivors:
A Service of the Center for Mental Health Services (CMHS) ◎ ◎ ◎

http://www.mentalhealth.org/links/advocacy.htm

An extensive listing of mental health advocacy Web sites are presented at this CMHS page. Useful links include Internet support groups, a bilingual mental health discussion list, and the consumer-run Justice in Mental Health Organization (JIMHO), which provides consumer-run alternatives for the mentally ill such as community drop-in centers. Links to information for health advocates and an online mental health magazine, 1st Person, are notable.

American Academy of Child and Adolescent Psychiatry (AACAP): Legislation ⊙ ⊙ ⊙

http://www.aacap.org/legislation

Visitors to this address will find legislative alerts, as well as links to information on current regulatory issues, state legislative issues, and important federal agency Web sites. Information about the State Children's Health Insurance Program (SCHIP) includes updates, benefit information by state, archived alerts, and CHIP state contact numbers. Visitors can also send specific messages to Congress, selecting Congressional recipients by zip code or member name.

American Academy of Psychiatry and the Law (AAPL) ⊙ ⊙ ⊙

http://www.emory.edu/AAPL

Dedicated to forensic psychiatry, the organization's Web site provides links to information about the organization and membership; publications, including the AAPL journal, newsletter, and ethics code; meetings, training programs, and fellowships in forensic psychiatry; information on board certification; other forensic resources and links; as well as a question forum.

American Psychiatric Association (APA) Public Policy Advocacy ⊙ ⊙ ⊙

http://www.psych.org/pub_pol_adv/index.html

This site offers information for psychiatrists on writing members of Congress, contacting the APA district branch in each state, and joining the APA's Grassroots Network. Information sources include action alerts and announcements, current issue briefs and fact sheets, transcripts of APA testimony, articles presenting current federal legislative and regulatory issues, APA regulatory comments, information on confidentiality issues, state law fact sheets, state testimony on mental health coverage and other issues, and newsletters offering state and federal policy updates.

Bazelon Center for Mental Health Law ⊙ ⊙ ⊙

http://www.bazelon.org

This nonprofit, legal advocacy organization provides legislative and law case updates at its Web site as well as a variety of online publication excerpts and ordering ability. Fair housing issues, children's rights, aging issues, mental health care, advance directives, and Americans with Disabilities Act resources are provided for attorneys and other advocates in the legal system.

Council for Exceptional Children (CEC) ⊙ ⊙ ⊙

http://www.cec.sped.org/ab

The Council for Exceptional Children is the largest international professional organization dedicated to improving educational outcomes for exceptional children. Learn more about the CEC at this Web site, which highlights the organization's current research endeavors and outlines its public policy positions. Current legislative information is provided directly and updated frequently. The professional development section tells of upcoming events and assists with software selection for developing Individualized Education Programs (IEPs). A Link to the Educational Resources Information Center (ERIC), which contains over 900,000 citations of educational documents and articles of the highest quality is easily accessible.

Council of Parent Attorneys and Advocates ⊚ ⊚ ⊚

http://www.copaa.net

The Web site of this independent, nonprofit organization of attorneys, advocates, and parents, outlines its mission and highlights many of the resources offered. Advocacy Training Program Development, information resources for parents of children with disabilities, and a complete annual conference synopsis are included. The membership brochure and application are available online.

Disability Rights Education and Defense Fund (DREDF), Inc. ⊚ ⊚ ⊚

http://www.dredf.org

The DREDF is a national law and policy center dedicated to advancing the civil rights of people with disabilities through legislation, litigation, and advocacy. At this site, find pertinent Court decisions and legislative information, a complete publication listing including comprehensive documents on the Americans with Disabilities Act. (ADA), and information on the ADA Technical Assistance Hotline, which provides businesses, governmental agencies, and consumers with informational materials regarding rights and responsibilities under Title II and III of the ADA.

Federation of Families for Children's Mental Health ⊚ ⊚ ⊚

http://www.ffcmh.org/enghome.htm

The Federation of Families for Children's Mental Health is a parent-run organization focusing on the needs of children with emotional, behavioral, or mental disorders. An in-depth mission statement along with links to further information are found at the Web site including local chapters and affiliates, details on managed care and children's health, a legislative update in connection with the Bazelon Center for Mental Health Law, and conference and membership material.

Institute of Law, Psychiatry, and Public Policy at the University of Virginia ⊚ ⊚ ⊚

http://ness.sys.virginia.edu/ilppp

Research activities at this University of Virginia institute include community and clinic based programs on mental health issues, such as adjudicative competence, the human genome project and its ethical, legal and social ramifications, serious juvenile offenders and their assessment, and violence in the workplace and on campus. Links to each program include faculty, related organizations, and comprehensive summaries of the program. Additional resources include a mental health law bibliography, online access to the publications of the Institute, including Developments in Mental Health and Law, as well as links to fact files on forensic evaluation services available at the Institute.

Knowledge Exchange Network: Advocacy/Consumers/Survivors ⊙ ⊙

http://www.mentalhealth.org/links/advocacy.htm

Visitors to this site will find links providing access to organizations, consumer groups, support groups, and advocacy resources related to mental health. Thirty-six sites are currently listed at the address.

MacArthur Research Network on Mental Health and the Law ⊙ ⊙

http://ness.sys.virginia.edu/macarthur

This Research Network aims to obtain new information on relationships between mental health and the law, and to develop improved tools and criteria for individual evaluation. Papers describing research findings are available at the site, on topics including adjudicative competence, violence risk, coercion, treatment competence, and additional research topics. The site also provides a directory of Network members.

National Alliance for the Mentally Ill (NAMI) ⊙ ⊙ ⊙

http://www.nami.org

The National Alliance for the Mentally Ill is the preeminent advocacy voice for those facing mental illness. The NAMI Web site provides comprehensive, up-to-date information on the latest developments in national mental health public policy initiatives and current legislation. Pertinent medical and legal information is reviewed and an array of position papers are easily accessed. Also provided are interesting book reviews, NAMI research information, and local NAMI affiliates.

National Association for Rights Protection and Advocacy (NARPA) ⊙ ⊙ ⊙

http://www.connix.com/~narpa

The NARPA exists to expose abuses and promote real alternatives to the current mental health system. The organization's Web site provides readings on mental health advocacy including current case decisions and legislative information, excerpts from the NARPA's Annual Conference and Annual Rights Conference, and an online version of *Rights Tenet* newsletter are available. Interesting links such as the history of mental health advocacy are easily accessed. Online membership information and application is provided.

National Association of Psychiatric
Health Systems (NAPHS) ◎ ◎ (some features fee-based)

http://www.naphs.org

The National Association of Psychiatric Health Systems advocates for health systems providing mental health and substance abuse services. The site provides a description of the organization and services, links to NAPHS and other sites offering consumer information, details of marketing opportunities, membership and contact details, and news articles. A resource catalog offers details of publications, conferences, and services of the organization, including advocacy materials and projects, clinical resources and projects, behavioral health events, financial resources, administrative resources, directories, and mailing lists. One section is restricted to registered members.

National Center for Kids Overcoming Crisis ◎ ◎ ◎

http://www.kidspeace.org

KidsPeace, the National Center for Kids Overcoming Crisis, is a not-for-profit organization that serves more than 2,000 children, providing a comprehensive continuum of mental health treatment programs. KidsPeace advocates for intervention services and educates children and parents around the globe on how to avert crisis. Information on round-the-clock telephone counseling and the National Referral Network database are available at the KidsPeace Web site. Other site features include an electronic version of the semiannual *Healing* magazine, topical index of articles for kids in crisis, a virtual cybermuseum, and a multimedia, bilingual, interactive presentation of the KidsPeace Continuum of Care.

National Empowerment Center (NEC) ◎ ◎

http://www.power2u.org

This nonprofit self-help organization describes its workshop offerings and a list of interesting articles on the explanations of mental illness via the empowerment vision of recovery. The NEC newsletter, with articles past and present, is available online as is the NEC chat room with a full schedule of live discussions. Articles, books, booklets, and videos are available for ordering online.

National Health Law Program (NHeLP) ◎ ◎ ◎

http://www.healthlaw.org

NHeLP is a national public interest law firm dedicated to improving healthcare for working and unemployed poor, minority, elderly, and disabled Americans. Resources at this valuable site include staff rosters, contact details, employment and internship listings, news, NHeLP publications, links to organizations and federal sites, and legal research resources. Topical resources are located under headings including private and federal advocacy, Medicaid, Medicare, public accountability, child health, racial/cultural issues, consumer resources, reproductive health, immigrant health, state and regional resources, managed care, and technology. Visitors can also subscribe to a mailing list alerting members about site updates.

National Information Center for Children and Youth (NICHCY) with Disabilities ◎ ◎ ◎
http://www.nichcy.org

NICHCY is a national referral center providing information on disabilities and related issues for families, educators, and other professionals with a special focus on children and youth. The organization's award-winning Web site describes its referral services and offers online publications in text-only or PDF format. (Acrobat Reader is downloadable from the Web site.) Publications include Basics for Parents and Education Rights, as well as parent guides, research briefings, and multiple fact sheets. Materials are also available in Spanish.

National Mental Health Association ◎ ◎ ◎
http://www.nmha.org/index.cfm

The National Mental Health Association works to increase tolerance and awareness, improve mental health services, prevent mental illness, and promote mental health. At this site, interested individuals will find updates on state and federal legislative actions, employment opportunities, an events calendar, and an information center providing links to referrals and educational materials. Informative links to discussions of topics including mental health disorders, advocacy issues, public education, and healthcare reform are found at the site, as well as links to the Association's affiliate and membership network.

National Mental Health Consumers Self-Help Clearinghouse ◎ ◎ ◎ (free registration)
http://www.mhselfhelp.org

The National Mental Health Consumers Self-Help Clearinghouse on the Web provides consumers with the ability to plan, provide, and evaluate mental health and community support services. Information about starting self-help groups, political material, and organization conference announcements are available to support the growing movement of mental health consumers. An online newsletter as well as several technical assistance guides are downloadable from the Web site after a brief registration process.

Psychiatry and the Law ◎ ◎ ◎
http://mentalhelp.net/law

This site, created by the Medical Director of the Taylor Hardin Secure Medical Facility in Alabama, is devoted to the disciplines of psychiatry and law. There are links to the National Forensic Hospital Database, general information regarding legal issues and psychiatry, links to mental health experts and attorneys, conference information, the

American Psychiatric Association's relevant position papers, and other related Web pages.

Psychiatry.com: Mental Health Advocacy ◎
http://www.psychiatry.com/directory/ment_health_advoc.html

Links are provided at this site to advocacy resources for patients with amyotrophic lateral sclerosis (ALS), AIDS/HIV, and other disabilities.

Rights—A Service of the Center for Mental Health Services ◎ ◎
http://www.mentalhealth.org/links/rights.htm

Included in this interesting list of Web sites are links to various organizations and agencies focusing exclusively on the rights of the mentally ill. Included are the National Association for Rights Protection and Advocacy (NARPA), the National Mental Health Association, and the Bazelon Center for Mental Health Law. All are dedicated to improving the lives of those affected by mental illness by advocating for patient rights, providing legal information, and promoting real alternatives to coercive or dangerous practices.

State Advocacy and Assistance Organizations ◎ ◎ ◎
http://www.mentalhealth.org/publications/stateresourceguides.cfm

The Center for Health Services, a federal agency, has assembled an extremely important and useful guide to state by state agencies that focus on issues of mental health advocacy and assistance. Hundreds of agencies across the country are profiled with complete descriptions, names of directors, addresses, telephone numbers, fax numbers, and statewide or national toll-free numbers. Many of the agencies within each state have their own Web sites.

State Protection and Advocacy
Agencies for Persons with Developmental Disabilities ◎ ◎ ◎
http://www.protectionandadvocacy.com/atoh.htm

Contained at this Web site is a state-by-state, comprehensive listing of contact information for advocacy programs around the country. Assistance program entries encompass those for people with disabilities as well as for the mentally ill, and include address, fax, e-mail, and Web sites where applicable.

7.5 **Antipsychiatry**

Antipsychiatry Coalition ☺ ☺

http://www.antipsychiatry.org

Articles at this site were written by psychiatrists and a lawyer representing former psychiatric patients. The publications offer criticisms of biologic psychiatry, psychiatric drugs, Ritalin and attention deficit hyperactivity disorder, electroconvulsive therapy, psychotherapy, and involuntary psychiatric commitment. Additional articles attempt to refute the existence of schizophrenia and biological depression. News, announcements, links to related sites, and a mailing list for messages from other site visitors are also found at this site.

Antipsychiatry Reading Room ☺ ☺

http://www.cjnetworks.com/~cgrandy/idx_main2.html

This address presents links to Web sites and articles related to psychiatric errors, psychiatric drugs and adverse effects, psychiatric practice and patients' rights, evidence of abuse, and electroconvulsive therapy. Poetry, illustrations, and other non-informational materials are also found at the site.

Antipsychiatry Web Site ☺ ☺ ☺

http://ourworld.compuserve.com/homepages/Duncan_Double

The understanding that mental illness is a myth with the argument that illness is a physical concept inapplicable to psychological disorders alone, is explored at The Antipsychiatry Web site. Articles critical of psychiatry, the Antipsychiatry Bulletin Board, and various links to Web sites critical of psychiatry are available including Successful Schizophrenia, Pseudoscience in Psychology, and the Critical Psychiatry Network.

Mental Health Facts ☺

http://www.mentalhealthfacts.com

This Web site is described as a "source of factual, unbiased information on Mental Heath, Mental Illness, and Treatment Options." There are links to articles on mental health, psychiatry, and related topics. Most articles are composed as anti-psychiatric editorials, but there are a few links to articles and Web sites that may prove informative to both professionals and the public.

What You Should Know About Psychiatry and Psychiatric Drugs ☺

http://www.geocities.com/HotSprings/3568/index.html

Books reviewed at this site offer scathing criticism of psychiatric drugs and the psychiatric profession. Links are also available to related sites.

7.6 **Child and Adolescent Psychiatry**

American Academy of Child and Adolescent Psychiatry (AACAP)   ⊙ ⊙ ⊙

http://www.aacap.org

The AACAP assists parents and families in understanding developmental, behavioral, emotional, and mental disorders affecting children and adolescents. The site offers general information about the organization, news, fact sheets, press releases, legislation resources, meetings details, awards information, a publications catalog and access to abstracts from the *Journal of the American Academy of Child and Adolescent Psychiatry,* membership information, employment opportunities, and links to related sites. Clinical practice, research and training resources are also available. The site offers resources for parents, including a section of suggestions and articles on helping children and adolescents after a disaster, teen violence management, children and the media, and school safety issues. Summaries and ordering information for parent handbooks published by the Academy are available, and users can search the site by keyword. An extensive resources section links to organizations related to child and adolescent psychiatry or pediatrics. Home pages of other national and international organizations, research and support groups, and government agencies are listed in this section.

Association for Child Psychoanalysis (ACP)   ⊙ ⊙

http://www.westnet.com/acp

The Association for Child Psychoanalysis (ACP) is an international not-for-profit organization providing a forum for the interchange of ideas and clinical experience in order to advance the psychological treatment and understanding of children and adolescents and their families. This site was designed to promote the association and its programs. Links to a searchable roster, referral information, the ACP archives, psychoanalysis related sites, and a comprehensive list of programs developed by ACP members are available at the site.

Child and Adolescent Psychiatry Online   ⊙ ⊙

http://www.pol-it.org/psychild.htm

Resources at this site are mainly for patients and caregivers, and include articles on specific topics, professional articles, a database of residential treatment units in the United Kingdom, a bulletin board, and links to additional sites offering child and adolescent psychiatry information, reviewed by Psychiatry Online editors. Visitors can search the site by keyword for specific information.

Child Neurology Home Page ☺ ☺ ☺

http://www.waisman.wisc.edu/child-neuro/index.html

Created to coordinate the available Internet resources related to child neurology for consumers and professionals, this site contains lists of links to organizations, books, journals, child neurology research projects, teaching products, an online course, parent resources, MEDLINE, and other Internet resources.

Child Psychiatry Pamphlets ☺ ☺

http://www.klis.com/chandler

This Web site, created by a pediatric psychiatrist, provides access to psychiatric pamphlets providing in depth information on the diagnosis and treatment of many child and adolescent psychiatric disorders, including attention-deficit/hyperactivity disorder, conduct disorder, bipolar disorder, social phobia, panic, depression, and oppositional defiant disorder. The information contained in these pamphlets came from textbooks, scientific articles, or the creator's clinical experiences.

ChildPsychiatry.Net ☺ ☺

http://www.childpsychiatry.net

The mission of ChildPsychiatry.Net is to provide help to children, families and mental health professionals. The site offers access to MEDLINE, links to related psychiatry and children's sites, self-questionnaires, medical seminar information, primary care guidelines for psychiatric referral, literature reviews, fact sheets for medication reactions in children, and contact information. Important subjects related to child and adolescent psychiatry are also discussed.

Childswork/Childsplay ☺ ☺ ☺

http://www.childswork.com

This site is for teachers, parents and others involved with helping children cope with their psychological disorders. There are lists of links to sites for parents, presenting topics such as divorce issues, learning problems, and for teachers, with topics on multiple intelligence and conflict issues. There are also links to current newsgroups, books, discussion groups and sites related to children's mental health. Included are sites to common childhood disorders, a list of products, training resources and contact information.

Glossary of Symptoms and Mental Illnesses Affecting Teenagers ☺

http://www.aacap.org/Web/aacap/about/glossary/index.htm

Common mental illnesses and emotional problems affecting teenagers are listed at this site, including alcohol and drug abuse, anorexia nervosa, anxiety, attention-deficithyperactivity disorder, bulimia nervosa, conduct disorder, depression, obsessive-compulsive disorder, physical abuse, posttraumatic stress disorder, psychosis, schizophrenia, sexual abuse, suicide, and Tourette's disorder. Descriptive information and symptoms are available for each problem.

Indiana University School of Education: Adolescence Directory Online ◎ ◎ ◎
http://education.indiana.edu/cas/adol/adol.html

A service of the Center for Adolescent Studies at Indiana University, this award-winning site serves as an online directory of Internet resources on adolescent issues. Topics include conflict and violence, mental health issues, health and health risk issues, resources for counselors, and resources for teens.

Indiana University School of Education: Mental Health Risk Factors for Adolescents ◎ ◎
http://education.indiana.edu/cas/adol/mental.html

Internet resources are listed at this site related to mental health risk factors in adolescents. Subtopics include abuse, adolescent development, alcohol and other drugs, attention-deficit/hyperactivity disorder, autism, bipolar disorder, conduct disorder, depression, eating disorders, grieving, obsessive-compulsive disorder, panic disorder, retardation, sexual abuse, stress, and suicide. General resources and support groups are also found through the site. Short site descriptions are provided with each link.

Maternal and Child Health Bureau ◎ ◎
http://www.mchb.hrsa.gov/index.html

This Bureau is dedicated to improving the health of mothers and children in the United States. This site offers a history and mission of the organization, directories of staff and regional offices, grant resources, newsletters and other publications, and links to specific divisions within the Bureau and to related sites. Visitors can also search the site by keyword.

Online Psych: Children's Issues ◎ ◎ ◎
http://www.onlinepsych.com/home.html/Childrens_Issues

Resources available through links at this site include a list of questions to ask prior to hospital treatment of children and adolescents, information related to attention-deficit/hyperactivity disorder, adolescent depression, adolescent violence, anxiety disorders, Asperger's syndrome, autism, bed wetting, child abuse, schizophrenia, sleep apnea, and many other topics. Many additional resources are offered concerning child and adolescent mental and physical health. Visitors can also order related books through Amazon.com at the site.

Pediatric Psychiatry Page ◎ ◎

http://pubweb.acns.nwu.edu/~gjw569/pedpsych/homepage.htm

A board-certified child and adolescent psychiatrist developed this home page, which describes professional interests, provides bibliographies for pediatric psychiatry topics, and offers information on workshops, conferences and links to related sites.

Portland State University: Research and Training Center on Family Support and Children's Mental Health ◎ ◎ ◎

http://www.rtc.pdx.edu

This Research Center aims to improve services for families of children with serious mental, emotional, or behavioral disabilities. The site describes current projects, training activities, and dissemination of knowledge by the Center. Specific research themes include family participation in services, family participation at the policy level, families and out-of-home care, evaluation of family organizing efforts, and interventions in professional education. Publications, including an online newsletter, mailing lists, faculty and staff directories, employment opportunities, a site search engine, and conference details are also found at the address.

Stanford University Child and Adolescent Psychiatry ◎ ◎

http://www-cap.stanford.edu

This site offers information on current projects in Stanford's Child and Adolescent Psychiatry Department. Subjects include neuroimaging, behavioral neurogenetics, violence prevention, eating disorders, autism, mood disorders, pediatric posttraumatic stress disorder, and anxiety disorders. Recruitment information is available for those wishing to volunteer in current research studies, with responsibilities including data coding, transcription, observations, and interviews. Additional information on patient services, training, research, and staff listing are also available.

TLTP Project: Child Development ◎ ◎

http://www.ccc.nottingham.ac.uk/~mczwww/tltp/child.htm

At this site, downloadable Windows and Macintosh versions of this program displaying the key stages of development form birth to six years are available. Topics introduced and discussed include motor and speech development, play, communication, and social behavior development. Users can access information either by selecting an age, which displays milestones typically achieved by that age, or by selecting an individual subject area, chronologically displaying different milestones in that subject area.

University of Texas Southwestern
Department of Psychiatry: Child Psychiatry Research ◎ ◎
http://www.swmed.edu/home_pages/psych/ResearchChild.html

The Department of Psychiatry lists nine current research projects relating to Child Psychiatry at this address. The title of the study, principal investigator, co-investigators, funding source, and research summaries are available for each project.

University of Virginia Curry
School of Education: Office of Special Education ◎ ◎
http://curry.edschool.virginia.edu/go/cise/ose/categories

This address contains directories of site links related to attention-deficit/hyperactivity disorder, autism, cerebral palsy, communication disorders, hearing impairment, learning disorders, mental retardation, serious emotional imbalance, traumatic brain injury, and visual impairment. Visitors can find organizations, educational resources, information on medications, conference and forum details, and general resources related to each topic through this site.

University of Wisconsin
Madison Waisman Center: Child Neurology Home Page ◎ ◎ ◎
http://www.waisman.wisc.edu/child-neuro/index.html

Many valuable Internet resources can be found through this online directory. Resource categories include academy sites, online books, clinical service information, Continuing Medical Education online, mailing lists for child neurologists, journals, MEDLINE search engines, parent information, pharmaceutical information, professional information, research in child neurology, teaching resources, general medical Web portals, and online courses. Major sources for information are also listed, including PubMed, full-text online journals, government resources, and professional organizations.

Virtual Hospital:
Patient Information by Department: Child Psychiatry ◎ ◎
http://www.vh.org/Patients/IHB/Psych/Peds/PedsPsychiatry.html

Interested professionals and consumers can access resource materials from informative links, including topics in attention-deficit/hyperactivity disorder, Tourette's disorder, Trichotillomania, and children and family moves.

World Association for Infant Mental Health (WAIMH) ◎ ◎
http://www.msu.edu/user/waimh

WAIMH is an interdisciplinary and international association promoting education and research on all aspects of infant mental health. Included are links to the association's mission statement and membership information, conference listings, and affiliates.

Internet resources include training information and online access to the table of contents for the *Infant Mental Health Journal.*

7.7 Cultism

American Family Foundation (AFF)
Information about Cults and Psychological Manipulation ⊙ ⊙ ⊙
http://www.csj.org

Provided by the American Family Foundation (AFF), a professional organization devoted to public education about cults, this Web site provides consumers and professionals with links to online journals and their articles, essays, support and research information, a directory of specialized professionals, guides on cults and related topics, and meeting information. Links are provided to information about specific cult organizations by group or topic type. Topic listings assist in finding information for specific uses or audiences, including children, educators, psychology, social influence, civil rights, medical, recovery, substance abuse, women, and others. Consumer information, media, educational, mental health, government, religious studies, and law enforcement agencies are listed at the site for additional resources. In addition, current news and information about the organization is included.

Information About Cults and Psychological Manipulation ⊙ ⊙ ⊙
http://www.csj.org/index.html

This complete cult resource page of the American Family Foundation offers support as well as professional assistance in dealing with cults. Through a combination of publications, programs, and services, those who have been adversely affected by a cult will find valuable information, and professionals and educators, too, are offered a foundation of scholarly study and research in the area. The latest in news about cultic studies, essays by guest columnists, and standard checklists for cult identification are available. A cult information line provides confidential information and referrals and a wealth of resources for the professional and lay person, including study guides, periodicals, and article abstracts of cultic study may be accessed.

Social Psychology of Cults ⊙ ⊙ ⊙
http://www.fmdc.calpoly.edu/libarts/cslem/Cults/Cults.html

This psychology resource contains detailed links regarding the powerful social forces associated with cults and the social psychological effects that these groups have had and can produce. Obedience and conformity, alterations in personality, and posttraumatic stress disorder are examined. Journals covering the impact of cults, anti-cult organizations, and interesting article abstracts discussing sects and cults are all found in addition to an index of cult and anti-cult movements and cult-specific news coverage.

7.8 **Deinstitutionalization**

Deinstitutionalization: What will it Really Cost? ◎ ◎
http://www.mentalhealth.com/mag1/p51-sc02.html

This article on deinstitutionalization appeared in the *Schizophrenic Digest*. It is an editorial by a schizoaffective patient who compares the quality of life in an institution to the quality of life in a community. He finds the former more conducive to the health and well-being of the patient and articulates his reasons.

Trends in Chronic Care: Deinstitutionalization ◎ ◎
http://www.rwjf.org/library/chrcare/p2pg21.htm

Prepared by the Institute for Health & Aging at the University of California San Francisco for the Robert Wood Johnson Foundation, this site concerns the chronic care delivery system. It discusses the history of institutionalization and deinstitutionalization and the issues surrounding the homeless and mentally ill.

7.9 **Disabilities and Rehabilitation**

About.com: Parenting Special Needs ◎ ◎ ◎
http://www.specialchildren.about.com/home/specialchildren

This valuable Internet directory contains links to sites offering information on parents' special needs for children with physical, mental, or emotional disorders, including AD/HD, autism, cerebral palsy, cystic fibrosis, Down syndrome, epilepsy, muscular dystrophy, reactive attachment disorder, spina bifida, visual impairment, and many related disorders. Special articles are available on featured topics, and the site also offers a chat forum, newsletter, and an online bookstore and video store.

Center for Information Technology Accommodation (CITA) ◎ ◎ ◎
http://www.itpolicy.gsa.gov/cita

The Center for Information Technology Accommodation works with a network of public and private sector partners to create "a nationally recognized model demonstration facility influencing accessible information environments, services, and management practices." The site provides information on services and partnerships, current projects, the Universal Access Working Group, people with disabilities and the national infrastructure, resources for hearing-impaired and deaf persons, federal accommodation programs and initiatives, legislation and policies, assistive technology providers, and upcoming conferences. Information is also available on creating a more universally accessible Web site. Users can access a staff directory, the *CITA Handbook,* and the Department of Justice federal agency self-evaluations and checklists.

Disability and Medical Resource Mall ⊙ ⊙ ⊙

http://www.coast-resources.com

This directory contains links to over 400 companies offering disability and medical products, resources and services. Categories include augmentative communication computer and electronics, assistance animals products and services, vehicles, and services for the blind and visually-impaired, deaf, hearing, and speech-impaired, books and magazines, brochures and catalogs, canes, crutches, standers, walkers, children and parenting products and services, clothing, furniture, elevators, medical equipment, pharmaceuticals, and other related products and services.

Disability Resources Monthly Guide to Disability Resources on the Internet ⊙ ⊙ ⊙

http://www.geocities.com/~drm

This colorful Web site, available also in text-only version, is a comprehensive Internet resource to important disability-related material and was developed to promote awareness and accessibility to independent living. Interesting departments include a "State of the Week" in which disability organizations and resources in a particular locale are reviewed, in addition to its regional resource directory, updated topics of the week, disability news, past features, a list of FAQs, and an award-winning online newsletter, *Disability Resources Monthly (DRM),* which reviews resources for independent living. A variety of disability resources on the Internet are reviewed at the DRM Webwatcher and favorite pages can be accessed. New visitors are encouraged to read the online user guide, in order to take full advantage of all the site has to offer.

Disability/Exceptionality Web Resource Library ⊙ ⊙

http://www.pgh.auhs.edu/CFSP/brochure/library.htm

More than 125 sites are listed at this address offering sources for disability information and support. Categories include sites related to education, family issues, legal issues, medical information and therapies, specific disabilities, and general resources.

Disabled Peoples' International: Links ⊙ ⊙ ⊙

http://www.dpi.org/links.html

Disability resources found in the links section at this address include many national and international organizations support services and information, disability studies, and personal pages and stories. Topical sites are included under equal rights and advocacy, sports and leisure, travel, independent living and housing, and employment and education. All sites are listed by host country.

Educational Resources Information Center
Clearinghouse on Disabilities and Gifted Education (ERIC EC) ○ ○ ○

http://ericec.org

Sponsored by the U.S. Department of Education, Office of Educational Research and Improvement, and administered by the National Library of Education, ERIC EC "gathers and disseminates the professional literature, information, and resources on the education and development of individuals of all ages who have disabilities and/or who are gifted." The ERIC database, available through this site, offers journal articles, conference proceedings, papers, speeches, research reports, teaching guides and curriculum, and books related to educational issues. This site also offers instructions on submitting documents to ERIC and information on special projects, research details, fact sheets, answers to frequently-asked questions, mailing lists, links to similar information resources, conference calendars, and access to the National Parent Information Network and the "AskEric" question-answering Service.

Equal Access to Software and Information (EASI) ○ ○ ○

http://www.isc.rit.edu/~easi

Equal Access to Software and Information is a group committed to providing resources to the education community on access-to-information technologies. Specific activities include seminars and online workshops, an electronic journal, mailing lists, and other publications and videos. The site offers links to information and sources for adaptive resources, libraries, distance learning, science and math education, and other related sites. The group's journal and other publications are available from the site.

Integrated Network of
Disability Information and Education (INDIE) ○ ○ ○

http://laurence.canlearn.ca/english/learn/accessguide/indie/index.html

Available in text-only and French versions, the INDIE site may be searched for links by keyword or by clicking on any one of 15 available categories relating to disability information and education. Disability subtopics include rehabilitation, transportation, employment, organizations, recreation, and social development and legislation. Web addresses and direct connections are provided along with brief descriptions of the URLs.

International Center for Disability Resources on the Internet ○ ○ ○

http://www.icdri.org

A large collection of disability-related Internet resources are consolidated at this site where assisting the disability community is the primary mission. The latest in news, accessible travel resources, Internet guides, and disability publications can be viewed and important ramifications of the American with Disabilities Act regarding Internet usage are discussed.

Job Accommodation Network (JAN)
on the Web: Americans with Disabilities Act (ADA) Links ◎ ◎ ◎

http://janweb.icdi.wvu.edu

Links at this site provide valuable resources on ADA law, accessibility guidelines, ADA technical assistance manuals, ADA enforcement, and other ADA materials and Web sites.

Kansas Commission on Disability Concerns ◎ ◎

http://adabbs.hr.state.ks.us/dc

This site lists numerous resources, including more than 25 links to sites offering specific information on assistive technologies. Public service groups, companies providing assistive technologies, software sources, and state-based programs are included at the site. Over 20 links to general disability resources on the Internet are also provided. Specific topical resources are found on assistance dogs, independent living, and particular disabilities.

Knowledge Exchange Network: Assistive Technology ◎ ◎

http://www.mentalhealth.org/links/assistive.htm

This site lists 19 valuable Internet sources for information, products, and support-related to assistive technology. Resources include personal sites, databases of information, government organizations, state and international organizations, and research centers.

National Early Childhood Technical Assistance System ◎ ◎ ◎

http://www.nasdse.org/national_early_childhood_techn.htm

This technical assistance consortium provides services and information on and for children with disabilities and their families. Information on related organizations, and a staff directory is available, as well as current news items, legal information, archives, government links, such as a link to the Individuals with Disabilities Act and the Department of Education, and a publications list. Of interest to professionals is a project database, searchable by a variety of methods, and a link to resources on developmental delay in children, which includes project information, state and national support information, scientific articles on the subject, and a concept paper. Links to related sites are included, as well as contact information.

National Information Center for
Children and Youth (NICHCY) with Disabilities ◎ ◎

http://www.nichcy.org

This national referral center serves professionals and nonprofessionals by providing information on children and adolescents with disabilities. At this site, one can access the Center's publications, including fact sheets, summaries, news articles, parent and student guides, reference lists, and other information. There are links to state resource documents, an FAQ section, training information, a newsletter, related organizations and centers, conference information, and contact listings.

National Institute on Disability and Rehabilitation Research (NIDRR) ◎ ◎ ◎
http://www.ed.gov/offices/OSERS/NIDRR

The National Institute on Disability and Rehabilitation Research "conducts comprehensive and coordinated programs of research and related activities to maximize the full inclusion, social integration, employment, and independent living of disabled individuals of all ages." The site offers information about the organization, projects, research topics, programs, the Institute's Switzer Fellowship Program, and a calendar of events. Specific programs include model spinal cord injury systems, Rehabilitation Engineering Research Centers (RERC), Rehabilitation Research Training Centers (RRTC), and traumatic brain injury model systems. Research topics include assistive/adaptive technologies, burn rehabilitation, disability and health, emerging disability, employment, transition to post-secondary school for students with disabilities, universal design, and women with disabilities.

Occupational Therapy Internet World— Disability Related Information: Related Resources ◎ ◎
http://www.mother.com/~ktherapy/ot/otherpages/contest.htm

Links to sites offering information on disabilities are listed under many descriptive subtopics at this address, such as aging issues, HIV/AIDS, amputation, art therapy, assistive technology, cerebral palsy, cognitive therapy, Down syndrome, genetic diseases, mental health and retardation, research, special education, and many others. Sites are sometimes listed with short descriptions. Seventy-two electronic mailing lists related to a wide range of disabilities are also provided. Subscribers to mailing lists receive e-mail communications from fellow subscribers, and discussions focus on a specific topic. Newsgroups related to general disability and mental health issues are also described.

U.S. Department of Justice: Americans with Disabilities Act (ADA) Home Page ◎ ◎ ◎
http://www.usdoj.gov/crt/ada/adahom1.htm

Resources at this site include sources and instructions for obtaining publications, the toll-free telephone number for an information line, new or proposed regulation documents, information on certification of state and local building codes, and details of other ADA mediation activities. Enforcement information includes status reports, settlements, details of the ADA Litigation Project, and instructions on filing complaints. Visitors can search the site, the Freedom of Information Act ADA Information, and the Department of Justice press releases for additional resources.

University of Minnesota
Disability Services: Disability—Specific Web Sites ◎ ◎ ◎

http://disability/index.html

More than 150 categories are available in this directory of Internet sites offering information, support, legal, and product services related to a wide range of disabilities. A short description accompanies each site link.

University of Wisconsin
Trace Research and Development Center ◎ ◎

http://trace.wisc.edu/about

This Research Center aims to make computers, the Internet, and information kiosks more accessible to everyone through universal (accessible) design. The site offers information about the Center, project areas and activities, collaborators, and research and development history. Specific descriptions are available of the Center's projects in underlying technologies research, applied research and development, transfer and industry support, and dissemination, education, and user support. Contact details are also available at the site, and users can access links to sites of academic and industry collaborators.

Virtual Assistive Technology Center ◎ ◎ ◎

http://www.at-center.com

Visitors to this address will find articles and links to Internet sources for general information, commercial vendors, projects, and research related to assistive technologies. Shareware for Macintosh, Windows, and DOS operating systems can also be found through the site. Related books can be ordered at the site through Amazon.com.

Weaver's Web site for Parents of Children with Brain Disorders ◎ ◎

http://www.ioa.com/~d-g-weaver

Hosted by the mother of a child with mental disabilities, this site offers parents in similar situations valuable suggestions for coping with mental illness in a child. Each of 16 suggestions is offered with links to Internet resources for further information. Suggested coping strategies relate to self-education about the disorder, communication with the child, therapy, stress reduction, and support sources.

7.10 **Divorce**

Children of Divorce:
Psychological, Psychiatric, Behavioral Problems, and Suicide ◎ ◎ ◎
http://www.divorcereform.org/psy.html

This section of the Divorce Statistics Collection from Americans for Divorce Reform highlights the major aspects of the psychological effects of a broken family on children. Links to literature from the National Institute of Mental Health and the *Journal of Marriage and Family* are accessible, as is material and citations derived from major researchers in the field.

Divorce, Clinical Disorders, Childhood Depression ◎ ◎
http://www.divorcedoc.com/depressio.htm

Examining the distinction between depressed mood and clinical disorders, suggestions are offered on recognizing the important differences. Links to divorce articles, professional contact listings, psychological testing information, and the site's discussion/message board can be found.

Divorce Online ◎ ◎ ◎
http://www.divorceonline.com/ffindex.html

Resources on divorce at this site include articles related to financial, legal, psychological, ownership, and other issues common to the process of divorce. Recent articles offer advice on child custody, choosing a matrimonial lawyer, dating, and other relevant topics. A bulletin board, site search engine, and professional referral directory are also available for use by site visitors. Professionals can list a practice in the referral section. Consumers confronting divorce will find this site a valuable reference.

7.11 **Dream Research**

Association for the Study of Dreams ◎ ◎
http://www.asdreams.org

This nonprofit organization is dedicated to the "pure and applied investigation of dreams and dreaming." Conference information, a magazine, education resources, discussion forums, membership details, on online bookstore, details of current projects, a membership directory, and contact details are all found at the site. Abstracts of articles and other details of the Association's journal, *Dreaming*, are available at the site, as well as some full-text articles. A search engine is available for more specific information.

International Institute for Dream Research ⊙ ⊙ ⊙
http://psych.ucsc.edu/dreams

From the University of California at Santa Cruz, technical information regarding methodology and findings via a method of objective and quantitative dream research is explained. Discoveries pertaining to cross-cultural similarities, gender influences, and age differences are analyzed with the approach, and the consistency and continuities between waking life and dreams lead the researchers to conclude that accurate predictions about the dreamers concerns and interests may be made with the method. Content analysis, representative samples, and statistical approach are completely explained, and a spreadsheet for quantitative dream data may be downloaded. Scientists and students with further interest in the field may find links to additional information regarding quantitative dream study.

Lucidity Institute ⊙ ⊙ ⊙
http://www.lucidity.com

This Web site, dedicated to the understanding of lucid dreaming, research in the area, and the application of the research to the betterment of human health, offers resources for lucid dreaming including scientific publications, books, and tapes—all at an online catalog. Lecture and workshop listings and practical excerpts from lucid dreaming literature are accessible. Research articles and abstracts may also be viewed, and the Institute discussion forum and mailing list keep visitors up-to-date regarding the physiology and philosophy of lucid dreaming, new Web sites, events, and dream experiments.

7.12 Emotions

Forsyth's Motivation and Emotion Page ⊙ ⊙ ⊙
http://www.vcu.edu/hasweb/psy/psy101/forsyth/zmoemo.htm

Subjects such as nonverbal expressions, personal motivation, happiness, anger, autonomic nervous system and emotions, emotional intelligence and related sexual topics are discussed in comprehensive and detailed documents available at this site. In addition, there are links to resources on various aspects of psychology, such as intelligence, learning, personality, social psychology, and other related sites.

Limbic System: The Center of Emotions ⊙ ⊙ ⊙
http://www.epub.org.br/cm/n05/mente/limbic_i.htm

This Web site reviews the anatomy and function of the limbic system, offers a review of different theories on limbic system function and emotions, explains the evolution of emotions, and provides detailed information on specific brain structures and emotions. Informative illustrations are present.

7.13 **Ethics and Psychiatry**

Abuse, Memory, Science, Therapy Ethics, & Malpractice ◎ ◎
http://www.idealist.com/memories/sitemap.shtml

Full-text articles, book reviews, tables of research findings, research studies, and peer-reviewed article abstracts are found at this site devoted to issues of therapy ethics. Users can request free reprints of 10 selected articles from the site.

American Psychiatric Association (APA) Principles of Medical Ethics with Annotations Especially Applicable to Psychiatry ◎ ◎ ◎
http://www.psych.org/psych/htdocs/apa_members/ethics_index.html

This site provides the current *Principles of Medical Ethics with Annotations Especially Applicable to Psychiatry.* Many of the current annotations are based on the American Medical Association's *Principles of Medical Ethics.* Resources include the full-text *Principles with Annotations,* and procedures for handling complaints of unethical conduct. Addendums offer guidelines for ethical practice in organized settings, and questions and answers about procedures for handling complaints of unethical conduct.

Forensic Psychiatry and Medicine: Professional Ethics ◎ ◎
http://www.forensic-psych.com/catProfEthics.html

This site offers a short discussion of professional ethics, and links to relevant professional associations, court rulings, articles, and major sites offering professional ethics resources.

7.14 **Forensic Psychiatry**

Forensic Psychiatry: Medicine and Psychiatry Expert ◎ ◎
http://www.forensic-psych.com

This site is hosted by the co-director of the Program in Psychiatry and the Law at Harvard Medical School. Subjects discussed at the site include managed healthcare and medical malpractice, employment issues, emotional and physical damages, important court rulings on standards for experts, product liability, criminal justice and public safety, family and custody issues, testamentary and contractual capacity, professional ethics, trial consulting, organizational consulting, and risk management. Discussions are accompanied by general and professional articles. Links are available to Internet resources and articles related to telemedicine and other related sites. A profile of the medical director and news stories related to Forensic Psychiatry are also found at this address.

Forensic Psychiatry Online ◎ ◎

http://www.priory.com/forpsy.htm

Presented by Psychiatry Online, this site offers full-text professional articles relating to forensic psychiatry. Psychiatry Online provides brief and case reports, an archive of professional documents, transcultural mental health resources, news, and a bulletin board, current research articles, Continuing Medical Education materials, a forum for students, a side-effect registry, and links to worldwide psychiatry resources and other related sites. Links are also provided to similar resources produced from Italy and Brazil. Users can search the site for specific information and order books and other products at the site. This site is supported by an unrestricted educational grant from AstraZeneca.

Forensic Psychiatry Resource Page ◎ ◎ ◎

http://mhnet.org/law/about.html

This site, created by a professor and Medical Director of the Taylor Hardin Secure Medical Facility, offers links to a wide range of forensic psychiatry resources. Visitors can access a database comparing forensic facilities, general psychiatry, and legal information for attorneys and psychiatrists, information on forensics in countries outside of the United States, position statements from the American Psychiatric Association, meeting and conference calendars, literature searches through MEDLINE, summaries of landmark cases in mental health law, and legal databases.

Forensic Psychiatry Resources ◎ ◎

http://www.umdnj.edu/psyevnts/forensic.html

A board-certified psychiatrist has compiled this list of Internet resources related to Forensic Psychiatry. Professional associations, additional Internet directories, legal resources, sites hosted by psychiatrists, Institutes, professional services resources, and educational materials are included.

Institute of Law, Psychiatry, and Public Policy at the University of Virginia ◎ ◎ ◎

http://www.bitlink.com/ilppp/ilppphome.html

This Institute at the University of Virginia is an interdisciplinary program in Mental Health Law, Forensic Psychiatry, and Forensic Psychology. The Institute offers academic programs, forensic clinical evaluations, professional training, empirical and theoretical research, and public policy consultation and review. Information at the site includes a description of the Institute, teaching programs, research activities, clinical evaluations and other services, and fellowship programs. Faculty biographies, publications, a directory of forensic evaluators in Virginia, and registration forms for conferences, training programs, and symposia are also found at the site.

New York Center for
Neuropsychology and Forensic Behavioral Science ⊙ ⊙
http://www.nyforensic.com

This Center, a combination of two New York mental health centers, offers diagnostic, assessment, treatment, and consulting services to patients, and medical and judicial professionals. Services include clinical evaluations and psychological testing; individual, group, couples, and family therapy; psychological and legal testimony; diagnostic services; sexual offender treatment; corporate consultations; and more. In addition, the Center offers workshops and seminars in the areas listed above.

Ultimate Forensic Psychology Database ⊙ ⊙ ⊙
http://flash.lakeheadu.ca/~pals/forensics/index.html

As its name implies, this site is home to a large database of different types of forensic psychology resources, including a library of books on various related topics, a journals list, a news bulletin, educational information, events index, consulting directory, employment, FAQ section, related links, and a large article database. In addition, there is an online newsgroup and information on Forensic Psychology.

7.15 Genetics and Psychiatry

Genetics of Depressive Illness ⊙ ⊙ ⊙
http://www.psycom.net/depression.central.genetics.html

Contained within are interesting archived article links covering the recent agenda in the field of genetics and psychiatry, heredity versus environment as a cause of depression, and the genetics of seasonal affective disorder, affective and schizophrenic disorders, and bipolar depression.

International Behavioural and Neural Genetics Society (IBANGS) ⊙ ⊙
http://www.ibngs.org

Formerly the European Behavioural and Neural Genetics Society (EBANGS), this international Society supports research in the field of Neurobehavioral Genetics. Membership information, Society information, rules, a member directory, meeting details, links to member societies, and past meeting transcripts are available at the site. Links are also available at the site to sources for meeting information, societies and networks, institutions and databases, and publications of interest in neurobehavioral and neural genetics.

International Society of Psychiatric Genetics ⚙

http://www.ispg.net

The International Society of Psychiatric Genetics promotes and facilitates research, education, and communication in the genetics of psychiatric disorders, substance abuse, and related traits. This address offers a Board of Directors listing, information on upcoming meetings, Society bylaws and mission statement, and links to several related sites.

National Institute on Drug Abuse
Genetics Workgroup: Genetics Web Resources ⚙ ⚙ ⚙

http://www.nida.nih.gov/genetics/genetics6.html

This address offers a comprehensive list of Internet sites related to human genetics and mental health. Links are included to major government and private sources for resources related to human genetics, genetics of animals used in research (mouse, rat, Caenorhabditis elegans, Drosophila, zebrafish), quantitative methods, organizations, journals, and publishers.

Psychiatric Genetics ⚙ ⚙ ⚙

http://www.unizh.ch/bli/BLI/Subhome/geneti.html

A comprehensive listing of links to genetic databases and projects seeking to reveal the genetic basis of diseases influenced by multiple genes can be found at this Web site. Current mathematical models that go beyond the standard segregation linkage research paradigm may demonstrate further insights into genetic etiology of psychiatric illness. The actual projects explore familial syndrome patterns, genetic maps, polynucleotide markers, and genotype-phenotype associations, and much more. Thirty-two genetic databases from prominent national and international laboratories and institutes are directly accessible.

Skeptical Psychiatrist: Genetics ⚙

http://home.gci.net/~dougs/genetics.htm

The psychiatrist presenting this site offers reviews of two articles presenting research on possible genetic components to schizophrenia, bipolar disorder, and attention-deficit/hyperactivity disorder. Bibliographical citations are available for both articles.

7.16 Geriatric Psychiatry and Gerontology

American Association for Geriatric Psychiatry (AAGP) ⚙ ⚙

http://www.aagpgpa.org/home.html

The AAGP is dedicated to promoting the mental health and well being of older people and improving the care of those with late-in-life mental disorders. The site offers national and AAGP news, calls for abstracts, fellowship information, and provides AAGP staff listings and contact information. The site also offers an online version of its bimonthly member newsletter. Full-text articles provide general news updates in the field.

American Psychological Association (APA): Division 20 ◎ ◎ ◎
http://www.iog.wayne.edu/APADIV20/APADIV20.HTM

This Division of the American Psychological Association studies the psychology of adult development and aging. The site offers information about the Division, including research and employment opportunities, programs of study, awards, and a directory of members. Educational resources include suggested videotape and book lists, graduate and undergraduate syllabi, and curriculum suggestions. Students can access a guide to graduate and post-doctoral study, and a list of student awards offered by the Institute. Conference details, including those offering Continuing Medical Education credits, and links to related sites are also found at this address.

American Society on Aging (ASA) ◎ ◎ (some features fee-based)
http://www.asaging.org

The American Society on Aging provides information resources on gerontology through educational programming, publications, and training. General resources at this site include membership and contact details, meeting information, conference and training schedules, and awards listings. Links are available to information on publications, including *Aging Today* and *Generations*. Visitors can also access news, links to related sites, job banks, and information on specific ASA networks, including business and aging; environments, services, and technologies; healthcare and aging; lesbian and gay aging issues; lifelong education; mental health and aging; multicultural aging issues; religion and spirituality; and aging. Databases containing information on conferences, training events, and resources on aging issues are available for members, as well as a chat forum, special offers, and member directories.

CanWest Therapeutics: Geriatric Institute ◎ ◎ (free registration)
http://www.geriatricinstitute.com/messenger.htm

Visitors to this site, presented by CanWest Therapeutics, can access a calendar of upcoming conferences, chat forums, patient education materials on anxiety and depression, links to related sites, a site search engine, and an online bookstore. Articles, presentations, case studies, and other resources are available only to professional members.

Gerontological Society of America ◎ ◎ ◎
http://www.geron.org

The Gerontological Society of America promotes research and disseminates information related to gerontological research. Site sections list awards, annual meeting details, press releases, employment opportunities, news, publications, Society divisions, and links to related sites. Related foundations, a referral service, useful sources for information, student organization details, and membership details are also found through the site. A discussion is available on social security and women. Visitors can search the site by keyword for specific information.

National Aging Research Institute, Incorporated ⊙ ⊙ ⊙
http://www.mednwh.unimelb.edu.au

This Australian institute for gerontology and geriatric medicine research offers general information about the Institute, current projects, research publications, educational resources, and links to related sites at this address. Visitors can search the site by keyword for specific information and access some full-text articles from official publications of the Institute.

National Institute on Aging (NIA) ⊙ ⊙ ⊙
http://www.nih.gov/nia

The National Institute on Aging promotes healthy aging, and supports public education and biomedical, social, and behavioral research. Press releases, employment opportunities, program announcements, and program updates are found at the site. The site describes extramural and intramural aging research programs, an international program, and provides news from the National Advisory Council on Aging. Researchers can access funding information, training information, and the NIA Draft Strategic Plan for Fiscal Years 2001–2005. Information for the general public includes resources on Alzheimer's disease, public education booklets, brochures, fact sheets, press releases, and public service advertisements. Assorted publications for health professionals are available on issues related to the care of older people.

Senior Sites ⊙ ⊙ ⊙
http://www.seniorsites.com

This site serves as a directory for senior citizens searching for information on nonprofit housing communities and other resources on the Internet. Resources at the site include a discussion on the benefits of choosing nonprofit housing, a calendar of upcoming events of interest to seniors by state, a directory of national and state associations, and links to other useful sites. Visitors can conduct detailed searches of the site's directory of nonprofit housing facilities, choosing from a wide range of options to include in the search. this site is presented by the California Associations of Homes and Services for the Aging and Creative Computer Services, Inc.

U.S. Administration on Aging—Department of
Health and Human Services Directory of Web Sites on Aging ◎ ◎ ◎
http://www.aoa.dhhs.gov/aoa/webres/mental.htm

This site contains links to resources specific to aging and general mental health sites. Specific topics listed with associated Web sites include elder abuse, primary healthcare, Alzheimer's, long-term care, long-term care ombudsman, wellness, nutrition, and exercise. A site search engine is available for locating site links by keyword, and a more specific topics menu is provided with associated Web sites.

7.17 Grief and Bereavement

Compassionate Friends ◎ ◎
http://www.compassionatefriends.org

The Compassionate Friends is a national nonprofit organization helping families cope with the death of a child of any age, from any cause. Visitors to the site can access chapter directories, brochures, conference details, links to chapter Web sites, news, and links to related Internet resources. An online catalog of publications and videotapes, general information about the organization, chat forums, and subscription information for the organization's magazine are also available at the site.

Crisis, Grief, and Healing ◎ ◎ ◎
http://www.webhealing.com

This site is hosted by a psychotherapist and author of several popular books on male grieving patterns. General information about the grieving process, book excerpts, an online bookstore, chat forums, and suggestions on grieving from other site visitors are all found at this address. Information about the site host, Tom Golden, LCSW, includes a description of his private practice, speaking schedule, workshops, and consultations.

Death and Dying ◎ ◎ ◎
http://www.death-dying.com

Primarily a support site, resources include a chat room and message boards, links to grief support articles, newsletters, and other related sites and organizations. Also, there are planners, many fact sheets on grief support and bereavement, near-death experience articles, terminal illness issues, legal subjects, and sites for online support, expert advice, and child and adolescent related subjects.

GriefNet ◎ ◎ ◎
http://rivendell.org

GriefNet, supervised by a practicing clinical psychologist, offers online grief support through more than 30 e-mail support groups. Visitors can join e-mail support groups for children, and those suffering the loss of a spouse or partner, child, parent, sibling, or friend. Special groups are devoted to losses due to health problems, support for men, losses of pets, deaths due to violence, suicide, and spiritual aspects of loss. One group offers discussion and support to professional counselors. Visitors can also access a companion site for children, an online bookstore, memorials, an online newsletter, and links to related resources, including suicide prevention and survivors' resources.

State University of New York (SUNY) University at Buffalo Counseling Center: Coping with Death and Dying ◎ ◎ ◎
http://ub-counseling.buffalo.edu/Grief/grief.html

Targeted to college students, this fact sheet offers information on typical reactions to death and dying. The site discusses stages of grief, including denial and shock, anger, bargaining, guilt, depression, loneliness, acceptance, and hope. Suggestions on coping with death and dying, and helping bereaved students are available, as well as contact information for University sources of help.

Teenage Grief (TAG) ◎
http://www.smartlink.net/~tag/index.html

This nonprofit organization is composed of professionals who train school personnel, health professionals, law enforcement officials, and organizations serving at-risk youth in grief support. The site discusses why ongoing support is necessary for grieving teens, in addition to grief and the adolescent, the spiritual dimension of grief, and anger. News, an online store for publications, and links to related sites are also available at this address.

7.18 Homelessness

Health Care for the Homeless Information Resource Center (HCH) ◎ ◎
http://www.prainc.com/hch/index.html

This Resource Center provides technical assistance and information to providers and program staff in an effort to improve the delivery of healthcare services to homeless individuals. Site resources include annotated bibliographies, clinical tools, including clinical intake, assessment, and screening topics, a video lending library, a quarterly bulletin, conference details, a directory of current HCH grantees and subcontractors, and a directory of organizations providing services to homeless individuals.

Knowledge Exchange Network: Homelessness ◎ ◎

http://www.mentalhealth.org/links/homelessness.htm

Six sites are listed at this address, offering the home pages of nonprofit organizations, government agencies, and service providers. Short site descriptions are provided with each link.

National Coalition for the Homeless (NCH) ◎ ◎ ◎

http://nch.ari.net

This national organization is an advocacy network of individuals, activists, and service providers working to end homelessness through public education, policy advocacy, grassroots organizing, and technical assistance. Visitors to the site will find facts and statistics on homelessness, including a discussion of homelessness and mental health, legislation and policy resources, news alerts, organization directories, information on NCH projects, a calendar of events, links to related Internet resources, an online newsletter, and NCH publications. The NCH online library offers a searchable bibliographic database with references to research on homelessness, housing, and poverty.

National Resources Center on Homelessness and Mental Illness ◎ ◎ ◎

http://www.prainc.com/nrc

The National Resource Center on Homelessness and Mental Illness provides policy makers, service providers, researchers, consumers, and other interested parties with technical assistance and research findings related to homelessness and mental illness. Resources offered at the site include a description of technical assistance services, directories of organizations and assistance resources, annotated bibliographies by subject, a periodic bulletin, events notices, monographs and papers, and links to related sites. Visitors can also submit information requests by e-mail or phone.

7.19 **Infertility**

Infertility Counseling and Support: From the American Society for Reproductive Medicine ◎ ◎

http://www.collmed.psu.edu/obgyn/infcouns.htm

This online fact sheet, courtesy of the American Society for Reproductive Medicine, outlines the emotional stresses associated with infertility and provides a checklist for depression and information on finding counseling and support.

Psychological and Coping Information ○ ○

http://www.thelaboroflove.com/forum/infertility/coping.html

Included at this Web site are educational tools designed to assist those coping with infertility. An in-depth article and online guide written by infertility specialists offers advice to family members and friends in understanding the emotional difficulties associated with infertility, and a list of FAQs attempts to to explain when psychological counseling may be useful as well as the general impact which infertility has on emotional well-being.

Psychological and Social Issues of Infertility ○ ○

http://www.ihr.com/infertility/psychosocial.html

Encouraging a balanced approach to infertility, this Internet resource guide to the psychological and social issues, provides useful strategies for managing the complex emotions associated with infertility. Survey results offer insight on depression and infertility and the stress of infertility compared to other factors and concludes that the Internet has great potential to help people faced with infertility. An article summarizing ways in which to balance infertility treatment and work-related responsibilities and an online brochure for preferred responses to insensitive family and friends are some of the features found.

7.20 Informatics

An Informatics Curriculum for Psychiatry ○ ○ ○

http://www.psych.med.umich.edu/Web/Umpsych/staff/mhuang/papers/infocurric.htm

This in-depth research article on the current state of information technology and its relation to the field of Psychiatry, outlines the components of medical informatics principles as applied to the field. Patient care, communication, education, and practice management are stressed. In conclusion, assessment of resources and other issues affecting program implementation are discussed.

National Library of Medicine: Research Programs ○ ○ ○

http://www.nlm.nih.gov/resprog.html

Visitors to this site will find links to National Library of Medicine centers for research, computational molecular biology resources, including molecular biology databases and other online molecular tools, and medical informatics resources. Additional materials available through this site are relevant to digital computing and communications, digital library research, interactive multimedia technology, and medical informatics training. The Visible Human Project and details of extramural funding opportunities are also available.

Psychiatric Society for Informatics   ◎ ◎ ◎
http://www.psych.med.umich.edu

The home page of the Psychiatric Society for Informatics serves to increase the understanding and use of informatics related to the field of Psychiatry. Information on the organization, its current news and upcoming meetings, online membership information and benefits, and the organization's electronic newsletter are all presented.

7.21 Insanity Defense

Insanity Defense   ◎ ◎
http://www.psych.org/public_info/INSANI~1.HTM

The subject of the insanity defense, including medical definitions and legal aspects, is explored at this American Psychiatric Association (APA) site. The article is an in-depth examination of the issues, the position of different states, the frequency of use, and other relevant topics related to the insanity defense.

7.22 Marriage

Coalition for Marriage, Family, and Couples Education   ◎ ◎ ◎
http://www.smartmarriages.com

In addition to links that provide general statistics about marriage and divorce rates, this site has links to fact files on divorce predictors, links to a large number of online articles both scholarly and popular, a directory for counseling and training programs, and conference information. A fact sheet on the coalition itself, a directory of children's courses, books, conference tapes, and other products are present as well.

Latest Research on Marital Adjustment and Satisfaction   ◎ ◎
http://www.apa.org/releases/marital.html

This report of the American Psychological Association briefly outlines the recent research regarding the relationship between psychological type and a couple's satisfaction with each other. Also presented is a summary on recent findings and overall trends related to marital adjustment and individuality from parents.

Psychology: Marriage and Family   ◎ ◎
http://www.filmakers.com/MARRIAGE.html

This interesting Web site describes current films, courtesy of the American Psychiatric Association, American Psychological Association, and other organizations, that document universal difficulties and themes within the context of marriage. Insightful explanations as to whom people fall in love with and why couples argue are addressed in these family relations documentaries that may be ordered online.

Whole Family: Marriage Center ⊙ ⊙ ⊙
http://www.wholefamily.com/maritalcenter/index.html

A consumer-oriented site, the Marital Center of the Whole Family Web site provides real-life situations and offers therapeutic coping formulas for couples. The crisis center presents difficult dilemmas encountered within the marital relationship and offers responses and opportunities for visitors to contribute their own advice. Self-tests, exercises, and surveys help partners to understand each other more completely. *The Family Fishbowl,* an electronic magazine, and *Meet the Family,* an online drama, both deal uniquely with a variety of marital issues including money, sensitivity, communication, fighting fairly, alcohol, children, and the secrets to successful marriages.

7.23 **Non-Treatment Consequences**

Non-Treatment Consequences ⊙ ⊙ ⊙
http://www.psychlaws.org/General%20Resources/Fact1.htm

Consequences of untreated mental illness are explored at this important site, offering statistics on homelessness, incarceration, episodes of violence, victimization, and suicide. The costs and community impact of untreated mental illnesses are included in this survey.

7.24 **Nutrition and Mental Health**

Mental Health and Nutrition Journal ⊙ ⊙ ⊙
http://www.minj.com

The *Mental Health and Nutrition Journal* is an online publication presenting information from recent studies investigating links between nutrition and several mental disorders, including schizophrenia, bipolar disorder, depression, Alzheimer's disease, and other dementias. Articles, notices of upcoming events, tutorials, links to related sites, a glossary of relevant terms, and contact details are all available at this address. Both professionals and consumers will find the articles presented at the site interesting and informative.

Nutrition Science News Online:
Natural Remedies for Depression   ◎ ◎

http://www.nutritionsciencenews.com/NSN_backs/Feb_99/depression.html

A report on altering the brain's chemistry through dietary changes is presented in this online issue of *Nutrition Science News*. The possible roles of amino acid supplementation, vitamin and mineral therapy, and herbal additions to the diet are all explored in terms of boosting neurotransmitters and elevating mood.

7.25 Organizational and Occupational Psychiatry

Academy of Organizational and Occupational Psychiatry (AOOP)   ◎ ◎

http://www.aoop.org

The Academy of Organizational and Occupational Psychiatry provides a forum for communication between psychiatric professionals and personnel in the workplace. The site offers annual meeting details, general Academy news items, and a description of the organization. Research papers, bulletins, membership details, descriptions of previous annual meetings, and links to related sites are all found at this address.

7.26 Patient Education and Support

ABC's of Internet Therapy   ◎ ◎ ◎

http://www.metanoia.org/imhs

This "consumers guide" to telepsychiatry provides links to fact sheets on online therapy and its related issues, therapists credentials, information on teletherapy, its ethics, confidentiality, legal aspects and effectiveness. The kinds of services available, therapist directory, a newsroom, and contact information is provided.

American Self-help Clearinghouse—Self-help Sourcebook Online   ◎ ◎ ◎

http://mentalhelp.net/selfhelp

Supported by Mental Health Net, this site primarily serves persons affected by mental health disorders searching for support groups and information. Links include an FAQ section, support group research, information on starting support groups; local, national, and international self-help clearinghouses and phone numbers, as well as contact information. Links to various disorders and online purchase of this guide are available.

Concerned Counseling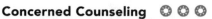

http://www.concernedcounseling.com/page2.htm

Consumers can interact with counselors, online support groups, view the events calendar, get information on eating disorders, and access fact sheets on over 40 psychiatric disorders and topics. Chat rooms, bulletin boards, and extensive support information are present.

Coping with Serious Illness

http://helping.apa.org/mind_body/haber.html

Written by a clinical psychologist, this article gives answers to common questions about medical illness and mental health. Topics include the importance of mental health, psychological therapy, emotional support, coping issues, support information, and how to choose the best therapy.

CYPHERNet: Children, Youth, and Families Education, and Research Network

http://www.cyfernet.org

Part of the National Children, Youth, and Families at Risk Initiative, this site has links to scientific information on children, adolescents, families, and the community. Each subject area contains a number of links to information on support and information resources. In addition, there is a chat room and a section for professionals, containing links to databases, funding information, training information, as well as other topics. This site is searchable and provides information for kids, current events, and a number of links to community project information.

Focusing on Bodily Sensations

http://www.netvision.net.il/php/gshalif

This page on biofeedback and the theory of emotional feedback in psychology was created by a psychologist and provides facts on these topics, as well as links to related sites, links to an electronic book on biofeedback, scientific research studies on emotions, theory of emotions, biofeedback equipment, and more.

Handling your Psychiatric Disability in Work and School

http://www.bu.edu/sarpsych/jobschool

Described as the only site devoted to supplying information about the Americans with Disabilities Act and related issues, this site provides consumers and professionals with links to fact sheets on accommodations and psychiatric disabilities, legal support for affected persons, discrimination in school and work, mental illness and work issues, disclosing your disability, learning and mental illness topics, documenting your disability, and other resources. This site was supported by the Tower Foundation.

InteliHealth.com ☺ ☺ ☺

http://www.intelihealth.com/IH/ihtIH/WSIHW000/408/408.html

Primarily directed toward the general public, the mental health subsection provides a number of links to mental health disorders, such as anxiety, personality and depressive disorders, child and adolescent psychiatric disorders, schizophrenia, physical, sexual and emotional abuse, and somatoform disorders. There is also a clinical directory and numerous links for those seeking mental healthcare support.

Internet Mental Health: Booklets ☺ ☺ ☺

http://www.mentalhealth.com/book/fr40.html

Online patient education booklets and related resources are listed at this important site. Links are listed by topic, including anxiety disorders, childhood disorders, eating disorders, impulse-control disorders, mood disorders, personality disorders, schizophrenia, sleep disorders, substance disorders, medications, treatment and therapy, and general interest.

Mental Help: Procedures to Avoid ☺ ☺

http://www.quackwatch.com/01QuackeryRelatedTopics/mentserv.html

Primarily for consumers, this document, written by a clinician, lists 11 therapies of dubious merit, and reviews their therapeutic procedures and scientific value. References are provided.

Mentalwellness.com ☺ ☺

http://www.mentalwellness.com

In addition to providing resources for finding support groups and therapists, this site has links to mental illness and economic issues, support issues, books, mental health definitions and links, as well a link to fact sheets on various psychiatric disorders.

National Network of Adult and Adolescent Children who have Mentally Ill Parent(s) ☺ ☺

http://home.vicnet.net.au/~nnaami

Created by adult children of mentally ill parents, this Web site offers many links to articles and other documents that provide information and support, and other Internet sources of information.

Patient UK ☺ ☺

http://www.patient.co.uk

This site lists a large number of links (mostly for resources in the United Kingdom) to organizations, personal pages, Web sites, fact sheets, and support groups related to mental health topics. In addition, information on diseases, medicine, books, alternative treatments and self-help topics can be found.

Psychiatric Disability Management Page ☉ ☉ ☉

http://start.at/occupational.psychiatry

Sponsored by PRS Disability Management, this site provides links to many fact files and articles on various topics related to reducing the damages and effects of workplace-related mental health disability. At this site, there are links to a brief overview of psychiatric disability management, information and case study summaries of stress and psychiatric illness in the workplace, and a comparison of medical treatment versus disability management of workplace mental illness issues. There are special links sections for disability management professionals, including informative links for disability claims and human resource managers and benefits administrators. In addition, there is a links section for consumers and professionals, which includes information on career and mental health management and recovery from mental health disability. The site provides a search engine for keyword searches and a list of other disability links.

Self-Help and Psychology Magazine ☉ ☉ ☉

http://www.shpm.com

This site offers a large number of links to questions and answers for a range of mental health issues, such as children's behavior, dreams, depression, stress disorders, addiction, grief, divorce, Internet psychology, men's and women's topics, relationships, aging, and seasonal issues. There are links to discussion forums, online products, lists of related articles on various topics, telehealth resources, a newsletter for professionals, and links to other Web sites of interest.

Support-Group.com ☉ ☉ ☉

http://www.support-group.com

Support-Group.com allows people with health, personal, and relationship issues to share their experiences through bulletin boards and online chats and provides plenty of links to support-related information on the Internet. The A to Z listing offers hundreds of connections to disease-related support, bereavement assistance, marriage and family issue groups, and women's/men's issues, to name a few. The Bulletin Board Tracker lists the most recent messages and provides a complete cross-reference of topics. By visiting the Support-Group.com Chat Schedule page, dates, times, and group facilitators for upcoming chat events can be viewed. Users have the option of participating in real time chat groups via Internet Relay Chat or JavaChat using a Java-capable Web browser. Complete instructions are available at the Web site.

Therapy/Counseling on the Net ☉ ☉

http://ourworld.compuserve.com/homepages/selfheal/net.htm

This site contains a number of links to sites related to online mental illness or psychiatric therapy and counseling.

World Federation for Mental Health ◎ ◎

http://www.wfmh.com

This international organization is devoted to preventing mental illness, promoting mental health, and providing education and support to those affected by mental illness. There are links to conference information, the Eastern Mediterranean branch of the Federation, programs sponsored by the Federation, access to the newsletter, links to related organizations, consumer and survivor information, and contact information. General information about the Federation and membership is also included.

7.27 Patient Exploitation

A Thin Line: Patient/Therapist Sexual Contact ◎ ◎

http://www.ect.org/shame/dateline.html

Sexual misconduct in medical settings is a major ethical issue that is explored through this Dateline NBC discussion. Statistical incidence, warning signs, and methods of filing complaints are all discussed.

Patient Exploitation ◎ ◎

http://www.psych.org/public_info/PATIEN~1.HTM

Patient/therapist sexual conduct is explored at this American Psychiatric Association (APA) site, which explores issues related to medical ethics and the position of the APA. A listing of state psychiatry associations is provided to report incidences of sexual exploitation by therapists.

Sexual Abuse in Professional Relationships ◎ ◎

http://www.kgrs.com/info/abuse.htm

Ethical and legal aspects of patient sexual exploitation are explored at this site which examines the extent of the problem, issues of ethical conduct, and warning signs.

7.28 Religion and Mental Health

Psychology and Religion Pages ◎ ◎ ◎

http://www.psywww.com/psyrelig/index.htm

Pages accessible at this site were developed as a resource for those interested in the psychological aspects of religious belief and behavior. This general introduction to the psychology of religion describes all that psychologists have learned regarding the influence of religion. Conference listings, a message board, information on the future of the field, and an essay from a psychoanalytically trained psychiatrist are all found along with feature books, organizations, and an index of primary journals in the field.

7.29 Sexuality

Kinsey Institute for Research in Sex, Gender, and Reproduction ◉ ◉
http://www.indiana.edu/~kinsey/index.html

This nonprofit corporation is affiliated with Indiana University and "promotes interdisciplinary research and scholarship in the fields of human sexuality, gender, and reproduction." Information about the Institute, an online library catalog, descriptions of archives and art collections at the Institute, details of special events and exhibitions, reference services, links to related sites, and lists and ordering information for recent Institute publications are available through the site. Information on the Institute's Sexual Health and Menstrual Cycle Clinics is also found at this address.

Mental Health Net: All About Sexual Problems ◉ ◉
http://mentalhelp.net/sexual

Resources related to sexual problems are found at this site, including lists and descriptions of symptoms and related diagnoses. Links are available to many related resources, including patient education brochures, commercial sites, support resources, information sources, newsgroups, articles, publications, and organizations.

Resources in Sexuality ◉ ◉ ◉
http://www.sexualhealth.com

This Web site, a service of the Sexual Health Network, comprehensively covers the area of sexuality in relation to physical and mental health including plenty of fundamental and unique information. Sexuality following disability, antidepressants and sexual functioning, discussions on love, libidos, and possible physical and mental obstacles to sexual fulfillment are discussed. A special Sex Over 40 section, a chat room, and the complete Sexual Health Network library are all available online for professionals, students, teachers, and anyone interested in further exploring hundreds of topics in the area of sexual health.

Sexual Health InfoCenter ◉ ◉ ◉
http://www.sexhealth.org/infocenter

Everything from sexual difficulties to sexual techniques is covered at the Sexual Health InfoCenter. Search the InfoCenter for the desired information or click on one of 12 departments, including safer sex, sex and aging, or better sex. A listing of favorite links, and a sex tip of the week are regularly featured, as are a monthly educational quiz and the Web circle grouping of addresses geared toward sex education.

7.30 **Software**

Computers in Mental Health ◎ ◎ ◎
http://www.ex.ac.uk/cimh

As a subsection of the Internet Mental Health Web site, this site provides the latest news and technological advances in software and mental health. Software information is divided into lists such as diagnosis, child psychology, clinical education, medical records, disorders, and several other useful sections. There is a discussion forum, online access to articles relating to software and mental health, a list of reference materials, and links to other related sites.

Mental Health Software ◎ ◎ ◎
http://magellan.excite.com/health/mental_health/psychiatry/software

Magellan's Internet Guide provides a listing of 10 Web sites that offer downloadable software and links to other mental health software sites. The Family Therapy Genogram Generator program generates flowcharts outlining family emotional pattern processes throughout generations, and the Mental Health Speechwriter, a voice recognition system for mental health professionals, is also available. In addition, products are included that may assist practitioners with diagnostic decision making and computerized documentation.

Psychiatry Software ◎ ◎ ◎
http://psychwrite.com/rx.html

PsychWrite Pro, a clinical case management software program, may be downloaded directly from the Web site, and is designed for psychiatrists and other clinicians who wish to easily maintain clinical records and have access to medication and managed care databases. Information on voice recognition programs to be used in conjunction with the software is available, and an online help screen answers frequently-asked questions and provides a forum for e-mail support.

7.31 **Stigma/Mental Illness**

Report from Stigma Plank: National Summit of Mental Health Consumers ◎ ◎ ◎
http://www.mhselfhelp.org/rstigma.html

At this site, the Report on the Stigma Plank is presented by panelists from the University of Chicago who shared information about internalized stigma as well as external stigma. Stigma Plank goals, 10 action steps, and steps for overcoming internal and external stigma are outlined.

7.32 **Surrogacy**

Psychological and Emotional Aspects of Surrogacy ⊚ ⊚ ⊚
http://www.surrogacy.com/psychres/article/index.html

Links to nine articles regarding the psychological and emotional aspects surrounding surrogacy are available at this address including material on the motivations of surrogate mothers as well as the psychological experiences of recipients. A personal experience synopsis concerning the components of a successful surrogate arrangement is outlined, and the grief and shame linked to the infertility experience are examined— all provided by the American Surrogacy Center.

Surrogacy-Related Viewpoints ⊚ ⊚ ⊚
http://www.opts.com/articles.htm

The Organization of Parents Through Surrogacy, Inc.'s Web site offers extensive information surrounding the psychological components of the surrogacy experience. The Surrogate's Point of View contains personal thoughts and discussions regarding the decision to become a surrogate mother, and the family stories section describes common conceptions and misperceptions on the decision to pursue a gestational carrier. The Counselor's Corner contains articles by specialists in the field regarding the emotional insights of surrogacy. A special section on siblings' and the adopted childrens' experiences is included.

7.33 **Theoretical Foundations**

A Glossary of Freudian Terminology ⊚ ⊚
http://www.haverford.edu/psych/ddavis/p109g/fgloss.html

This site, compiled by a professor of psychology at Haverford College, offers detailed explanations and definitions of terms used or developed by Freud in his published works. Links to additional Internet resources on Freud and assorted publications are also available.

Albert Ellis Institute ⊚ ⊚
http://www.rebt.org

Previously listed as the Institute for Rational-Emotive Therapy, this nonprofit educational organization's Web site provides background information on the Institute and its founder, provides access to papers by Dr. Ellis, and has professional services, educational training and products information. Consumer information available includes workshops and lectures for the public, therapist referrals, and self-help and support. The Institute's publications and products are cataloged for sale at this site.

Alfred Adler Institute of San Francisco ◉ ◉

http://www.behavior.net/orgs/adler

This site describes in detail the approaches and concepts behind classical Adlerian psychology, and discusses how this system differs from other psychological approaches. More detailed information is available on basic principles of classical Adlerian psychology, the 12 stages of classical Adlerian psychotherapy, and the Institute's professional training program and seminars. Several related articles are available, and contact information is provided.

Association for the Advancement of Gestalt Therapy (AAGT) ◉ ◉

http://www.g-g.org/aagt

The Association for the Advancement of Gestalt Therapy provides a professional forum dedicated to the preservation and advancement of gestalt therapy. This site describes the Association and its special interest groups, and offers a simplified summary of gestalt therapy, conference information, an online newsletter, and several links to related sites.

B. F. Skinner Foundation ◉ ◉

http://www.lafayette.edu/allanr/skinner.html

The B. F. Skinner Foundation publishes literary and scientific works in behavioral analysis and educates professionals and the public about behavioral science. The site describes continuing and upcoming activities, and offers a brief autobiography of Skinner, reviews of books by Skinner and others, a full bibliography of Skinner's publications, and contact details.

C. G. Jung Institute, Boston ◉ ◉

http://members.aol.com/~cgjungbos1

Dedicated to the discipline of analytical psychology, the C. G. Jung Institute–Boston is chartered by the New England Society of Jungian Analysts. Descriptions and admissions criteria for the Analyst Training Program are available, as well as information on public education programs, a directory of members, and a calendar of events. Contact information is also available.

C. G. Jung Page ◉ ◉ ◉

http://www.cgjung.com

This page was created to encourage education and dialog. Readings offering an introduction to Jung, chat forums and bulletin boards, Jungian articles, an editorial page, editorial, news, and seminars archives, and a search engine are available at the address. Links are available to psychology and psychiatry sites, general Jungian sites, Jungian training institutes, collected works, institutes, professional ethics resources, and sources for books and other publications. Jungian essays on psychology and culture are found at the site, offering psychological commentaries on technology and film. Visitors searching for information on Jung and Jungian analysis will find this site to be an excellent resource.

Classical Adlerian Psychology ◎ ◎ ◎
http://ourworld.compuserve.com/homepages/hstein

This site provides a wealth of information on classical Adlerian psychology and is searchable, providing links to fact sheets on distance training courses and educational materials, graphics, biographies of interest, tapes and books, workshop information, readings in classical Adlerian psychology theory and practice, and a questions and answers section. Additional resources are available in philosophy, theology, parenting, and teaching. Interviews, quotes, and biographies are provided for insight into how professionals chose the field of Adlerian psychology.

Gestalt Growth Center of the San Francisco Bay Area ◎
http://www.gestaltcenter.net

This site describes the Center and director, offers general information on gestalt therapy, and provides contact information for the Center.

Gestalt Therapy Page ◎ ◎
http://www.gestalt.org

This Web page, a joint project sponsored by *The Gestalt Journal* and the International Gestalt Therapy Association, offers a catalog of books, conference information, academic articles, contact information, and ordering information for the Web site on CD-ROM. A worldwide directory of Gestalt therapists in private practice is also available.

JungWeb ◎ ◎
http://www.onlinepsych.com/jungweb

For those interested in specifically Jungian psychology, this Web site offers a number of links to resources on Jungian conferences and workshops, national and international organizations, related forums, Web sites devoted to Jungian psychology, related articles and Jungian links, and many links to information on dreams and personality.

Philosophy of Psychiatry Bibliography ◎ ◎ ◎
http://www.uky.edu/~cperring/PPB4.HTM

This site contains a bibliography of psychiatry publications, covering many specific topics, with links to Amazon.com ordering information. Topics include ethics and philosophy, law, gender and antipsychiatry, psychoanalysis, criminal responsibility, genetics, classification, and antipsychiatry and critical theory.

Sigmund Feud and the Freud Archives ◎ ◎ ◎

http://plaza.interport.net/nypsan/freudarc.html

This site provides links to Internet resources related to Freud and his works. Biographical materials, museum sites, general information about Freud, Freud texts on the Internet, transcripts of Freud letters, and writings on Freud are all available through the links at this site.

8. ORGANIZATIONS AND INSTITUTIONS

8.1 **Associations and Societies**

Directories of Associations

Mental Health InfoSource: Association Address Book ⊙ ⊙ ⊙

http://www.mhsource.com/hy/address.html

This site contains a directory of professional associations related to mental health. Information includes a street address, telephone number, and a Web site address if available. Visitors can also find annual association meetings listed by date.

Mental Health Net: Professional Associations and Organizations ⊙ ⊙ ⊙

http://mentalhelp.net/guide/pro80.htm

Links to home pages of more than 350 professional associations and organizations related to mental health are available at this address. A short summary and rating is available for each listed address. Organizations include professional societies, academies, support groups, research institutes, and other groups.

Mental Health Services Database ⊙ ⊙ ⊙

http://www.cdmgroup.com/Private/Ken/kenindexnew.htm

This database includes information on over 1,800 organizations and government offices that provide mental health services. The database, searchable by keyword, organization, state, or city, returns contact information, abstracts, and additional keywords to help the visitor find similar organizations.

Individual Association Web Sites

Introduction

Below are profiles of more than 80 associations and societies in the field of Psychiatry. Those organizations that have a specific focus appear a second time in this volume under particular diseases and disorders or under an appropriate topical heading.

Academy for the Study of the Psychoanalytic Arts ⊙

http://www.academyanalyticarts.org

This site provides professionals with free online access to program papers, articles, and other reference materials on the topics of psychoanalysis and related fields. The organization's background, meeting, and membership information is also provided.

Academy of Eating Disorders ⊙ ⊙ ⊙

http://www.acadeatdis.org/mainpage.htm

This multidisciplinary professional organization focuses on anorexia nervosa, bulimia nervosa, binge eating disorder, and related disorders. Divisions of the Academy specialize in Academic Sciences, Human Services, Primary Medicine, Psychiatry, Psychology, Dietetics, Nursing, and Social Work. Visitors to the site can access membership information, annual conference details, facts on all eating disorders, and a bibliography of information sources. Specific topical discussions include the prevalence and consequences of eating disorders, courses and outcome of eating disorders, etiology, and treatment.

Academy of Organizational and Occupational Psychiatry (AOOP) ⊙ ⊙

http://www.aoop.org

The Academy of Organizational and Occupational Psychiatry provides a forum for communication between psychiatric professionals and personnel in the workplace. The site offers annual meeting details, general Academy news items, and a description of the organization. Research papers, bulletins, membership details, descriptions of previous annual meetings, and links to related sites are all found at this address.

Academy of Psychological Clinical Science ⊙ ⊙

http://w3.arizona.edu/~psych/apcs/apcs.html

The Academy of Psychological Clinical Science is an alliance of leading and scientifically oriented doctoral training programs in clinical and health psychology in the United States and Canada. The site includes links to the various academic members, a list of officers, a mission statement, membership information, a history of the Academy and a link to related Web sites.

Al-Anon/Alateen Organization ⊙ ⊙ ⊙

http://www.al-anon.org

Al-Anon and Alateen are part of a worldwide organization providing a self-help recovery program for families and friends of alcoholics. Resources available at this official site include meeting information, the 12 steps, traditions, and concepts of the programs, information on Alateen, pamphlets, suggested readings and videotapes, an online newsletter, a calendar of events, and information on a television public service announcement developed by the organization. Professional resources include information on the organization, reasons people are referred to Al-Anon/Alateen, a description of group activities and how they help, and details of how Al-Anon/Alateen cooperates with professionals.

Alzheimer's Association ◎ ◎ ◎

http://www.alz.org

The Alzheimer's Association offers information and support on issues related to the disease. Patients and caregivers can access general facts about Alzheimer's disease, and detailed discussions of medical issues, diagnosis, expected lifestyle changes, treatment options, clinical trial participation, planning for the future, and contact information for special programs and support. Caregiver information and professional resources are also available. Resources for investigators include a summary of current research, lists of grant opportunities, lists of past grant awards, progress report forms, and information on the Reagan Institute. The Association also offers news, program, and conference calendars; publications; and information on advocacy activities at this site.

Alzheimer's Disease Society ◎ ◎

http://www.alzheimers.org.uk

Created to provide information about Alzheimer's disease and other dementias, this site has links to descriptive fact sheets on these disorders, their symptoms, and physical causes and consequences, treatment and prognosis. In addition, there are summaries of current research theories on these dementias. For caregivers, there is general support advice and related topics, as well as current news, information about the society itself, as well links to other related societies.

American Academy of Addiction Psychiatry ◎ ◎

http://www.aaap.org/index.html

Informational links on the academy and membership, as well as the different committees and policy statements are provided. Links to previous, present, and future annual meetings, Accreditation Council for Graduate Medical Education (ACGME) information, as well as a Web store for reference tapes and other materials are present.

American Academy of Child and Adolescent Psychiatry (AACAP) ◎ ◎ ◎

http://www.aacap.org

The AACAP assists parents and families in understanding developmental, behavioral, emotional, and mental disorders affecting children and adolescents. The site offers general information about the organization, news, fact sheets, press releases, legislation resources, meetings details, awards information, a publications catalog and access to abstracts from the *Journal of the American Academy of Child and Adolescent Psychiatry,* membership information, employment opportunities, and links to related sites. Clinical practice, research and training resources are also available. The site offers resources for parents, including a section of suggestions and articles on helping children and adolescents after a disaster, teen violence management, children and the media, and school safety issues. Summaries and ordering information for parent handbooks published by the Academy are available, and users can search the site by keyword. An extensive resources section links to organizations related to child and adolescent psychiatry or pediatrics. Home pages of other national and international organizations, research and support groups, and government agencies are listed in this section.

American Academy of Clinical Neuropsychology (AACN) ◎ ◎

http://www.med.umich.edu/abcn/aacn.html

This site presented by the American Academy of Clinical Neuropsychology allows users to search the AACN directory of members, view the articles and bylaws of the Academy, view current AACN news, and access continuing education materials. Links to other neuropsychology sites are present.

American Academy of Doctors of Psychology ◎ ◎ ◎

http://www.doctorsofpsychology.org

This site allows access to a directory of psychologists in the United States, and a large number of links to information about psychology and psychological disorders and treatment. In addition, there are links of interest to doctors, including specialties, media and literature information, as well as academy membership information. Graduates and students will find links to related organizations, as well as license, training, and employment information. Selected articles from the *Psychological Letter* are available online. Numerous online services, such as newsgroups and other listservers are present.

American Academy of Experts in Traumatic Stress ◎ ◎

http://www.aaets.org

American Academy of Experts in Traumatic Stress membership includes health professionals, as well as professionals from emergency services, criminal justice, forensics, law, and education committed to the advancement of intervention for survivors of trauma. The Academy's Web site provides extensive informational links for professionals in the field. A description of the academy, links to membership information, credentials, certifications, education credits, searching the national registry, the administration, board of advisors are present. Free access to selected articles from *Trauma Response* is provided. Also, ordering instructions for the *Practical Guide for Crisis Response in Our Schools* (3rd edition) are available.

American Academy of Psychoanalysis ◎ ◎

http://aapsa.org

The American Academy of Psychoanalysis represents the National Academy of Professional Medical Psychoanalysists. Informative links to the *Journal of the American Academy of Psychoanalysis*, selected articles from the *Academy Forum*, related meetings, member roster, organization information, publications, and research details are available at the site.

American Anorexia Bulimia Association ◎ ◎

http://www.aabainc.org

The American Anorexia Bulimia Association is a national nonprofit organization dedicated to the prevention and treatment of eating disorders. This site contains a number of links to informative pages on eating disorders, such as anorexia, bulimia, and binge eating. Information on symptoms, support, medical consequences, risk factors, a list of references about these disorders, as well as membership information is included.

American Association
for Geriatric Psychiatry (AAGP) ◎ ◎ ◎ (some features fee-based)

http://www.aagpgpa.org

The AAGP Web site includes numerous links to various issues of interest for both professionals and interested laypersons. There are news reports, the AAGP bookstore, meeting information, consumer information, including brochures and a question/answer section, advocacy and public policy section, a link to the *American Journal for Geriatric Psychiatry*, a health professional bulletin, member meeting place, staff listing, and a link to the AAGP Education and Research Foundation.

American Association of Community Psychiatrists ◎ ◎

http://www.comm.psych.pitt.edu/find.html

The American Association of Community Psychiatrists promotes excellence in inpatient mental healthcare, solves common problems encountered by psychiatrists in a community setting, establishes liaisons with related professional groups for advocacy purposes, encourages psychiatrist training, improves relationships within community settings between psychiatrists and other clinicians and administrators, and educates the public about the role of the community mental health system in the care of the mentally ill. This site provides information on the mission of the Association, board members, and membership information. The present and previous newsletters and issues of *Community Psychiatrist* are available, as well as links to relevant training and research programs in the discipline.

American Association of Marriage
and Family Therapists (AAMFT) ◎ ◎ ◎ (fee-based)

http://www.aamft.org

The American Association for Marriage and Family Therapy is the professional association for the field of marriage and family therapy, representing the professional interests of more than 23,000 marriage and family therapists throughout the United States, Canada and abroad. This site allows professionals and other interested parties to search directories for therapist listing and provides information on the Association. General information includes clinical updates on various marriage and family mental health issues; the link for practitioners lists information on conferences and conference highlights, resources, a referral section, publications, education, training, licensing links, and membership information.

American Association of Psychotherapists ⊙ (fee-based)

http://www.angelfire.com/tx/Membership/index.html

The American Association of Psychotherapists is a national nonprofit, multidisciplinary professional organization of certified clinicians dedicated to the support and development of psychotherapy. This Web site was created to provide networking opportunities for professionals. The site provides a message board, chat room, and online membership application.

American Association of Suicidology ⊙ ⊙ ⊙

http://www.suicidology.org

This nonprofit organization is dedicated to the understanding and prevention of suicide. The Web site includes information regarding the Association, conference information, links to other relevant sites, internship information, and a directory for support groups and crisis centers. In addition, there are links to sources for books and other printed resources, links to legal and ethical issues, treatment, assessment and prediction, and certification/accreditation manuals.

American Association on Mental Retardation (AAMR) ⊙ ⊙

http://www.aamr.org

"AAMR promotes global development and dissemination of progressive policies, sound research, effective practices, and universal human rights for people with intellectual disabilities." Site resources include information about the AAMR, current news, bookstore, membership information, reference materials from the annual meeting, free access to the *American Journal on Mental Retardation* and *Mental Retardation*, a list of the divisions of the AAMR, and links to the discussion group and chat rooms.

American Family Therapy Academy ⊙

http://www.afta.org

This nonprofit professional organization fosters an exchange of ideas among family therapy teachers, researchers, and practitioners. The site presents the organization's objectives, policy and press releases, membership details, a membership directory, excerpts of the organization's newsletter, and lists of recent awards with recipients.

American Group Psychotherapy Association ⊙ ⊙ ⊙

http://www.groupsinc.org

The American Group Psychotherapy Association works to enhance the practice, theory, and research of group therapy. The Association offers information about group therapy, a directory of group therapists for interested patients, news, contact information, a meetings and events calendar, and publications details at this site. Specific resources for group therapists and students include ethical guidelines for group therapists, training opportunities information, certification details, government reports, advanced principles of psychotherapy, and links to affiliated societies.

American Hyperlexia Association ◎ ◎

http://www.hyperlexia.org

"The American Hyperlexia Association is a nonprofit organization comprised of parents and relatives of children with hyperlexia, speech and language professionals, education professionals, and other concerned individuals with the common goal of identifying hyperlexia, promoting and facilitating effective teaching techniques both at home and at school, and educating the general public as to the existence of the syndrome called hyperlexia." This Web site includes links to pages describing hyperlexia and treatment options, as well as links to the mailing list, membership information, materials order list, organizations and therapist directories, other hyperlexia sites, and a guestbook.

American Neuropsychiatric Association (ANPA) ◎ ◎

http://www.neuropsychiatry.com/ANPA/index.html

Resources offered by the ANPA at this site include program and registration information for the group's 2000 Annual Meeting, contact information, membership applications, an e-mail news subscription service, a directory of members, an online newsletter, journal information, and links to related sites of interest to neuroscientists. Internet access for this site is made available by Butler Hospital, and the site is supported by an unrestricted educational grant from Hoechst. A list of ANPA officers is also provided.

American Occupational Therapy Association, Inc. ◎ ◎ ◎

http://www.aota.org

This organization offers information on occupational therapy, news, membership details, details of events, products and services, academic accreditation resources, continuing education resources, publications, and information on academic and fieldwork education. Student resources include journals and information on educational programs, fieldwork, and careers. Consumers can access information on occupational therapy, fact sheets, case studies, a directory of practitioners, and links to related sites. Conference details and links to related sites are also found at this address.

American Professional Society on the Abuse of Children (APSAC) ◎ ◎

http://www.apsac.org

The mission of APSAC is to ensure that everyone affected by child maltreatment receives the best possible professional response. This professional society's site provides information on the society itself, membership information, legislative activities, professional education, state chapters, and public affairs, and current news. Information on the society's publications, such as the APSAC Advisor, the APSAC Guidelines for Practice, the APSAC Handbook on Child Maltreatment and Child Maltreatment are available online. There is also information for those interested in donating to the society.

American Psychiatric Association (APA) ☉ ☉ ☉

http://www.psych.org

The American Psychiatric Association is a national and international association of psychiatric physicians. The site includes updates, public policy and advocacy information, clinical and research resources, membership information, medical education, related organizations, governance, library and publications, events schedule, psychiatric news, APA catalog, and a link to APPI (APA Press, Inc.).

American Psychiatric Nurses Association ☉ ☉ ☉

http://www.apna.org

The American Psychiatric Nurses Association is devoted to providing leadership to psychiatric and mental health nursing professionals. This Web site has links to information on membership, conferences, the association, advocacy updates, legislative news, APNA chapters, and a calendar of events. With respect to publications, there is access to the table of contents to the APNA journal, as well as position papers, APNA news articles, graduate programs in psychiatric nursing, and other related links.

American Psychoanalytic Association ☉ ☉ ☉

http://apsa.org

The American Psychoanalytic Association is a professional organization of psychoanalysts throughout the United States. Press releases, a calendar of events and meetings, general information about psychoanalysis, fellowship details, an online book store, a directory of psychoanalysts, *Journal of the American Psychoanalytic Association* abstracts, and an online newsletter are all available at the site. An extensive catalog of links to related online journals, institutes, societies, organizations, libraries, museums, and general sites are offered through the site. The Jourlit and Bookrev databases are also available, together constituting a formidable bibliography of psychoanalytic journal articles, books, and book reviews. Information on obtaining journal reprints is supplied.

American Psychological Association (APA) ☉ ☉ ☉ (fee-based)

http://www.apa.org

The American Psychological Association Web site provides numerous links including reference materials, publications, national and international research sites, education, conferences, government information, and help centers. Comprehensive information regarding the Association itself is present.

American Psychological Society (APS) ⊙ ⊙ ⊙

http://www.psychologicalscience.org

The American Psychological Society aims to provide a forum for research and application to the science of psychology. The site offers information regarding membership, current news, conventions, and APS publications. Updates on funding opportunities and legislative events relevant to psychology are provided.

American Psychotherapy and
Medical Hypnosis Association (APMHA) ⊙ ⊙ ⊙

http://fourohfour.xoom.com/Members404Error.xihtml

The APMHA was founded in 1992 for State Board Licensed and Certified Professionals in multi-disciplines of Medicine, Psychology, Social Work, Family Therapy, Alcohol and Chemical Dependency, Professional Counseling, Dentistry, and Forensic and Investigative Hypnosis. The site provides a description of hypnosis, membership information and application, professional referrals, training and certification program information, links to related sites, ordering information for professional video training tapes, and contact details.

American Sleep Disorders Association (ASDA) ⊙ ⊙ ⊙

http://www.asda.org

The professional section of the site provides links to information on membership, ASDA history and goals, directory of accredited centers, educational products, ASDA staff, accreditation information and policy, board certification, funding opportunities, position papers, professional education, free online access to publications from the National Center on Sleep Disorders (NCSDR), abstracts from the 1998 meeting, and the journal Sleep. Links to other sleep-related sites are included. The patient and public area provides links to answers of common questions about sleep disorders, diagnoses and treatment, patient support groups, resources from (NCSDR) and other related links.

American Society of Addiction Medicine (ASAM) ⊙ ⊙ ⊙

http://www.asam.org

The American Society of Addiction Medicine aims to educate physicians and improve the "treatment of individuals suffering from alcoholism and other addictions." Medical news items related to addiction treatment, clinical trials, practice guidelines, and other topics are available at the site. Publications offered at the site include practice guidelines, Chapter One of ASAM's *Principles of Addiction Medicine*, newsletters, patient placement criteria, and the table of contents and abstracts for the *Journal of Addictive Diseases*. General information about ASAM, activities of the AIDS and HIV

Committee of ASAM, a physician directory, annual meeting details, membership information and directory, certification resources, discussion forums, news, resources on nicotine addiction, pain management information, contact information, state chapter details, and links to related sites are all found at this address.

American Society of Psychoanalytic Physicians ⊙

http://pubweb.acns.nwu.edu/~chessick/aspp.htm

This Society and Web site were created to provide a forum for psychoanalytically-oriented psychiatrists and physicians. The purpose of the Society, as well as a list of the officers and editorial board are available.

American Society on Aging (ASA) ⊙ ⊙ (some features fee-based)

http://www.asaging.org

The American Society on Aging provides information resources on gerontology through educational programming, publications, and training. General resources at this site include membership and contact details, meeting information, conference and training schedules, and awards listings. Links are available to information on publications, including *Aging Today* and *Generations*. Visitors can also access news, links to related sites, job banks, and information on specific ASA networks, including business and aging; environments, services, and technologies; healthcare and aging; lesbian and gay aging issues; lifelong education; mental health and aging; multicultural aging issues; and religion, spirituality; and aging. Databases containing information on conferences, training events, and resources on aging issues are available for members, as well as a chat forum, special offers, and member directories.

Angelman Syndrome Association ⊙ ⊙

http://www.australianholidays.com/asa/frames/asahome-f.htm

The Australian Angelman Association provides general information at its Web site pertaining to the diagnosis, research, and treatment of the rare, neuro-genetic disorder. The Angelman syndrome LISTSERV is provided for communication via e-mail as are past issues of the Association's newsletter.

Anorexia Nervosa and Bulimia Association ⊙ ⊙ ⊙

http://www.ams.queensu.ca/anab

Primarily a supportive organization for those affected by or interested in eating disorders, this Web site has extensive links to support groups, as well as lots of information on eating disorders in general, including an overview of the biology of eating disorders, treatment and diagnosis, as well as predisposing factors. There is a list of reference materials as well as online access to the association's newsletter.

Anxiety Disorders Association of America (ADAA) ⊙ ⊙ ⊙

http://www.adaa.org

The Anxiety Disorders Association of America, comprised of health professionals, researchers and others interested in these disorders, "promotes the prevention and cure of anxiety disorders." The site offers ordering information for patients suffering from anxiety disorders, including self-help publications, participation information for research studies, membership details, conference information, an online bookstore, news, and speech transcripts. Fact sheets are available, with titles including Consumers Guide to Treatment, Social Phobia, Social Anxiety Disorder Information, Generalized Anxiety Disorder (GAD), Specific Phobias, Obsessive-Compulsive Disorder, Posttraumatic Stress Disorder (PTSD), Panic Disorder and Agoraphobia, Anxiety Disorders and Medication, Anxiety Disorders in Children and Adolescents, Anxiety Disorders: Helping a Family Member, and A Journey to Recovery from Anxiety Disorders. Consumers can also find resources related to support groups and links to related sites.

Association for Academic Psychiatry ⊙ ⊙

http://www.aapsych.org/index.html

This Association focuses on education in psychiatry. The Web site includes links to the Association's officers, full online access to the bulletin and Academic Psychiatry, membership information, teaching resources, annual conference information, and a link to Collaborative Academic Resources (CAR).

Association for Applied
Psychophysiology and Biofeedback (AAPB) ⊙ ⊙ ⊙ (fee-based)

http://www.aapb.org

This nonprofit organization of clinicians, researchers, and educators is dedicated to advancing the "development, dissemination and utilization of knowledge about applied psychophysiology and biofeedback to improve health and the quality of life through research, education, and practice." General information at the site includes a description of biofeedback and psychophysiology, a list of common health problems helped by biofeedback, meetings and workshop information, membership information, a bibliography of recent research articles related to biofeedback and psychophysiology, links to related sites, an online bookstore, and content lists of AAPB publications. The site offers a directory of biofeedback practitioners and a forum for asking questions of biofeedback experts. Submission instructions are available for the AAPB 2000 Annual Meeting.

Association for Behavior Analysis ⊙ ⊙

http://www.wmich.edu/aba/contents.html

The Association for Behavior Analysis, an international organization based at Western Michigan University, promotes experimental, theoretical, and applied analysis of behavior. Visitors to the site can access a job placement service, lists of affiliated chapters, student committees, special interest groups, annual convention details, membership details, a member directory, Association publications, and links to related Web sites.

Association for Child Psychoanalysis (ACP) ◎ ◎
http://www.westnet.com/acp

The Association for Child Psychoanalysis (ACP) is an international not-for-profit organization providing a forum for the interchange of ideas and clinical experience in order to advance the psychological treatment and understanding of children and adolescents and their families. This site was designed to promote the association and its programs. Links to a searchable roster, referral information, the ACP archives, psychoanalysis related sites, and a comprehensive list of programs developed by ACP members are available at the site.

Association for Medical Education and Research in Substance Abuse ◎ ◎
http://www.amersa.org

The Web site for this multidisciplinary organization of professionals interested in substance abuse has links to the mission statement, organization and membership information, conference information, an online discussion group, and a link to the table of contents for the journal, *Substance Abuse*.

Association for Psychoanalytic Medicine ◎ ◎
http://cpmcnet.columbia.edu/dept/pi/psychoanalytic/APM

The Association for Psychoanalytic Medicine (APM) is a nonprofit organization, and is an affiliate society of both the American Psychoanalytic Association and the International Psychoanalytic Association. Most members are graduates of the Columbia University Center for Psychoanalytic Training and Research, participating in professional development and community outreach activities. An extensive list of the association-sponsored lectures, held at the New York Academy of Medicine, as well as online access to publications, such as *The Bulletin—the Journal of the APM,* and *The Shrink*. There is information on awards, and a membership roster. Other links include postgraduate education information, and mental health resources.

Association for Research in Nervous and Mental Disease (ARNMD) ◎
http://cpmcnet.columbia.edu/www/arnmd

The Association for Research in Nervous and Mental Disease is the oldest society of neurologists and psychiatrists. The site provides links to the history and mission of ARNMD, the board of trustees, ARNMD publications from 1920, an events calendar, 1998 meeting abstracts, and a list of program speakers and talks from the 1998 annual course.

Association for the Advancement of Gestalt Therapy (AAGT) ◉ ◉

http://www.g-g.org/aagt

The Association for the Advancement of Gestalt Therapy provides a professional forum dedicated to the preservation and advancement of gestalt therapy. This site describes the Association and its special interest groups, and offers a simplified summary of gestalt therapy, conference information, an online newsletter, and several links to related sites.

Association for the Advancement of Philosophy and Psychiatry ◉ ◉

http://www.swmed.edu/home_pages/aapp

The mission of the Association for the Advancement of Philosophy and Psychiatry is to encourage interdisciplinary activity in philosophy and psychiatry and to advance knowledge, promote research, and facilitate understanding in both fields. The Association's mission statement is provided at the site, as well as links to the officers and executive council members, meetings and conferences, local and special interest groups, and free access to the official journal of the Association, *Philosophy, Psychiatry, and Psychology.*

Association for the Study of Dreams ◉ ◉

http://www.asdreams.org

This nonprofit organization is dedicated to the "pure and applied investigation of dreams and dreaming." Conference information, a magazine, education resources, discussion forums, membership details, on online bookstore, details of current projects, a membership directory, and contact details are all found at the site. Abstracts of articles and other details of the Association's journal, *Dreaming,* are available at the site, as well as some full-text articles. A search engine is available for more specific information.

Association for the Treatment of Sexual Abusers (ATSA) ◉ ◉

http://www.atsa.com

The Association for the Treatment of Sexual Abusers is an international organization focused specifically on the prevention of sexual abuse through effective management of sex offenders. The site provides membership information, *Sexual Abuse* journal table of contents, 1999 graduate research awards and ATSA research grants, position statements, conference information, internship and fellowship opportunities, employment opportunities, and book lists.

Association for Treatment and Training in the Attachment of Children ⊙ ⊙ ⊙

http://www.attach.org

This coalition of parents and professionals exchanges information on attachment and bonding issues. Information on healthy attachment, membership details, events and training notices, a newsletter, recommended reading lists, book reviews, assessment instrument reviews, and clinical notes are found at this address. Details of the organization's structure, research reviews, links to related sites and contact details for non-Internet resources, and lists of suggested professional resources are also available.

Association of Traumatic Stress Specialists (ATSS) ⊙ ⊙

http://www.atss-hq.com

This international nonprofit organization provides professional education and certification to those actively involved in crisis intervention, trauma response, management, treatment, and the healing and recovery of those affected by traumatic stress. The site provides information on the organization, membership benefits, certification as a trauma specialist, an events calendar, links to other trauma-related sites, and a resource guide.

Autism Society of America (ASA) ⊙ ⊙ ⊙

http://www.autism-society.org

The mission of the Autism Society of America is to promote lifelong access and opportunities for persons within the autism spectrum and their families, to be fully included, participating members of their communities through advocacy, public awareness, education, and research related to autism. This site contains a large amount of information and links pertaining to all aspects of autism. There are links to advocacy and government action alerts, the ASA and membership information, legislative action news, conference information, and a searchable directory of the Web site and mailing list. A link to research in autism, including articles from autism research professionals, and numerous links including reference materials, glossary, treatment and diagnosis, medical and insurance information, and links to other related organizations and sites are provided.

Canadian Psychiatric Association ⊙ ⊙ ⊙ (free registration)

http://cpa.medical.org

This voluntary professional association for psychiatrists encourages communication and collaboration both within psychiatry and with other professions, consumers, and government agencies. Visitors to the site will find links to associated academies (including the Canadian Academy of Geriatric Psychiatry and the Canadian Academy of Psychiatry and the Law), continuing professional development, annual meeting and other program details, employment listings, membership information, and news releases. A chat forum is available to members and registered users. Full-text articles from the *Canadian Journal of Psychiatry,* position papers, guidelines and statements, newsletters, annual reports, and patient education brochures are all found at the site.

Cyclic Vomiting Syndrome Association ◎ ◎
http://www.beaker.iupui.edu/cvsa/index.html

This organization's site provides basic information about the disorder, lists upcoming events and conferences, provides information about membership, and offers a list of related links to Web sites. In addition, there is ample research information, as well as support resources.

Depression and Related
Affective Disorders Association (DRADA) ◎ ◎
http://www.med.jhu.edu/drada

This site provides information about DRADA, links to research reports and other reference materials, book reviews, an online store for videos and books, support groups and other related organizations, as well as a link to clinical research studies seeking participants.

Dyslexia—The Gift: Davis Dyslexia Association International ◎ ◎ ◎
http://www.dyslexia.com

The Davis Dyslexia Association International offers workshops and training to teachers and professionals on helping individuals with dyslexia and other learning disabilities. A resource library at the site includes articles, questions and answers about dyslexia, book excerpts, and links to other information sources. Educational materials, professional resources, chat forums, a Davis Program provider directory, and workshop calendars are all found at the site. Resources are provided in English, Spanish, German, French, Dutch, and Italian.

Gerontological Society of America ◎ ◎ ◎
http://www.geron.org

The Gerontological Society of America promotes research and disseminates information related to gerontological research. Site sections list awards, annual meeting details, press releases, employment opportunities, news, publications, Society divisions, and links to related sites. Related foundations, a referral service, useful sources for information, student organization details, and membership details are also found through the site. A discussion is available on social security and women. Visitors can search the site by keyword for specific information.

Harry Benjamin International Gender Dysphoria Association, Inc.

http://www.tc.umn.edu/nlhome/m201/colem001/hbigda

This professional Association is committed to the understanding and treatment of gender identity disorders, with members from the fields of Psychiatry, Endocrinology, Surgery, Psychology, Sociology, and Counseling. Site resources include general information about the Association, details of the Association's biennial conference, membership information, the full text of the Benjamin Standards of Care for Gender Identity Disorders (5th version), links to related sites, and contact details for those seeking more specific information.

International Angelman Syndrome Association (IASO)

http://www.asclepius.com/iaso

The organization's mission and member countries are enumerated at this site along with information on joining the IASO electronic mailing list. The Web site's conference announcements are also available and may be viewed in English, French, Spanish, or German.

International Association of Eating Disorders Professionals (IAEDP)

http://www.iaedp.com

The International Association of Eating Disorders Professionals offers a certification process for health professionals seeking specialized credentials in the treatment of patients with eating disorders. The Web site provides information regarding the Association, membership and certification information, and registration details for symposium events.

International Association of Group Psychotherapy

http://www.psych.mcgill.ca/labs/iagp/IAGP.html

The Association is dedicated to the development of group psychotherapy as a field of practice, training, and scientific study and by means of international conferences, publications, and other forms of communication. The Web page consists of membership information and a directory of the executive and board of directors. The site also offers links to conference information, an electronic forum, and links to other sites of interest. Upcoming links include abstracts of scientific articles relating to group psychotherapy.

International Behavioural and Neural Genetics Society (IBANGS)

http://www.ibngs.org

Formerly the European Behavioural and Neural Genetics Society (EBANGS), this international Society supports research in the field of neurobehavioral genetics. Membership information, Society information, rules, a member directory, meeting details, links to member societies, and past meeting transcripts are available at the site. Links are also available at the site to sources for meeting information, societies and networks, institutions and databases, and publications of interest in neurobehavioral and neural genetics.

International Dyslexia Association ◎ ◎ ◎

http://www.interdys.org

This nonprofit Association is devoted to the study and treatment of dyslexia. Site resources include information about the organization, position papers, descriptions of branch services, membership details, conference and seminar calendars, an online bookstore, technology resources, legal and legislative information, research discussions, press releases, and a bulletin board for site visitors. The site also offers a detailed discussion of dyslexia, including information and links to Internet resources for adolescents, college students, parents, adults, and educators and other professionals.

International Psychoanalytical Association (IPA) ◎ ◎ ◎

http://www.ipa.org.uk

Described as the world's primary psychoanalytic accrediting and regulatory body, the Association's Web site has numerous links to the various conferences and congresses organized by the Association, as well as links to special committees' synopses, a message forum, access to IPA newsletters, and other related links.

International Society for the Study of Dissociation (ISSD) ◎ ◎ ◎

http://www.issd.org

This nonprofit professional organization advocates research and professional training in the diagnosis, treatment and education of dissociative disorders, as well as serving to promote international communication among scientists and professionals working in this area. There are links to conference information, membership and society information, a link to the *Journal of Trauma and Dissociation,* the ISSD newsletter, education resources, including articles on related topics, and a list of dissociation disorder treatment guidelines. In addition, there is a set of professional and self-help links, and contact information.

International Society for Traumatic Stress Studies (ISTSS) ◎ ◎

http://www.istss.org

A professional society created for the sharing of scientific information and strategies on traumatic stress, this Web site has links to conference information, other affiliates of the ISTSS, membership information, related links, and access to articles from the *Journal of Traumatic Stress,* as well as critical reviews and treatment guide.

International Society of Psychiatric Genetics ⊙

http://www.ispg.net

The International Society of Psychiatric Genetics promotes and facilitates research, education, and communication in the genetics of psychiatric disorders, substance abuse, and related traits. This address offers a Board of Directors listing, information on upcoming meetings, Society bylaws and mission statement, and links to several related sites.

International Society of Psychosomatic Medicine, Obstetrics, and Gynecology ⊙ ⊙

http://www.ispog.org

The International Society of Psychosomatic Obstetrics and Gynaecology promotes the study and education of the psychobiological, psychosocial, ethical, and cross-cultural problems in the fields of Obstetrics and Gynecology. This site presents the objectives of the Society, as well as a newsletter and links to local chapters. Free online access to the abstracts of the *Journal of Psychosomatic Obstetrics and Gynecology* is available, as well as links to information on international meetings and congresses. Related links and a keyword search engine are available.

Learning Disabilities Association (LDA) ⊙ ⊙ ⊙

http://www.ldanatl.org

This nonprofit organization advances the education and general welfare of children and adults with learning disabilities. Visitors to the site will find a mission statement, resources on specific conditions, position statements, suggested reading lists, news, a calendar of upcoming events, membership information, contact details, links to state affiliates, fact sheets, an online bookstore, and contact information for support organizations, educational resources, and publication sources.

Mood Disorders Association of British Columbia ⊙ ⊙

http://www.lynx.net/~mda

This association's Web site has links to general information about certain mood disorders, and offers an information request form and links to related sites.

National Association for Rights Protection and Advocacy (NARPA) ⊙ ⊙ ⊙

http://www.connix.com/~narpa

The NARPA exists to expose abuses and promote real alternatives to the current mental health system. The organization's Web site provides readings on mental health advocacy including current case decisions and legislative information, excerpts from the NARPA's Annual Conference and Annual Rights Conference, and an online version of *Rights Tenet* newsletter are available. Interesting links such as the history of mental health advocacy are easily accessed. Online membership information and application is provided.

National Association of
Anorexia Nervosa and Associated Disorders ◎ ◎ ◎
http://www.anad.org

This national nonprofit organization helps eating disorder victims and their families through hotline counseling, support groups, and referrals to healthcare professionals. The site offers information about the organization, eating disorder definitions, fact sheets, warning signs, therapy information, statistics and demographics, and suggestions on confronting someone with an eating disorder. Visitors will also find information on insurance discrimination and eating disorders, legislative alerts, and links to related useful sites.

National Association of Cognitive-Behavioral Therapists ◎ ◎ ◎
http://www.nacbt.org

Up-to-date information and news is provided at the official site of the National Association of Cognitive-Behavioral Therapists, including back issues of the *Rational News* newsletter. A referral database sends you to the organization's National Database of Certified Cognitive-Behavioral Therapists. Professional certifications offered by the organization are outlined, and a professional and self-help resources store is provided online. Products for professionals include home study courses, books, and audiovisual materials. Likewise, self-improvement courses, and multimedia materials are available to the lay community.

National Association of Psychiatric
Health Systems (NAPHS) ◎ ◎ (some features fee-based)
http://www.naphs.org

The National Association of Psychiatric Health Systems advocates for health systems providing mental health and substance abuse services. The site provides a description of the organization and services, links to NAPHS and other sites offering consumer information, details of marketing opportunities, membership and contact details, and news articles. A resource catalog offers details of publications, conferences, and services of the organization, including advocacy materials and projects, clinical resources and projects, behavioral health events, financial resources, administrative resources, directories, and mailing lists. One section is restricted to registered members.

National Association of Social Workers (NASW) ◎ ◎
http://www.naswdc.org

This international organization of professional social workers is devoted to the professional growth of its members, the creation and maintenance of professional standards, and the advancement of social policies. Membership details, chapter listings, publications information, a directory of social workers, continuing education resources, employment notices, an online store, news, and advocacy activities are listed at the site. Links are available to state chapters, professional organizations, government and advocacy resources, child abuse prevention and child welfare resources, health, mental health, substance abuse resources, and commercial partners.

National Attention Deficit Disorder Association ⊙ ⊙ ⊙
http://www.add.org

The National Attention Deficit Disorder Association helps people with AD/HD lead happier, more successful lives through education, research, and public advocacy. Membership information, conference details, articles, news, guiding principles for diagnosis and treatment, and a directory of professionals treating AD/HD are available at the site. Research, treatment, and general information about AD/HD is offered, as well as links to sites offering resources on work, family, education, and legal issues associated with AD/HD. Support group sites and sites for children and teens are also listed. Visitors can read personal stories and interviews, and search the site by keyword.

National Coalition of Arts Therapies Associations (NCATA) ⊙ ⊙
http://www.ncata.com/home.html

This alliance of professional associations dedicated to the advancement of art therapy represents six organizations. Art therapy, dance/movement therapy, drama therapy, music therapy, psychodrama, and poetry therapy are defined and discussed at this site. Information on upcoming conferences and contact details for professional organizations are available.

National Depressive and Manic-Depressive Association ⊙ ⊙ ⊙
http://www.ndmda.org

The National Depressive and Manic-Depressive Association strives to educate patients, families, professionals, and the public concerning the nature of depressive and bipolar disorders as treatable medical disorders, foster self-help, eliminate discrimination, improve access to care, and promote research. The site contains extensive information on the Association and links to general information on depression and bipolar disorder and related issues. Links to support groups, patient assistance programs, education, advocacy, clinical trials, and reference materials are listed.

National Mental Health Association ⊙ ⊙ ⊙
http://www.nmha.org/index.cfm

The National Mental Health Association works to increase tolerance and awareness, improve mental health services, prevent mental illness, and promote mental health. At this site, interested individuals will find updates on state and federal legislative actions, employment opportunities, an events calendar, and an information center providing links to referrals and educational materials. Informative links to discussions of topics including mental health disorders, advocacy issues, public education, and healthcare reform are found at the site, as well as links to the Association's affiliate and membership network.

New England Society for the Study of Dissociation ◎ ◎
http://www.nessd.org

This Society, an affiliate of the nonprofit International Society for the Study of Dissociation (ISSD), serves professional members from Connecticut, Maine, Massachusetts, New Hampshire, Rhode Island, and Vermont. Quarterly meetings offer professional presentations, discussion groups, consultation clinics, networking opportunities, and the Society sponsors educational workshops on the treatment of dissociative disorders and other topics. This site provides visitors with a mission statement, membership information, a calendar of events, recent newsletter articles, a bulletin board, and links to related sites.

Psychiatry Society for Informatics ◎ ◎ ◎
http://www.psych.med.umich.edu

The home page of the Psychiatric Society for Informatics serves to increase the understanding and use of informatics related to the field of psychiatry. Information on the organization, its current news and upcoming meetings, online membership information and benefits, and the organization's electronic newsletter are all presented.

Safer Society Foundation ◎ ◎
http://www.safersociety.org

This national nonprofit organization provides advocacy, referrals, and research for the prevention and treatment of sexual abuse. At this site, professionals and consumers can find news updates, learn about the Foundation's information and referral services, training and consulting information, research resources, and order books, and other reference materials provided by the Safer Society Press. Contact information and links to related organizations are also provided.

Social Phobia/Social Anxiety Association Home Page ◎ ◎ ◎
http://www.socialphobia.org

The purposes and goals of the Social Phobia/Social Anxiety Association (SP/SAA), informational articles, and current news are enumerated at the Association's Web site. Social anxiety links, fact sheets, and mailing lists may be accessed. The Anxiety Network bookstore page allows users to choose and order books securely over the Internet. Professional literature and a subscription to the quarterly publication, *SP/SAA Journal* is available through a mail-in registration process.

Society for Manic Depression ◎ ◎

http://www.societymd.org

Online patient support forums, including a remission program, and a detailed description of bipolar disorder are available at this address. Topics include open communication with a psychiatrist, diagnosis, denial, manic and depressive states and medications. Some chat forums, allowing individual online communication with specialists, are available to those with a membership, which requires a fee.

Society for Neuronal Regulation (SNR) ◎ ◎

http://www.snr-jnt.org

This organization consists of professionals interested in neurofeedback training and research. Site resources include a glossary, a reference center, a listing of neurofeedback providers, conference information, and a neurofeedback archive of online abstracts and papers from selected SNR meetings. There is also free access to the *Journal of Neurotherapy*.

Society for the Autistically Handicapped ◎ ◎ ◎

http://www.autismuk.com

The Society exists to bring an increased awareness of autism and expand patient's exposure to well-established and newly developed approaches in the diagnosis, assessment, education, and treatment of the disease. This site has many links describing autism, its treatment and diagnosis, including updated news on the latest research and treatment. There are large news and fact files, as well as informative links to topics such as sexuality, the culture and treatment of autism, and a list of worldwide conferences, workshops, and seminars relating to autism. There is also access to Europe's largest autism library, a message board, and related links. This site is a very informative resource for professionals and the public.

Society for the Exploration of Psychotherapy Integration (SEPI) ◎ ◎

http://www.cyberpsych.org/sepi.htm

"The primary objectives of SEPI are to encourage communication and to serve as a reference group for individuals interested in exploring the interface between differing approaches to psychotherapy." This site provides information on the society's mission, conference information, a list of influential books, training opportunities in psychotherapy integration, an online article, and links of interest.

Society for the Study of Ingestive Behavior ◎ ◎

http://www.jhu.edu/~ssib/ssib.html

This professional society's site includes links to current news and information on ingestive behavior topics, relevant journals, calendar of events, membership information, employment, access to the newsletter, awards and grants and links to related organizations and other sites. This site is searchable by keyword.

Society of Behavioral Neuroendocrinology ◎ ◎

http://www.sbne.org

This Society targets research professionals in the fields of behavior and neuroendocrinology. The site includes conference information, membership information, society officers, goals and bylaws of the Society, a link to related meetings. Publications resources include access to the official journal of the Society, *Hormones and Behavior*, and related journals, namely the *Journal of Neuroscience and Neuropeptides*.

Stress and Anxiety Research Society (STAR) ◎ ◎

http://star-society.org

This professional multidisciplinary organization of researchers promotes the exchange of information on anxiety and stress. At this site, the society's mission and history is presented, as well as membership information, STAR members, conference information, national and international representatives, and a list of publications from STAR. A list of related organizations, academic departments, journals, databases, employment opportunities, and online newsgroups and mailing lists is also provided.

Tourette's Syndrome Association (TSA), Incorporated ◎ ◎ ◎

http://tsa.mgh.harvard.edu

Described as the only national organization dedicated to providing information on Tourette's syndrome (TS), the Tourette's Syndrome Association's Web site includes links to public service announcements and a chat room. The site contains numerous general facts about TS, as well as scientific links, such as a publications list, research grant awards and TS diagnosis and treatment. Interested persons will find links to national chapters of the association, and international contacts. There are links to order TSA publications, and online access to selected relevant articles.

United States of America Transactional Analysis Association ◎ ◎

http://usataa.org

This organization is a community of professionals utilizing transactional analysis in "organizational, educational, and clinical settings, and for personal growth." A history of the organization, membership details, events notices, and articles are available at the site. Links are provided to transactional analysis associations, online publications, and educational sites.

World Association for Infant Mental Health (WAIMH) ◉ ◉

http://www.msu.edu/user/waimh

WAIMH is an interdisciplinary and international association promoting education and research on all aspects of infant mental health. Included are links to the association's mission statement and membership information, conference listings, and affiliates. Internet resources include training information and online access to the table of contents for *Infant Mental Health Journal*.

World Psychiatric Association (WPA) ◉ ◉ ◉

http://www.wpanet.org

This organization of professional psychiatric societies is devoted to the advancement of psychiatric and mental health education, research, clinical care, and public policy initiatives. Proceedings and conclusions of the most recent general assembly, ethical guidelines related to psychiatric practice, and descriptions of official Association publications are available at the site. Educational activities of the Association are presented at the site, with a calendar of upcoming educational events, information on Continuing Medical Education and general public education, and links to other psychiatry education sites. A list of WPA scientific sections and chairs, a calendar of general meetings, and a description of the organization's structure are also found at the address.

8.2 Research Centers

Directories of Research Centers

Centerwatch: Profiles of Centers Conducting Clinical Research ◉ ◉ ◉

http://www.centerwatch.com/procat17.htm

This site is ordered geographically by state. It provides an in-depth profile of hundreds of clinical institutions and research centers engaged in psychiatric research. The contact information of each center is provided along with an overview, research experience description, information on facilities, staff expertise, and patient demographics.

Centerwatch: Profiles of Industry Providers ◉ ◉ ◉

http://www.centerwatch.com/provider/provlist.htm

Centerwatch has cataloged an extensive listing of preclinical and clinical research, laboratory, monitoring, project management, trial design, patient recruitment, post-marketing services and regulatory services providers in the U.S., organized topically and geographically. For each industry provider, Centerwatch has prepared an in-depth profile listing services, facilities, and contact information.

Laboratories at the National Institute of Mental Health (NIMH), Division of Intramural Research Programs ⊙ ⊙ ⊙

http://intramural.nimh.nih.gov/research

Connections to 28 laboratories/branches may be accessed at the National Institute of Mental Health's Intramural Research site. The research roles of each section and its subdivisions are enumerated as are key division personnel and contact information. Research divisions include the Laboratory of Neurochemistry, the Behavioral Endocrinology Branch, the Laboratory of Brain and Cognition, and the Section on Pharmacology.

Research, Training, and Technical Assistance Centers ⊙ ⊙ ⊙

http://www.mentalhealth.org/publications/allpubs/KEN95-0010/KEN950010.htm

These research, training, and technical assistance centers are supported by the Center for Mental Health Services. Services may include technical assistance, information and referrals, on-site consultation, training, library services, publications, and annotated bibliographies, among other resources. Contact information on individual research centers as well as brief outlines of the information, conferences, and other services they provide are included.

Individual Research Centers

Center for Mental Health Policy and Services Research ⊙ ⊙

http://www.med.upenn.edu/~cmhpsr

A component of the University of Pennsylvania's Health System, this Center provides general overviews of the ongoing and completed research projects in topics including aging, forensics, serious mental illnesses, homeless issues, substance abuse, and prevention. A list of the Center's publications, presentations, and managed care consensus reports, a faculty, staff, fellows, and student directory, as well as fellowship information are included.

Center for Mind-Body Medicine ⊙ ⊙

http://www.healthy.net/othersites/mindbody/index.html

This educational organization promotes the recognition and study of all aspects of health and illness, including mental, emotional, social, and physical. The Center encourages new paragons in care, including education of professionals and students and service-oriented personnel. Current programs include research in mind-body awareness, school wellness, and professional and community education. A variety of workshops, comprehensive conference information, references, staff information, and other links are included.

Center for the Study of Issues in Public Mental Health ◎ ◎

http://www.rfmh.org/csipmh

This Center exists as a collaboration of various New York State mental health organizations and institutes. The Center's mission is to research severely mentally ill adults in a community and multidisciplinary fashion. Projects of the Center include studies that focus on the development, organization, finance, and evaluation of assistance to adults with severe mental illness. Overviews of specific projects are provided, in topics such as homelessness, managed care, drug abuse, recovery, and innovative treatment. Online access to the Center's newsletter, current events, links to faculty and research partner sites, and references to other related publications are included.

Chicago Institute for Psychoanalysis ◎ ◎

http://chianalysis.org

This Web site features information on the Institute's clinic and offers answers to common questions about psychoanalysis. There is also information on the Child and Adolescent Clinic, the Barr-Harris Clinic, and the Fluency Readiness Program. Information on the various educational programs offered at the Institute, conferences, current news, and links to other related Web sites are provided.

Clinical Neuroscience Research Unit ◎ ◎ ◎

http://info.med.yale.edu/psych/cnru

Located within Yale University's School of Medicine, this Research Unit is currently studying and operates clinics in the areas of depression, the neurobiology of cocaine addiction, postpartum depression, mood disorders, menstrual disorders, obsessive-compulsive disorder, and schizophrenia. Links to each of these mental disorders provides information on the services at the clinic, diagnosis and treatment, as well as other basic information. Training opportunities and information, as well as general information about the Center is provided.

Crisis Prevention Institute's
Violence Prevention Resource Center ◎ ◎

http://www.crisisprevention.com

This Center provides training information and other resources in violence and crisis intervention. Intervention techniques and information are provided in the areas of education, healthcare, mental health, security, corrections and police, business, human service and government, and youth services.

Institute for Behavioral Genetics ◎ ◎

http://ibgwww.colorado.edu

Located within the University of Colorado, Boulder, this multidisciplinary Institute focuses on performing research on the genetic and environmental factors that contribute to individual differences in behavior. At this site, lists of publications from the Institute are available, and computer programs written by and courses taught by the faculty are listed. Faculty, staff, scientists, and students home page links are included at the site.

Institute for Behavioral Healthcare ◎ ◎

http://www.ibh.com

This California-based Institute, a division of the Institute for the Advancement of Human Behavior, provides continuing medical and general education to professionals in the mental health fields. The site contains clinical workshop information, and home study courses on various topics such as substance abuse, pain control, and attention-deficit/hyperactivity disorder. Upcoming conference information, and a link to the National Leadership Council, which consists of over 170 behavioral healthcare organizations, are provided.

Institute for Mathematical Behavioral Sciences ◎ ◎

http://aris.ss.uci.edu/mbs

Located at University of California, Irvine, the Institute's mission is to facilitate communication between scientists interested in creating and testing human behavior theories. There is a comprehensive faculty list, information on the doctoral program and students, online access to technical report abstracts, and information on the upcoming workshop. A list of related university sites is also available.

Institute for Psychological Study of the Arts ◎ ◎

http://www.clas.ufl.edu/ipsa/intro.htm

This University of Florida Institute site provides links to seminars, in topics such as psychoanalytic psychology and criticism, a staff list and brief summaries of their interests, online abstracts and bibliography of the Institute, and a link to the *Journal for the Psychological Study of the Arts*. The site also offers links to relevant sites and other associations, as well as conference information.

Institute of Psychiatry and the
Department of Psychiatry and Behavioral Sciences ◎ ◎ ◎

http://www.musc.edu/psychiatry

Located within the Medical University of South Carolina in Charleston, this Institute provides psychiatric and drug abuse treatment, rehabilitation, and prevention assistance. Clinical psychiatric services include adult, general, and special services, such as eating disorders, crime victims research and treatment, family bonding, and geropsychiatry programs. In addition, there are programs designed for youth, such as the Tic and Tourette's Program, eating disorders treatment, and the adolescent dual diagnosis program. Alcohol and drug rehabilitation programs are also offered. Research program information is available at the site in topics including Alzheimer's research, anxiety, drug and alcohol abuse, clinical psychopharmacology, and more. A referral service as well as other general information about the Institute are also available.

Los Angeles Institute and Society for Psychoanalytic Studies ◎ ◎
http://home.earthlink.net/~laisps

The Los Angeles Institute and Society for Psychoanalytic Studies is a division of the Society of the International Psychoanalytical Association. At this site, the latest publications of the Institute are available in full, as well as a bibliography of publications by the Institute's members. Seminar and workshop information, as well as extension courses and training program details are present.

Louis de la Parte Florida Mental Health Institute ◎ ◎ ◎
http://www.fmhi.usf.edu

A component of the University of South Florida, this Institute is described as the primary research and training center for mental health services in Florida. Current research focuses on various issues regarding aging and mental health, such as cognitive aging, and mental health needs of senior citizens. In addition, there is a link to research that examines the mental health of children and families, such as autistic children, special risk children, and families with children that have serious emotional disturbances. There are also projects that focus on the law and mental health, including criminal competence assessment, child abuse, substance abuse in prisons, and drug court programs. A comprehensive list of publications by the faculty at the center is available in abstract and full text form. Information on educational opportunities and upcoming events are also present at this site.

Mental Health Research & Training Agencies ◎ ◎ ◎
http://www.mentalhealth.org/publications/allpubs/KEN95-0010/KEN950010.htm

Twenty separate government agencies focused on mental health research, training, and technical assistance are profiled at this useful site established by the Center for Mental Health Services, a federal agency. The agencies cover children's mental health, family support, psychiatric disabilities, psychiatric rehabilitation, empowerment, consumer self-help, homelessness, government planning, transitional assistance, networking in the field of mental health, and technical assistance in many forms.

Nathan Kline Institute for Psychiatric Research ⊙ ⊙ ⊙

http://www.rfmh.org/nki

This Institute, a constituent of New York State's Office of Mental Health, is described as one of the nation's foremost centers of excellence in mental health research. Each link to a research topic provides an overview of the topic, ongoing studies, collaborators, achievements, and a publications list. Research topics include Alzheimer's disease, analytical psychopharmacology, basic neuroimaging, cellular and molecular neurobiology, clinical neuroimaging, issues in public mental health, cognitive neuroscience and schizophrenia, co-occurring disorders, dementia, movement disorders, homelessness research, addiction and dual diagnosis, neurobehavioral and genetics, neurochemistry and neurobiology, quantitative EEG, violence and the mentally ill, and others. A description of the Institute's facilities, a faculty list, upcoming events, and other related links are provided.

National Center for Stuttering ⊙ ⊙

http://www.stuttering.com

This Center performs research studies in many different aspects of stuttering. The mission of the Center is to provide facts about stuttering, offer a hotline, conduct research, provide treatment, and supply continuing education for professionals. An overview of the research findings, as well as the treatment programs, and a summary of the Center's model of stuttering are provided.

National Technical Assistance
Center for State Mental Health Planning ⊙ ⊙ ⊙

http://www.nasmhpd.org/ntac

This Center provides technical aid and training to professionals. The site provides information on its meetings, research, and publications. Users can search for information on specific projects by topic or state. There are over 30 topics, from advocacy and support, to telecommunications technology. Selected project highlights, a comprehensive resource list, links to state assistance centers, current events, and online access to the Center's publications are all available at this comprehensive site.

New York Psychiatric Institute ⊙ ⊙ ⊙

http://www.nyspi.cpmc.columbia.edu

Described as the nation's first psychiatric research institute, over 300 psychiatry-related studies are currently performed at this center. Links to research areas provide professionals with a comprehensive project background and summaries, as well as extensive information about the involved faculty and departments. Research areas include psychiatric genetics, neuroscience, depression evaluation, clinical pharmacology, anxiety disorders (such as phobias and panic disorder), developmental psychobiology (such as maternal deprivation), molecular neurobiology, child psychiatry, epidemiology, and mental illness in children. Links are offered to details of current treatment programs for a variety of psychiatric disorders. Information on education and training opportunities is available, as well as details of clinical services.

Perceptual Science Laboratory ◎ ◎

http://mambo.ucsc.edu

Part of the University of California, Santa Cruz, this Laboratory performs research in the areas of perception and cognition. A major focus of research is on speech perception by ear and eye, as well as facial animation, and professionals and other interested individuals can access research news and updates on this research. Links to the faculty home pages, a publications list, and downloadable demonstrations of current research are provided. There are numerous links to related sites, in topics such as facial animation and analysis, speech reading, and computer graphics.

Psychoanalytic Institute of New England, East ◎

http://www.analysis.com/pine

The mission of this Institute is to study psychoanalysis and its evolution over time, especially in reference to current theory and treatment. Educational information, current programs and seminars, and a list of faculty are provided at the site.

San Francisco Psychoanalytic Institute and Society ◎ ◎

http://www.sfpi.org

This nonprofit Institute provides educational and training services for professionals, conducts seminars for consumers and professionals, and provides psychoanalytic services for the public. Included are links to introductory information on psychoanalysis, an events calendar, clinic information, and a referral service, as well as links to child development programs, such a child psychotherapy and divorcing parents support groups.

University of California, Los Angeles Center for Research of Treatment and Rehabilitation of Psychosis ◎ ◎

http://www.npi.ucla.edu/irc

This research center conducts experiments, and provides consulting and technical support to other professionals interested in severe psychiatric illnesses, like schizophrenia. Research activities and laboratories at the Center study topics including cognition, psychophysiology and neuropsychology, diagnostic and psychopathology assessment, psychopharmacology, and psychosocial assessment and treatment. Detailed overviews of these programs, summaries of important findings of the Center, and a faculty directory are offered at the site.

University of Southern Mississippi
Psychophysiology Research Laboratory ○ ○ ○
http://ocean.st.usm.edu/~gejones/psyphylab.html

This Laboratory performs research in the area of human psychophysiology, with primary emphasis on visceral perception and related topics. Site resources include complete texts of conference presentations, overviews of current research projects, recent and upcoming publications lists, and abstracts and presentations. A reference list for visceral perception articles and links to other related sites are included at the site.

8.3 Selected Hospital Psychiatry Departments

Barnes-Jewish Hospital, Washington University Medical Center ○ ○ ○
http://www.bjc.org

The site provides a general overview of facilities available, hospital statistics, support groups, events, contact information, and specific hospital services and programs.

Research	A wide range of techniques were pioneered at the Hospital, including the first double-lung transplant and the first laparoscopic nephrectomy. Specialized techniques include multiple organ transplantation, in-vitro fertilization, osteoporosis treatment, lung volume reduction surgery, minimally invasive surgery, diabetes treatment, eye treatment, cancer treatment, and cardiology. Services related to psychiatry include research and care for sleep disorders and Alzheimer's disease, electroconvulsive therapy, and a full range of behavioral health services, including a crisis response center and individual, group, and family therapy.
Patient Resources	Lodging suggestions, general information about St. Louis, physician referral service, and health risk appraisal will be of interest to patients.
Location	St. Louis, Missouri

C. F. Menninger Memorial Hospital ○ ○ ○
http://www.menninger.edu

Detailed information about the types of services offered for children and adults with learning disorders are provided. Guidelines are listed for parents to help determine if their child suffers from a learning disorder. Information about the Institute's Summer Teacher Training program, and development and educational services offered to public and private schools, clinics, professional organizations and families is also given.

Research	Research carried out at the Child and Family Center include delineating patterns of psychological and behavioral disturbance in

infants, designing interventions to foster the bonding of fathers to their newborn infants, designing interventions with parents of disturbed infants to ameliorate the infant's disturbance, studying the relation between attachment patterns and conduct disorder in children and studying the early childhood factors that contribute resilience and risk for disturbance in adolescence and early adulthood. The Menninger Center for Clinical Research conducts clinical trials involving the comprehensive testing of the efficacy and safety of investigational drugs. Such studies have been carried out in Alzheimer's disease, anxiety disorders, child and adolescent mental disorders, duodenal ulcer, hypertension, mood disorders, migraine headaches, menstrual problems, obesity, pediatric headaches, schizophrenia, and related psychotic disorders.

Patient Resources   The site contains referral information and a comprehensive list of psychiatric services offered to adults, children and adolescents, as well as corporations. The various programs of the hospital that have been described in detail are the Child and Family Center, Center for Learning Disabilities, Institute for Psychoanalysis, continuing education, Center for Clinical Research, and training programs for mental health professionals. General information about the hospital including history, location, governance and staff, mission statement, clinical staff, employment opportunities and benefits, news releases, telephone directory, library, bookstore, and subscription information for the hospital's bulletin are provided.

Location   Topeka, Kansas

Children's Hospital, Boston ⊙ ⊙ ⊙

http://www.childrenshospital.org

Children's Hospital, Boston is the pediatric teaching hospital of Harvard Medical School. Patient care services, research activities, training opportunities, contact information, employment opportunities, community services, department Web sites, and directions for visitors are offered at this site. Users can find specific information with a site search engine.

Research   Research news, administration, and facilities information, and links to departments and laboratories are offered for details of current research. Research and services of psychiatric interest in Neurology are offered through the Behavioral Neurology Program, the Mental Retardation Research Center, and the Division of Clinical Neurophysiology and Epilepsy. The Department of Psychiatry integrates cognitive, behavioral, psychoeducational, psychodynamic, family, group, developmental, and biological methods in the treatment of disorders and preventative interventions. The Division of Psychology provides patient evaluation, education, psychodiagnostic testing, and therapy.

Patient Resources   The site provides detailed informational resources from each division, department, and program, inpatient hospital visit details, explanations of a patient's healthcare team at the hospital, hospital resources, international patient services, and associated specialty and primary care locations.

Location   Boston, Massachusetts

Duke University Medical Center
Department of Psychiatry and Behavioral Sciences ◎ ◎
http://niles.mc.duke.edu

Research   Current areas of research include behavioral medicine, biological psychiatry, child and adolescent psychiatry, medical psychology, geriatric psychiatry, community psychiatry, and personality disorders.

Patient Resources   Detailed information is presented about the department's administrative structure and Grand Rounds conferences. Links are provided for psychiatrically oriented institutions, online journals, newsgroups, and other Internet resources. Information about continuing medical education and educational programs for physicians, medical residents, and psychologists is presented. Several clinical programs and their descriptions and an alphabetical listing of research activities is presented.

Location   Durham, North Carolina

Johns Hopkins Hospital
Department of Psychiatry and Behavioral Sciences ◎ ◎ ◎
http://www.med.jhu.edu/jhhpsychiatry/master1.htm

Information on depressive disorder and bipolar disorder is well presented. Research reports, books and video information, support group information, and links to other organizations are provided. Book reviews are also available at this site.

Research   Obsessive-compulsive disorders, child and adolescent psychiatry, neuropsychiatry and memory, genetics of schizophrenia, and psychiatric neuroimaging are the main foci of investigation. Specific psychiatric disorders being studied in the child and adolescent psychiatry division include attention-deficit/hyperactivity disorder, anxiety disorders, major depression and bipolar disorder, autism, developmental disorders, and fragile X-linked mental retardation. The neuropsychiatry group's investigation mainly involves the study and treatment of Alzheimer's disease and its related illnesses. The epidemiology and genetics program is involved in the identification of schizophrenia susceptibility genes.

Patient Resources — Information is provided about the hospitals clinical services, fellowships and training programs, educational programs, faculty, research programs, patient resources, and directions and parking at the hospital. Links to other Johns Hopkins Web sites are also provided.

Location — Baltimore, Maryland

Massachusetts General Hospital ○ ○

http://www.mgh.harvard.edu/depts/allpsych/HomePage.html

Information is available for participation in several research programs in the areas of women's mental health and depression. Several links to depression resource centers are provided.

Research — Studies are being conducted in the areas of clinical pharmacology and psychotherapy, drug abuse behavioral pharmacology, neuroimaging, substance abuse epidemiology, bipolar mood disorders, alcohol and drug dependence, eating disorders, gerontology, HIV infection, pediatric psychopharmacology, psychiatric oncology and trauma, neurobiology, and schizophrenia. Research studies carried out at the Center for Women's Mental Health include identification of effective treatments for women suffering from premenstrual dysphoric disorder, postpartum psychiatric illness, and menopause-associated depression.

Patient Resources — The site provides extensive information about the various departments in the psychiatry division of the Massachusetts General Hospital. These departments include Analytic Psychotherapy, Center for Women's Mental Health, a child and adolescent psychiatry residency training program, a depression clinical and research program, an obsessive-compulsive disorders clinic and institute, pediatric psychopharmacology, psychotic disorders, telepsychiatry, and a law and psychiatry service. Information about psychiatry fellowships and psychiatry residency training programs is also provided. A physician location service is also featured at this site.

Location — Boston, Massachusetts

Mayo Clinic ○ ○

http://www.mayo.edu/mcr

This site provides details of services offered at the Clinic, including care by specialty, educational programs, and typical procedures for patient testing and treatment. The site also presents general information on lodging, directions, and amenities available to patients and visitors.

Research   All major areas of medicine are investigated at the Clinic, including research in Psychiatry and Psychology, but information on this program is not provided at the site.

Patient Resources   Detailed descriptions of services offered to patients and families during treatment are found at the site.

Location   Rochester, Minnesota

McLean Hospital ◎ ◎ ◎

http://www.mcleanhospital.org

Information about participation in research studies of Alzheimer's, attention deficit hyperactivity disorders, depression and other psychiatric disorders is provided for patients and their families.

Research   The McLean Hospital's research program in neuroscience and psychiatry is the largest of private psychiatric hospitals in the United States. Research is being carried out in drug and alcohol abuse, bipolar and psychotic disorders, schizophrenia-related changes in brain microcircuitry, psychotic depression, treatment of adult survivors of childhood trauma, degenerative diseases of the nervous system including Alzheimer's, Parkinson's, and Huntington's diseases. Research at the brain-imaging center involves the monitoring of changes in brain chemistry to document the course of illness or the effects of medication. The Brain Bank at McLean collects and distributes human brain tissue for research.

Patient Resources   The McLean Hospital is a teaching facility of the Harvard Medical School and an affiliate of the Massachusetts General Hospital. The site contains detailed information about the hospital's clinical programs, research, educational and professional training programs, and library resources and services. Extensive links to other psychiatric organizations, institutes, information centers, and libraries are also provided. Employment opportunities at the hospital are listed.

Location   Belmont, Massachusetts

Mount Sinai Medical Center Department of Psychiatry ◎ ◎

http://www.mssm.edu/psychiatry/home-page.html

Research   Extensive research is being conducted in Alzheimer's disease, autism, mood and personality disorders, post-traumatic stress disorders, schizophrenia, anxiety disorders, molecular neurobiology and neurogenetics, neuroinflammation, molecular neuropsychiatry, psychopharmacology, neuropathology, neurochemistry, neuroscience positron emission tomography, and neuroanatomy and morphometrics.

Patient Resources   This page offers information about the various research programs and laboratories in psychiatry and clinical programs and services available for patients including emergency services, electro-convulsive therapy, and psychological and neurological testing. Training information for psychiatric residents is also presented in detail.

Location   New York, New York

New York Presbyterian Hospital Columbia University Campus ⊙ ⊙ ⊙

http://cpmcnet.cpmc.columbia.edu/dept/pi/psych.html

Important links to several psychiatric organizations and hospitals are provided at this site for patient perusal.

Research   More than 300 biological, behavioral and social research studies are being conducted at the psychiatric institute. Studies in neuroscience, depression evaluation, clinical psychopharmacology, bulimia, anxiety disorders, developmental psychobiology, molecular neurobiology, and child psychiatry are currently in the forefront of research at the psychiatric institute.

Patient Resources   This Web page contains a profile of the Psychiatry Department, its administrative structure, list of faculty members, and description of clinical, research, and affiliated centers training programs. Departmental components including the Presbyterian Hospital psychiatric services, departmental clinical services, and the New York State Psychiatric Institute are described in detail. Links to the Columbia University home page and affiliated institutions, namely, the Harlem Hospital Center, the Creedmoor Psychiatric Center, and St. Luke's Roosevelt Hospital are provided. Links can also be found to other psychiatry departments in the U.S., and psychiatric associations, institutes, and agencies. In addition, a long list of psychiatric references including journals, Internet resources, and the National Library of Medicine may be accessed.

Location   New York, New York

UCLA Neuropsychiatric Hospital ⊙ ⊙

http://www.npi.ucla.edu

Two online resource directories are available: 1) The California Developmental Disabilities Netlink provides information about services and programs for children and adults with developmental disabilities 2) The Women with Developmental Disabilities link provides several informative resources on housing, health and wellness, books, and links to related Web sites for women.

Research   Studies are aimed at understanding the biological mechanisms of and treatment of anxiety disorders. Specific projects in the child and adolescent anxiety program focus on selective mutism, Tourette's disorder, and other Tic disorders. Severe mental illnesses such as schizophrenia are under investigation at the UCLA Center for Research on Treatment and Rehabilitation of Psychosis. Other research areas include mental retardation and managed care for psychiatric disorders.

Patient Resources   This Web site offers information about the various psychiatric departments and their programs, the Women's Life Center, which offers mental health treatment during pregnancy, menopause, etc., and presents a guide to literature on qualitative research methods and qualitative and quantitative research integration methods. Links are provided to other UCLA departments and UCLA related Web sites as well as other neuropsychiatric and healthcare related Web sites.

Location   Los Angeles, California

UCSF Stanford Health Care ◎ ◎
http://www-med.stanford.edu

This site offers general health information for patients and the public, links to associated hospitals and clinics, and specific information on services offered at the general and children's hospitals.

Research   Continuing Medical Education information, and clinical highlights are available at the site. Specialty services in Psychiatry and Behavioral Sciences are offered through the Aging Clinical Research Center, Bipolar Disorders Clinic, Center for Narcolepsy, Child and Adolescent Psychiatry Program, Eating Disorders Research Studies, Psychosocial Treatment Laboratory, and the Stanford/VA Alzheimer's Center.

Patient Resources   Health and medical news, health tips, and clinical highlights are available for patients. Overviews of medical services available for adults and children, international patient resources, and referral resources are also found at the site.

Location   Stanford, California

University of California San Francisco
Medical Center Langley Porter Psychiatric Institute ◎ ◎
http://itsa.ucsf.edu/~lppi

Research   Studies are focused on innovative treatments for substance abuse, and the pharmacology, physiology, and psychology of commonly abused drugs in humans.

Patient Resources   This site provides extensive information about the hospital's clinical services, training programs, research divisions, and links to affiliated sites. Insurance and intake and referral information is provided.

Location   San Francisco, California

University of Chicago Hospitals & Health System ⊙ ⊙ ⊙

http://www.uchospitals.edu/index_js.html

The site provides an introduction and history of the Health System, location and directions, patient checklist, news releases, events, community outreach programs, resources for physicians, employment opportunities, links to departments and specialties, online video presentations, and contact information.

Research   The Department of Psychiatry offers assessment and treatment programs for disorders of mood, emotion, cognition, perception, memory, intellect, and behavior. A full range of child and adolescent psychiatry services is also provided at the System's facilities. News releases, online hospital publications, and contact details are available for additional research information.

Patient Resources   A section of the site is devoted to patients, and provides suggestions for appointment preparations, directions to the hospitals, resources available during a visit, and additional issues to consider before an appointment.

Location   Chicago, Illinois

University of Michigan Medical Center Department of Psychiatry ⊙ ⊙

http://www.med.umich.edu/psych

Information is presented on electroconvulsive therapy and women's health and anxiety issues. The *Schizophrenia Consultant*, a quarterly newsletter of the schizophrenia program containing information for patients, families, and providers is also accessible.

Research   Under research scrutiny in the ambulatory and hospital services division are areas such as evolutionary biology, unconscious processes, women's health, mood disorders, schizophrenia, Cushing's disease, and adrenergic psychoneuroendocrinology. Basic science research includes regulation of signal transduction in the nervous system, noninvasive studies in the human brain using positron emission tomography, biochemical correlates of regeneration, molecular and integrative studies of stress, opioids and dopaminergic systems, mapping of genes that cause neurological and psychiatric disorders, regulation of inositol lipid hydrolysis and calcium signaling in human neurotumor cells, neurochemical imaging, etc.

Patient Resources   This site provides information concerning research and links to information on postdoctoral, residency, and fellowship training in the

Department of Psychiatry. Links are also provided to helpful Web resources.

Location   Ann Arbor, Michigan

University of Missouri Health Sciences Center ◎ ◎

http://www.hsc.missouri.edu

General information about the Center and its recent acquisition of Columbia Regional Hospital, clinic information and locations, a physician directory, links to specific hospital information, patient care details, research information, and information on education programs are available at this site.

Research   The Missouri Institute of Mental Health in St. Louis is associated with the Center, offering the Policy Information Exchange online (at pie.org), a source of materials on issues affecting mental health policy in North America. Links to additional research information are available at the site, offering details of research facilities, current clinical trials, grants information, and other resources.

Patient Resources   Patients can access information on clinical programs and services at the Health Sciences Center through an alphabetical listing of topics. General facts about the Center, maps, and contact details are also provided.

Location   Columbia, Missouri

University of Pennsylvania Health System (UPHS) ◎ ◎ ◎

http://www.med.upenn.edu/health/vi_files/vi_hup/vi_hup.html

Resources at this site include visitor information, news, a description of medical services offered, a site search engine, a physician referral service, an events calendar, and basic health information.

Research   Research and services are offered by UPHS in addiction, geriatrics, mood and anxiety disorders, bipolar disorders, depression, neuropsychiatry, schizophrenia, sleep disorders, and weight and eating disorders. Specialty research and treatments are provided through the Center for Cognitive Therapy, the Center for Psychotherapy Research, the Child, Adolescent and Young Adult Psychiatry Program, Forensic Psychiatry, and the Brain and Behavior Program.

Patient Resources   Health topics are presented at the site, including discussions in preventative medicine, general health information, and managing chronic conditions. Other information useful to patients includes a physician referral service, educational seminars and support groups details, and a list of health insurance plans accepted at the facility.

Location   Philadelphia, Pennsylvania

University of Pittsburgh
Medical Center Western Psychiatry Institute and Clinic ◉ ◉

http://www.wpic.pitt.edu

Information is presented for those interested in rendering volunteer service in the field of mental health care, research, and elementary education.

Research	Work is being done in the areas of bipolar disorder, child and adolescent depression and anxiety, eating disorders, schizophrenia, alcohol research, and autism.
Patient Resources	This site features information about education and training opportunities at the Medical Center, programs for mental health providers, a faculty directory, and information about educational conferences and upcoming events. Extensive information about the clinical programs including those in child psychiatry and development, adult mood and anxiety disorders, schizophrenia, geriatrics, and eating disorders. Several important Internet links to libraries, journals, government organizations, and the University of Pittsburgh are also provided.
Location	Pittsburgh, Pennsylvania

University of Washington Medical Center
Department of Psychiatry and Behavioral Sciences ◉ ◉

http://depts.washington.edu/psychweb/index.html

Research	The Department has nationally recognized research programs in neurosciences, molecular biology, molecular genetics, endocrinology, neuroimaging, physiological psychology, as well as in psychosocial and socio-cultural areas, epidemiology, and health services.
Patient Resources	Information is available about the department's academic, clinical and research programs, and its faculty, lectures, and grand rounds.
Location	Seattle, Washington

Yale/New Haven Hospital Department of Psychiatry ◉

http://info.med.yale.edu/yfp/ref_new/psyc.html

Contact and referral information for various psychiatric services is offered.

Research	The Alzheimer's research unit conducts clinical trials for investigational treatments for Alzheimer's disease and age-related cognitive impairment. Clinical studies in the neuroscience research unit are designed to determine the neurobiological mechanisms underlying depressive, bipolar, obsessive-compulsive, and pervasive developmental disorders. Research on trauma and anxiety disorders is also under investigation.

Patient Resources   This Web page offers information about the various psychiatric services available for patients in the Adolescent, Adult, and Geriatric Psychiatry program, Substance Abuse Program, and the Psychiatry/Medical Comorbidity Program. Contact information for specialists within each of the programs is listed.

Location   New Haven, Connecticut

8.4 **Selected Medical School Psychiatry Departments**

Baylor College Department of Psychiatry and Behavioral Science
http://www.bcm.tmc.edu/psych

Boston Graduate School of Psychoanalysis School of Psychoanalysis
http://www.bgsp.edu

Boston University Department of Psychiatry
http://www.bumc.bu.edu/Departments/HomeMain.asp?DepartmentID=68

Columbia University Department of Psychiatry and Neurology
http://cpmcnet.columbia.edu/dept/pi/psych.html

Cornell University Department of Psychiatry
http://www.nycornell.org/psychiatry

Dartmouth Medical School Department of Psychiatry
http://www.dartmouth.edu/dms/academics.html

Duke University Department of Psychiatry
http://psychiatry.mc.duke.edu

Emory University Department of Psychiatry and Behavioral Sciences
http://www.emory.edu/WHSC/MED/PSYCHIATRY/home.htm

Florida Mental Health Institute Department of Community Mental Health
http://www.fmhi.usf.edu/cmh/statement.html

Georgetown University Department of Psychiatry
http://www.dml.georgetown.edu/schmed/depts/psychiatry.html

Harvard University Department of Psychiatry
http://www.hmcnet.harvard.edu/psych/index.html

Indiana University School of Medicine Department of Psychiatry
http://www.iupui.edu/~psych

Johns Hopkins University Department of Psychiatry and Behavioral Sciences
http://www.med.jhu.edu/jhhpsychiatry/master1.htm

Medical College of Ohio Department of Psychiatry
http://www.mco.edu/depts/psych

Medical College of Virginia Department of Psychiatry
http://views.vcu.edu/views/psych

Medical College of Wisconsin Department of Psychiatry and Behavioral Medicine
http://www.mcw.edu/psych

Michigan State University Department of Psychiatry
http://www.com.msu.edu/dept/departments.html#anchor1751341

Mount Sinai School of Medicine Department of Psychiatry
http://www.mssm.edu/psychiatry/home-page.html

New York University Department of Psychiatry
http://www.med.nyu.edu/Psych/NYUPsych.Homepage.html

Northwestern University Medical School
Department of Psychiatry and Behavioral Sciences
http://www.nums.nwu.edu/psychiatry

Southern Illinois University Department of Psychiatry
http://www.siumed.edu/psych

Stanford University Department of Psychiatry and Behavioral Sciences
http://www.stanford.edu/dept/PBS

Texas A&M University Department of Psychiatry and Behavioral Science
http://www.sw.org/depts/psych/dept.htm

Tufts University/ New England Medical Center Department of Psychiatry
http://www.tufts.edu/med/dept/clinical/psych.html

Tulane University Department of Psychiatry and Neurology
http://www.mcl.tulane.edu/departments/psych_neuro/psnra01.htm

University of Alabama, Birmingham Department of Psychiatry
http://www.uab.edu/psychiatry

University of California, Davis Department of Psychiatry
http://neuroscience.ucdavis.edu/psychiatry

University of California, Los Angeles
Department of Psychiatry and Biobehavioral Sciences
http://www.MentalHealth.ucla.edu/psychiatry

University of California, San Francisco Department of Psychiatry
http://itsa.ucsf.edu/~lppi

University of Chicago Department of Psychiatry
http://psychiatry.uchicago.edu

University of Cincinnati Department of Psychiatry
http://psychiatry.uc.edu

University of Colorado Department of Psychiatry
http://www.uchsc.edu/sm/psych/dept/index.htm

University of Connecticut Department of Psychiatry
http://marvin.uchc.edu

University of Florida Department of Psychiatry
http://www.med.ufl.edu/psych

University of Iowa Department of Psychiatry
http://www.uihc.uiowa.edu/pubinfo/psych1.htm

University of Louisville Department of Psychiatry and Behavioral Sciences
http://www.louisville.edu/medschool/psychiatry

University of Massachusetts—Worcester Department of Psychiatry
http://www.ummed.edu/dept/Psychiatry/index.html

University of Miami Department of Psychiatry & Behavioral Sciences
http://www.med.miami.edu/psychiatry/main.html

University of Michigan Department of Psychiatry
http://www.med.umich.edu/psych

University of Minnesota-Twin Cities Department of Psychiatry
http://www.med.umn.edu/psychiatry

University of North Carolina Department of Psychiatry
http://www.med.unc.edu

University of Pennsylvania Department of Psychiatry
http://www.med.upenn.edu/psych

University of Pittsburgh Department of Psychiatry
http://www.wpic.pitt.edu

University of Rochester Department of Psychiatry
http://www.urmc.rochester.edu/smd/Psych

University of South Florida Department of Psychiatry and Behavioral Medicine
http://www.med.usf.edu/PSYCH/psychome.html

University of Southern California Department of Psychiatry and Behavioral Sciences
http://www.usc.edu/schools/medicine

University of Texas, Galveston Department of Psychiatry and Behavioral Sciences
http://psychiatry.utmb.edu

University of Texas, Southwestern Department of Psychiatry
http://www.swmed.edu/home_pages/psych/Index.html

University of Utah Department of Psychiatry
http://www.med.utah.edu/psychiatry

University of Virginia Department of Psychiatric Medicine
http://www.med.virginia.edu/medicine/clinical/psychiatric/home.html

University of Washington Department of Psychiatry and Behavioral Sciences
http://depts.washington.edu/psychweb/index.html

University of Wisconsin, Madison Department of Psychiatry
http://www.psychiatry.wisc.edu

Virginia Commonwealth University Department of Psychiatry
http://griffin.vcu.edu/views/psych

Wake Forest University Department of Psychiatry and Behavioral Medicine
http://www.wfubmc.edu/psychiatry

Washington University Department of Psychiatry
http://www.psychiatry.wustl.edu

Wayne State University Department of Psychiatry and Behavioral Neurosciences
http://psychiatry1.med.wayne.edu

Yale University Department of Psychiatry
http://info.med.yale.edu/psych/

Yeshiva University (Albert Einstein)
Department of Psychiatry and Behavioral Sciences
http://quark.aecom.yu.edu/psychlab

9. PSYCHIATRIC DISORDERS

9.1 Adjustment Disorders

Adjustment Disorder With Anxiety ◎ ◎
http://www.healthinformatics.com/docs/english/BHA/adjdsanx.bha.asp

HealthInformatics.com offers this on-line information sheet regarding adjustment disorder with anxiety, as well as its etiology, symptoms, and diagnostic criteria. Spontaneous resolution of symptoms is explained, as well as several useful relaxation strategies.

Adjustment Disorder With Depressed Mood ◎ ◎
http://www.healthinformatics.com/docs/english/BHA/adjdsdep.bha.asp

This online information sheet on adjustment disorder with depressed mood provides information on its etiology, symptoms, and treatment. Symptoms occurring in reaction to life stressors are explained, and the feelings of sadness and hopelessness specific to this adjustment disorder are reviewed. Differentiation of this condition from major clinical depression is made, and a link to the more serious symptoms of the latter are found.

Adjustment Disorders in Childhood and Adolescence ◎ ◎ ◎
http://www.mentalhealth.com/fr20.html

This article first appeared in *The Harvard Mental Health Letter*. Fundamental information on the description of adjustment disorder, symptoms, related disorders, assessment issues, prevalence, therapeutic practices, and reference materials are available at this informative site.

Health Center.com: Adjustment Disorder ◎
http://jp1.health-center.com/db/TopicReq?SessionID=1918&TopicID=50&Action=view

Explanation of the disorder, details of predisposing factors, and treatment options are briefly and concisely explored at this Web site.

Help for Families: Stress-Related Problems ◎
http://www.helpforfamilies.com/stress1.htm

Help for Families is an interactive parenting guide developed by a clinical psychologist. Topics of discussion include family communication, discipline, and school problems. This address offers descriptions of adjustment and anxiety disorders in children. Therapy and parental communication suggestions are available to help alleviate these problems, and parents can follow links discussing specific communication strategies.

PSYweb.com: Adjustment Disorders ⊙

http://www.psyweb.com/Mdisord/adjd.html

Adjustment disorders are discussed at this site, including a definition, diagnostic criteria (DSM-IV), and common specifiers and subtypes. Links to descriptions of different schools of psychotherapy are available.

What Are Adjustment Disorders? ⊙ ⊙

http://site.health-center.com/brain/adjust/

The many different categories of adjustment disorders are reviewed at an online table, courtesy of Health-Center.com. Adjustment disorder with depressed mood, anxiety, mixed anxiety and depressed mood, disturbance of conduct, mixed disturbance of emotions and conduct, and unspecified disturbances are differentiated.

9.2 Anxiety Disorders

General Resources

About.com: Panic/Anxiety Disorders ⊙ ⊙

http://panicdisorder.about.com/health/panicdisorder

Many quality sites are found through links at this site, including professional organizations, personal home pages, and patient education resources. Sites are organized by topics, which include agoraphobia, fear of flying, generalized anxiety disorder, obsessive-compulsive disorder, panic disorder, posttraumatic stress disorder, social phobia, specific phobias, medications, anger management, breathing exercises, relaxation, self-help and maintenance, stress management, cognitive-behavioral therapy, general therapy issues, therapist directories, international resources, information for women, youth anxiety, personal stories and Web sites, and general Web sites. Feature articles and news items, support forums, online stores, subscription information for an online newsletter, and answers to frequently asked questions (FAQs) are also available at the site.

Anxiety.com ⊙ ⊙

http://anxieties.com/home.htm

Created primarily for consumers, this site offers general summaries of the more common anxiety conditions, such as fear of flying, generalized anxiety disorders, social phobias, panic attacks, and more. In addition, there is a fact sheet on anxiety medication, self-help books, a personal assessment link, and information about online consultation. This Web site is also keyword searchable and provides instructions and a fee schedule for online consultations.

Anxiety Disorders Association of America (ADAA) ◎ ◎ ◎

http://www.adaa.org

The Anxiety Disorders Association of America, comprised of health professionals, researchers and others interested in these disorders, "promotes the prevention and cure of anxiety disorders." The site offers ordering information for patients suffering from anxiety disorders, including self-help publications, participation information for research studies, membership details, conference information, an online bookstore, news, and speech transcripts. Fact sheets are available, with titles including Consumers Guide to Treatment, Social Phobia, Social Anxiety Disorder Information, Generalized Anxiety Disorder (GAD), Specific Phobias, Obsessive-Compulsive Disorder, Posttraumatic Stress Disorder (PTSD), Panic Disorder and Agoraphobia, Anxiety Disorders and Medication, Anxiety Disorders in Children and Adolescents, Anxiety Disorders: Helping a Family Member, and A Journey to Recovery from Anxiety Disorders. Consumers can also find resources related to support groups and links to related sites.

Anxiety Disorders Education Program ◎ ◎ ◎

http://www.nimh.nih.gov/anxiety/anxiety/whatis/objectiv.htm

As a service of the National Institute of Mental Health (NIMH), the site of the Anxiety Disorders Education Program provides information on its national campaign to increase awareness among the public and health care professionals regarding anxiety disorders. Links to disorder information including panic disorder, phobias, and posttraumatic stress disorder (PTSD), pertinent news, and the Anxiety Disorders Education Program Library are all readily accessible. A professional section supplies a list of scientific books, articles, and educational videotapes, a list of professional meetings, and ordering information for patient brochures.

Anxiety Disorders in Children and Adolescents ◎ ◎

http://www.adaa.org/4_info/4i_child/4i_01.htm

Short descriptions of generalized anxiety disorder, obsessive-compulsive disorder, panic disorder, posttraumatic stress disorder, separation anxiety disorder, social phobia, and specific phobia in children and adolescents are presented at this site. Visitors can also find information on the treatment of anxiety disorders at the site.

Anxiety Disorders Report ◎ ◎

http://www.hoptechno.com/anxiety.htm

This online report was written primarily for consumers and provides general information about anxiety, panic, phobic, obsessive-compulsive, and posttraumatic stress disorders. Included are descriptions of symptoms, consequences of the disorder, personal descriptions of the disorder, treatment and information about support groups. This report is provided by the National Institute of Mental Health (NIMH).

Anxiety Network International ◎ ◎ ◎

http://www.anxietynetwork.com

The Anxiety Network home page provides information, support, and therapy for the three largest anxiety disorders: social anxiety, panic/agoraphobia, and generalized anxiety disorder. Over 100 individual articles and the Anxiety Network bookstore provide a broad base of information, with some individual publication ratings provided. The Social Anxiety Mailing List along with recovery programs, anxiety help links, and multimedia materials are available.

Anxiety Panic Internet Resource (tAPir) ◎ ◎ ◎

http://www.algy.com/anxiety/index.shtml

The Anxiety Panic Internet Resource (tAPir) is a self-help network dedicated to the overcoming and cure of debilitating anxiety. Support, information, and the tools of self-empowerment and recovery are available from the Web's first and still premier grassroots anxiety resource. Information about tAPir, treatment information, and an online discussion group are available. Here you will also find one of the Web's largest indexes of anxiety resource links.

Anxiety-Panic.com ◎ ◎ ◎

http://www.anxiety-panic.com

This is a global Web guide to anxiety, panic, phobia, trauma, stress, obsession, depression, and much more; browsing the collection of links is simple at this well-organized, informative site. Anxiety-Panic.com provides the user with a site search engine for topic-specific information retrieval. General resources, books, journals, chats, mail lists and newsgroups, organizations, medications, spiritual alternatives, and much more can be found, while the educational anxiety-panic trivia game tests your knowledge of anxiety, panic, and related disorders.

Anxiety-Panic-Stress.com ◎ ◎

http://anxiety-panic-stress.com

Dedicated to serving the needs of those suffering from symptoms related to stress and anxiety, this Web site provides concise, interesting case descriptions of anxiety disorder, panic disorder, obsessive-compulsive disorder, social phobia, and posttraumatic stress disorder. General resources and referrals, excerpts from PRNewswire released by the National Mental Health Association, and a list of FAQs are presented.

Anxiety/Panic Resource Site ◎ ◎ ◎

http://www.anxietypanic.com

The Anxiety/Panic Resource Site offers information on the signs and symptoms of panic attacks and a comprehensive list of medications commonly prescribed for panic attacks, obsessive-compulsive disorder, depression, and generalized anxiety. Information is also offered on the understanding of the disorders, potential dangers of aspartame, and access to a message board where anyone can come and tell their story. Featured books of the month may be ordered online.

ASAP Dictionary of Anxiety and Panic Disorders ◎ ◎
http://www.netaxs.com/people/aca3/AD-ENG.HTM#Home

This site provides basic definitions for psychological and clinical terms related to anxiety disorders, including hormones, therapies and support mechanisms, alternative medications, phobias, and anxiety disorders. In addition, there is a separate listing of related disorders definitions, basic information on medications and drug treatments, abbreviations, a chronology, statistics, and a list of references.

Center for Anxiety and Related Disorders ◎ ◎ ◎
http://www.bu.edu/anxiety

Located within Boston University, the Center treats anxiety disorders such as panic disorder, generalized anxiety disorder, specific phobias, depression, obsessive-compulsive disorder, as well as sexual disorders. At this site, links to a disorder provide fact files on the disorder, the Center's program of treatment, as well as other symptom and treatment information. The Center also has information on their different programs, divided into the adult, adolescent/child, sexuality, and general information. A link to recent and upcoming events at the center is also present.

Center for Anxiety and Stress Treatment ◎ ◎
http://www.stressrelease.com

This Web site provides reviews for related publications, information on programs for anxiety and stress reduction and management, online personal stories, symptoms checklist, a question and answer forum, and other related workshops and publications.

CyberPsych Anxiety Disorders Links ◎ ◎
http://www.cyberpsych.org/anxlink.htm

Links are available at this site offering resources related to panic disorder, phobias, obsessive-compulsive disorder, social phobia, generalized anxiety disorder, posttraumatic stress disorder, and childhood phobias. Sites include home pages of patients' groups, parenting resources, professional associations, and general information sources.

National Anxiety Foundation ◎ ◎
http://lexington-on-line.com/nafmasthead.html

This nonprofit organization provides fundamental information on all aspects of anxiety disorders, including describing the different anxiety disorders, such as panic, and generalized anxiety disorders, their differential diagnosis, treatment information, a reading list, and support organization information. There is also a case history and a description of panic disorder, including symptoms, and physical and psychological consequences and treatment.

National Institute of Mental Health (NIMH): Library ◉ ◉ ◉
http://www.nimh.nih.gov/anxiety/library/brochure/anxbrch.htm

At this site, both professionals and consumers can obtain information on the most common types of anxiety disorders, such as panic or obsessive-compulsive disorders, phobias, generalized anxiety, and posttraumatic stress disorders. Consumers can get basic information on the symptoms, treatment, and treatment centers for these anxiety disorders. Professionals can view the NIMH consensus statement on panic disorder, view literature references on a variety of anxiety disorders, obtain conference information, and find links to current news pertaining to anxiety disorders.

Panic & Anxiety Education Management Services (PAEMS) ◉ ◉ ◉
http://www.paems.com.au

This comprehensive site provides information to the professional and lay person alike on anxiety disorders, and related research and treatment. With a focus on recovery from anxiety and panic, stories of personal experiences with panic/anxiety, the PAEMS panic and anxiety chat room, and interviews with experts in the anxiety/panic field are all available.

Social Anxiety Network ◉ ◉
http://www.social-anxiety-network.com

This online network provides fundamental information on social anxiety, symptoms, and treatment. In addition, there are personal examples of social anxiety, a list of support and professional organizations, the difference between social anxiety and other psychological disorders, links to related Web sites, references and other products for support and information about social anxiety, and news updates.

Support-Group.com Anxiety/Panic Disorders ◉ ◉ ◉
http://www.support-group.com/cgi-bin/sg/get_links?anxiety_panic

Support-Group.com provides an overview of general resources available to those coping with anxiety/panic disorders. In addition to the site's comprehensive, state-by-state listing of support groups and organizations, one will also find links to an anxiety/panic disorder bulletin board, national and international organizations, governmental agencies and information sites, and information for healthcare professionals from the National Institute of Mental Health (NIMH).

Update on Potential Causes and New Treatments for Anxiety Disorders ☉ ☉ ☉

http://www.mhsource.com/narsad/anxiety.html

Supported by the National Alliance for Research on Schizophrenia and Depression, this document provides an overview of the types of anxiety disorders, their frequency of occurrence, treatments, diagnosis issues, possible causes, including genetics, comorbidity, and psychotherapy. Information on specific drugs is included, as well as references.

Your About.com Guide to Panic/Anxiety Disorders ☉ ☉ ☉

http://panicdisorder.miningco.com/health/panicdisorder

At this About.com Guide, the user will find a comprehensive list of over 30 links to panic/anxiety topics including agoraphobia, medication, posttraumatic stress disorder (PTSD), and cognitive-behavioral therapy. Special sections include, In the Spotlight, which provides a notable news topic, the Soothing Sight of the Day, crisis and suicide help, and an e-mail support list. Additional features include a topical video store, the Panic/Anxiety Disorders Bookstore, FAQs, and the panic/anxiety chat room.

Agoraphobia

Agoraphobia ☉

http://www.cstone.net/users/maybell/agora.htm

Symptoms, treatment, and general resources are available at the site. Books, informational support groups, and a listing of relevant links are available including an Anxiety and Panic Internet Resource Page.

Generalized Anxiety Disorder

Internet Mental Health: Generalized Anxiety Disorder ☉ ☉ ☉

http://www.mentalhealth.com/dis/p20-an07.html

Generalized anxiety disorder descriptions found at this site include the American description, European description, and links to the United States Surgeon General reviews of the condition. Access to papers on the future of treatment and research of anxiety disorders is offered, as well as several booklets on the condition from reputable organizations. An online diagnostic tool assists patients and practitioners in making accurate assessments.

Obsessive-Compulsive Disorder (OCD)

Anxiety-Panic Attack Resource Site:
Obsessive-Compulsive Disorder ◉ ◉

http://www.anxietypanic.com/ocd.html

Visitors to this site will find a thorough definition of obsessive-compulsive disorder. Links available at this site guide users to treatment information, support groups, and other resources.

Awareness Foundation for
Obsessive-Compulsive Disorder (OCD) and Related Disorders ◉ ◉

http://members.aol.com/afocd/afocd.htm

This Foundation works to increase professional, educational, and public understanding of obsessive-compulsive disorder and related disorders through workshop speakers and films. The site provides general information about OCD and the organization, contact details for film and video resources, a downloadable brochure, links to related sites, and contact details.

Expert Consensus Guidelines: Obsessive-Compulsive Disorder ◉ ◉ ◉

http://www.psychguides.com/oche.html

This document provides useful information for consumers on the specific symptoms, time course of action for the disorder, heritability, etiology, differential diagnosis, treatment, educational information, support information, and sections on specific therapies and drugs used to treat this disorder. Related reading materials and organizations are listed.

HealthGate.com: Obsessive-Compulsive Disorder ◉ ◉

http://bewell.com/hic/OCD

This site offers a general description on obsessive-compulsive disorder, and answers questions related to causes, symptoms, diagnosis, treatment, duration, self-care, and when to contact a physician.

Obsessive-Compulsive Disorder Fact Page ◉ ◉

http://ucsu.Colorado.EDU/~cowanck

Descriptive details about obsessive-compulsive disorder, including patient behavior, neurobiology, and treatments are available at this site, as well as a bibliography of sources and links to related sites.

Obsessive-Compulsive Disorder
(OCD) Resource Center ◎ ◎ ◎ (free registration)
http://www.ocdresource.com/ocdresource.nsf

This site was designed to provide information to consumers, and has links to fact files on a description of OCD, its diagnosis and treatment, support groups and a physician referral network, links to other OCD-related Web sites, and detailed information about fluvoxamine maleate tablets. There is also a number of links for child and adolescent OCD information.

Obsessive-Compulsive Disorder Web Server ◎ ◎ ◎
http://www.fairlite.com/ocd

Devoted to this disorder, this Web site has many links to clinical definitions and treatment, references, fact sheets on treatments, doctor and therapist referral lists and directories, support information and groups, online forums and lists, a large list of books about this and related disorders, links to current news, a list of articles, and more.

Obsessive-Compulsive Foundation ◎ ◎ ◎
http://www.ocfoundation.org

This comprehensive Web site serves to provide information for all interested groups with respect to obsessive-compulsive disorder (OCD). There are links to the description of OCD and related disorders, treatment and medication, and a screening test. There are links to support groups, message board, research awards, newsletters, conference information, an online bookstore, membership information, a research digest listing, and a variety of other links related to OCD of interest to both professionals and the public.

Online Psych: Obsessive-Compulsive Disorder Books ◎ ◎
http://www.onlinepsych.com/psychshop/Obsessive-Compulsive_Disorder/Books

Visitors to this address can order books on obsessive-compulsive disorder and related topics, including Tourette's disorder, phobias, and specific compulsive behaviors. Users can also search for publications by title, author, or ISBN.

Panic Disorder

Answers to Your Questions about Panic Disorder ◎ ◎
http://www.apa.org/pubinfo/panic.html

Supported by the American Psychological Association, this informative document offers consumers facts related to panic disorder symptoms, diagnosis, causes, treatment options, and consequences of the disorder.

How to Treat Your Own Panic Disorder ◎ ◎ ◎

http://e2.empirenet.com/~berta

Divided into self-help, healing, and treatment aids sections, this site offers basic, but comprehensive information on all aspects of panic disorders and their treatment. Within self-help, there are links to informative pages describing panic disorders, case studies, breathing treatments, etc. The healing section provides access to researched treatment exercises, and allows online purchase of materials. Treatment aids, such as breathing pattern monitors are also available online. Informative links to diagnosis, treatment, and causes of these disorders, as well as referral links and a bibliography are included.

Panic Disorder Consensus Statement ◎ ◎ ◎

http://www.nimh.nih.gov/anxiety/resource/constate.htm

This consensus statement is provided by the National Institute of Mental Health and provides comprehensive information on, and reviews the incidence, causes, assessment, clinical signs, and current treatment practices for panic disorders. Consequences of treatment, future research questions, and concluding thoughts are included.

Treatment of Panic Disorder ◎ ◎

http://www.mhsource.com/hy/paniccon.html

This National Institutes of Health consensus statement on panic disorder reviews the definition of the disorder, current treatment options, and their efficacy. A review of the epidemiology, therapy options, and effects is included, as well as disorder symptoms, diagnosis, psychotherapy, and important psychiatric areas for future research.

Posttraumatic Stress Disorder (PTSD)

American Academy of Experts in Traumatic Stress ◎ ◎

http://www.aaets.org

American Academy of Experts in Traumatic Stress membership includes health professionals, as well as professionals from emergency services, criminal justice, forensics, law, and education committed to the advancement of intervention for survivors of trauma. The Academy's Web site provides extensive informational links for professionals in the field. A description of the academy, links to membership information, credentials, certifications, education credits, searching the national registry, the administration, board of advisors are present. Free access to selected articles from *Trauma Response* is provided. Also, ordering instructions for the *Practical Guide for Crisis Response in Our Schools* (3rd edition) are available.

Association of Traumatic Stress Specialists (ATSS) ◎ ◎
http://www.atss-hq.com

This international nonprofit organization provides professional education and certification to those actively involved in crisis intervention, trauma response, management, treatment, and the healing and recovery of those affected by traumatic stress. The site provides information on the organization, membership benefits, certification as a trauma specialist, an events calendar, links to other trauma-related sites, and a resource guide.

ChildTrauma Academy ◎ ◎
http://www.bcm.tmc.edu/civitas

Created from a partnership between Baylor College of Medicine, Texas Children's Hospital, and the CIVITAS Initiative, ChildTrauma Academy is dedicated to improving the systems that educate, nurture, protect and enrich children. The Academy's site provides links to scientific articles on child trauma, research projects, including current research activities, provides information for professionals and consumers. General information about the academy, the associated clinic, and other resources are also available.

Clinical Digital Libraries Project:
Posttraumatic Stress Disorder Patient/Family Resources ◎ ◎ ◎
http://www.slis.ua.edu/cdlp/WebCoreAll/patientinfo/psychiatry/ptsd.htm

Online pamphlets, fact sheets, and other educational resources for patients and families suffering from posttraumatic stress disorder are available at this address. Sources include the American Psychiatric Association, National Institute of Mental Health, American Academy of Child and Adolescent Psychiatry, American Academy of Family Physicians, MEDLINEplus, and Yahoo.

David Baldwin's Trauma Information Pages ◎ ◎ ◎
http://www.trauma-pages.com/index.phtml

This award-winning site, created by a licensed psychologist, focuses on emotional trauma and traumatic stress, including posttraumatic stress disorder. Links include information on supportive resources, a bookstore, disaster handouts, trauma-related articles, and other trauma resources. There is a local search engine, a translator providing site content in Spanish, French, and other languages, and information about Dr. Baldwin, as well as links to other relevant sites.

Gift From Within ◎ ◎
http://www.sourcemaine.com/gift

This site is the home page for the International Charity for Survivors of Trauma and Victimization, an organization devoted to providing information and support for those affected by posttraumatic stress disorder (PTSD). Articles and lectures on PTSD, as well as prevention programs, products, support information and other related links are included.

International Society for Traumatic Stress Studies (ISTSS) ○ ○

http://www.istss.org

A professional society created for the sharing of scientific information and strategies on traumatic stress, this Web site has links to conference information, other affiliates of the ISTSS, membership information, related links, and access to articles from the *Journal of Traumatic Stress,* as well as critical reviews and treatment guide.

Internet Mental Health: Posttraumatic Stress Disorder ○ ○ ○

http://www.mentalhealth.com/dis/p20-an06.html

Resources on posttraumatic stress disorder are available at this address, including American and European descriptions, access to online diagnostic tools, treatment information from the National Institute of Mental Health, online educational booklets, magazine articles, and links to sites offering additional trauma and anxiety resources. Disorder descriptions including diagnostic criteria, associated features, and differential diagnosis.

National Center for Posttraumatic Stress Disorder (NC-PTSD) ○ ○ ○

http://www.ncptsd.org/Index.html

The National Center for Posttraumatic Stress Disorder, a government agency under the U.S. Department of Veteran Affairs, carries out a broad range of multidisciplinary activities in research, education, and training in an effort to understand, diagnose, and treat PTSD in veterans who have developed psychiatric symptoms following exposure to traumatic stress. The site provides information about the organization and its activities, staff directories, employment and training opportunities, a searchable database of traumatic stress literature, reference literature, table of contents to *PTSD Research Quarterly* and *NC-PTSD Clinical Quarterly,* assessment instruments, and links to information about the disorder for the public.

Posttraumatic Stress Resources Web Page ○ ○

http://www.long-beach.va.gov/ptsd/stress.html

This page, sponsored by the Carl T. Hayden Veterans Affairs Medical Center in Phoenix, Arizona, offers links to sites with resources on the disorder, medications, and discussion conferences. Related government and other support agency sites are also included.

Sidran Foundation ◎ ◎ ◎
http://www.sidran.org

The Sidran Foundation is a nonprofit organization dedicated to providing education, advocacy and research related to trauma-related stress in children and adults. Resources include a list of Sidran books, a catalogue of related literature, and a trauma resource center, which provides online access to relevant scientific articles, and assessment scales. There are also links to several sites for trauma survivors and other related sites.

Specific Phobia

Open-Mind.org-Social Phobia/Anxiety ◎ ◎
http://www.open-mind.org/SP

In addition to providing a large bibliography of books for professionals and consumers interested in anxiety and panic disorders and phobias, this site also has a searchable archive of related articles, Web sties, support and professional organizations, newsgroups and LISTSERVs, a chat room, and quotations.

Phobia List ◎ ◎
http://www.sonic.net/~fredd/phobia1.html

This site contains an alphabetized list of phobias, both common and rare. Included are links to information on phobia nomenclature, categories, treatment of phobias, and links to sites for information and support with respect to phobic disorders.

Shyness Home Page ◎ ◎
http://www.shyness.com

This site provides links to online articles on shyness, newsgroups, related organizations, the Shyness Clinic, the Shyness Institute, and other related sites, as well as support information.

Social Phobia in Children and Adolescents ◎ ◎ ◎
http://www.klis.com/chandler/pamphlet/socphob/content.htm

In addition to defining this condition, this site offers information on incidence, causes, symptoms, and the most feared social circumstances. Facts on related disorders, consequences of social phobia, treatment options, drug effects and other drug issues are all found at the site.

Social Phobia: The Largest Anxiety Disorder ◉

http://www.angelfire.com/biz/socialphobia

The first page of this site offers a basic description of social phobia, its symptoms, and treatment strategies. There are links to more detailed information about this disorder, and a listing of social phobia and anxiety related links.

Social Phobia/Social Anxiety Association Home Page ◉ ◉ ◉

http://www.socialphobia.org

The purposes and goals of the Social Phobia/Social Anxiety Association, informational articles, and current news are enumerated at the Association's Web site. Social anxiety links, fact sheets, and mailing lists may be accessed. The Anxiety Network bookstore page allows users to choose and order books securely over the Internet. Professional literature and a subscription to the quarterly publication, *SP/SAA Journal* is available through a mail-in registration process.

Social Phobias ◉ ◉ ◉

http://www.rcpsych.ac.uk/public/help/socphob/soc_frame.htm

This online handout, provided by the Royal College of Psychiatry reviews what social phobias are, different types of social phobias, symptoms, related psychological disorders, self-esteem issues, incidence, consequences and causes, self-help advice, behavioral therapies, drug treatments, and supportive contacts.

Stress Disorders

Job Stress Network ◉ ◉ ◉

http://www.workhealth.org

This site serves as the home page for the Center for Social Epidemiology. Many fact sheets, articles and other resources are available in the subjects of job strain, risk factors, health outcomes, prevention, and related research projects. Links to relevant references, news, events, and a site search engine are available.

Stress and Anxiety Research Society (STAR) ◉ ◉

http://star-society.org

This professional multidisciplinary organization of researchers promotes the exchange of information on anxiety and stress. At this site, the Society's mission and history is presented, as well as membership information, STAR members, conference information, national and international representatives, and a list of publications from STAR. A list of related organizations, academic departments, journals, databases, employment opportunities, and online newsgroups and mailing lists is also provided.

Web Stress Management & Emotional Wellness Page

http://imt.net/~randolfi/StressPage.html

Dedicated to those interested in managing stress, maximizing performance, and enhancing emotional health, this Web site offers a comprehensive list of links, discussion forum, Optimal Health Concepts Bookstore online, and stress management lecture information.

9.3 **Attention-Deficit and Disruptive Behavior Disorders**

Attention-Deficit/Hyperactivity Disorder (AD/HD)

ADD and Addiction.com

http://www.addandaddiction.com

Provided by a specialist in the field, ADD and Addiction.com is dedicated to informing visitors of the relationship between attention-deficit/hyperactivity disorder and co-occurring conditions such as substance abuse, eating disorders, behavioral addictions, and criminal behavior. Current articles and books, recent news, helpful links, and ordering information on the publication by the site-author are included.

ADD/ADHD Categorized Links Page

http://user.cybrzn.com/~kenyonck/add/Links/links_categories_new.htm

Links to sites offering resources related to attention-deficit/hyperactivity disorder (AD/HD) are offered at this site. Site categories include AD/HD experiences, adult AD/HD, children's sites, education, support groups, humor, law, marriage, medications, organizations, parenting, personal finance, personal stories, relationships, time management, treatments, women's issues, and workplace issues.

Adders.org

http://www.adders.org

This attention-deficit/hyperactivity disorder online support group offers links to worldwide sources for information, support, news, personal stories, and general self-help resources on the Internet. Educational resources, research articles, natural remedies, chat forums, freeware, children's resources, and contact details are listed at the site.

ADDvance

http://www.addvance.com

An award-winning site, ADDvance is the only online resource dedicated specifically to the understanding of AD/HD in females. Selected articles, books, tapes, support group information, and valuable AD/HD links, including subscription information for ADDvance magazine, are all available online.

ADHDNews.com ✪ ✪ ✪ (free registration)

http://www.adhdnews.com

Available at this Web site are opportunities to access timely information and articles concerning AD/HD as well as communicate with others concerned with AD/HD through e-mail discussion groups. Contributed to by professionals and experts in the field of special education, free subscriptions are offered to the online newsletter, ADDed Attractions and ADHD Research Update through a simple, online registration process. E-mail discussion groups include ADDadults, focusing on the particular concerns of the adult diagnosed with AD/HD, ADDtalk, a discussion group for those with educational, advocacy, and parenting concerns, as well as a group geared towards alternative treatments.

Attention-Deficit Disorder WWW Archive ✪ ✪

http://www.realtime.net/~cyanosis/add

This archive of sites related to AD/HD contains links to personal Web sites, medical sites, support groups, government resources, and organizations. Some links are listed with short site descriptions.

Attention-Deficit Disorders ✪ ✪ ✪ (free registration)

http://www.add.idsite.com

Created to give both parents and educators insight, suggestions, and information on children diagnosed with AD/HD and ODD, this colorful, award-winning site offers users an AD/HD message board as well as a live chat room with special guest moderators. A considerable amount of up-to-date information can be found in Research Update and ADDed Edition newsletters available through free online registrations. Much unique information is available at this site, including homework hints for helpful parents, 23 strategies to enhance self-esteem in AD/HD kids, AD/HD medication information, programs, and camps, and the online "Wild Child's" bookstore.

Attention-Deficit/Hyperactivity Disorder: A Definition ✪ ✪ ✪

http://www.brightok.net/~dmcgowen/adhd.html

This fact sheet offered by Plainview Elementary School in Oklahoma offers a definition of attention-deficit/hyperactivity disorder, including DSM-IV subtype definitions, behavioral signals, and difficulties children with these disorders may encounter. Multimedia education programs are discussed as an alternative teaching method and therapy for children diagnosed with AD/HD.

Born to Explore: The Other Side of ADD ◎ ◎ ◎

http://borntoexplore.org

The purpose of this site is to provide resources relating to different perceptions of AD/HD. Resources include fact sheets containing information on alternate views of AD/HD, temperament, creativity, and intelligence issues, nutrition, mood changes, support information, books, and links to related sites.

Children and Adults with Attention-Deficit/Hyperactivity Disorder (CHADD) ◎ ◎ ◎

http://www.chadd.org

Created principally to provide information for the general public, resources at this site include background information on CHADD, membership information, disorder fact sheets, legislative information, conference information, news releases, and online access to selected articles from *Attention* magazine. In addition, links to current research synopses on these disorders, government sites, legislative and legal resources, state legislative resources, and international organizations, as well as sites related to coexisting disorders, special education, disability, and health issues are provided. Links include those specific to attention-deficit/hyperactivity disorder, mental health, anxiety disorders, learning disorders, depression, Tourette's disorder, and pediatrics.

National Attention Deficit Disorder Association ◎ ◎ ◎

http://www.add.org

The National Attention Deficit Disorder Association helps people with AD/HD lead happier, more successful lives through education, research, and public advocacy. Membership information, conference details, articles, news, guiding principles for diagnosis and treatment, and a directory of professionals treating AD/HD are available at the site. Research, treatment, and general information about AD/HD is offered, as well as links to sites offering resources on work, family, education, and legal issues associated with AD/HD. Support group sites and sites for children and teens are also listed. Visitors can read personal stories and interviews, and search the site by keyword.

National Institutes of Health (NIH): Consensus Statements, Diagnosis and Treatment of Attention-Deficit/Hyperactivity Disorder (ADHD) ◎ ◎ ◎

http://odp.od.nih.gov/consensus/cons/110/110_statement.htm

This consensus statement on the diagnosis and treatment of AD/HD includes an abstract and introduction, and describes scientific evidence supporting AD/HD as a disorder, the impact of AD/HD on individuals, families, and society, effective treatments, any risks of medications, diagnostic and treatment practices, barriers to appropriate identification, evaluation, and intervention, and directions for future research. The consensus development panel, speakers, planning committee, lead organizations, and supporting organizations are listed, and users can access a bibliography of references.

One A.D.D. Place ☉ ☉ ☉

http://www.oneaddplace.com

A virtual neighborhood of resources relating to attention-deficit/hyperactivity disorder, and learning disorders, One A.D.D. Place includes a wide variety of support and management resources. Pertinent research articles, a virtual community library, Internet links, a list of FAQs, and helpful organizations and support groups are included. A professional section offers current information on treatment options, seminars, and programs.

University of Georgia: Learning Disabilities Research and Training Center ☉ ☉ ☉

http://www.rit.edu/~easi/easisem/ldnoelbw.htm

This site describes research and training at the Center, and offers an information guide for and about adolescents and adults with learning disorders and AD/HD. A detailed discussion of the guide is followed by directories of AD/HD organizations, consumer support groups, general education and adult literacy resources, centers and organizations for general disability information, transition and life management resources, employment, assistive and adaptive technology, government agencies, Internet sites of interest, legal documents and information, publications and books, organizations offering toll-free information services, and learning disabilities research and training center products. Many valuable resources are located through this site.

Disruptive Behavior Disorders

At Health Mental Health: Disruptive Behavior Disorders ☉ ☉ ☉

http://athealth.com/FPN_3_7.html

Useful resources are available at this site devoted to disruptive behavior disorders, including links to related articles, practice parameters, fact sheets, assessment resources, prevention information, and a support site for parents and teachers. General site resources also include an online directory of mental health professionals, a sponsor newsletter, notices of Continuing Medical Education meetings, an online bookstore of relevant materials through Amazon.com, and an extensive directory of mental health resources.

Critical Pathways for Disruptive Behavior Disorders ☉ ☉ ☉

http://pwp.usa.pipeline.com/~fuzzymills/dirupt.htm

The article found at the site examines the commonalities between oppositional defiant and conduct disorder and their shared roots of origin. The DSM-IV diagnostic criteria for the disorders are listed, and the criteria for severity of the conditions is explained. Relevant clinical features, assessment issues, and coexisting conditions are reviewed, such as hyperactivity and academic deficiencies. Risks coexisting with the disorder, including suicide gestures and depression, are also mentioned. "Indicators for Levels of Care" include explanations of emergent, transitional, and episodic intervention, and the issues associated with residential and custodial environments are explored.

Oppositional Defiant Disorder and Conduct Disorder

Fact Sheet: Oppositional Defiant Disorder ◎ ◎
http://noah.cuny.edu/illness/mentalhealth/cornell/conditions/odd.html

The New York Hospital-Cornell Medical Center fact sheet on this behavioral disorder concisely defines the disorder, offers information on the symptoms, causes, process, treatment, self-help advice, and provides contact information.

Internet Mental Health: Oppositional Defiant Disorder ◎ ◎ ◎
http://www.mentalhealth.com/fr20.html

As part of the Internet Mental Health compilation of disorders, this Web page is dedicated to the description, research, treatment, and educational information pertaining to oppositional defiant disorder. The American and European diagnostic criteria are included as are relevant Internet links.

Oppositional Defiant Disorder (ODD) and Conduct Disorder (CD) in Children and Adolescents: Diagnosis and Treatment ◎ ◎ ◎
http://www.klis.com/chandler/pamphlet/oddcd/content.htm

Oppositional defiant disorder information at this site includes an introduction, definitions, causes, diagnosis, and prognosis for the disorder. A discussion of conduct disorder includes a definition, diagnosis, and prognosis. Coexisting mental conditions are discussed. Information is mainly nontechnical, but both professionals and parents may find the site useful. Strategies for these disorders and possible therapies are also presented.

9.4 Catatonia

Catatonia and Neuroleptic Malignant Syndrome (NMS): Recognition and Treatment ◎ ◎
http://www.schizophrenia.com/ami/diagnosis/catatonia.html

Appearing first in *Psychiatric Times,* this article reviews the disorder of catatonia, its diagnosis, symptoms, related disorders, assessment issues, and treatment. In addition, information on NMS, its description, causes, and treatment is provided. Information on Toxic Serotonin Syndrome is also available.

Virtual Hospital: Medical Emergencies in Psychiatry: Lethal Catatonia ◎
http://www.vh.org/Providers/Lectures/
EmergencyMed/Psychiatry/MedEmergCatatonia.html

This document (click on MedEmergCatatonia) comes from an Emergency Psychiatry Service Handbook, and offers detailed information on signs, symptoms, and treatment of this condition.

9.5 Childhood and Adolescent Disorders

See Attention-Deficit and Disruptive Behavior Disorders; Eating Disorders; Infancy, Childhood, or Adolescence Disorders, Other; Learning Disorders; Mental Retardation; Pervasive Developmental Disorders; and Tic Disorders.

9.6 Communication Disorders

Expressive Language Disorders

Apraxia ◎ ◎
http://www.isn.net/~jypsy/apraxia.htm

A short description and links to information resources are available at this address devoted to apraxia. One link sends users to Amazon.com and a list of books on apraxia, and many autism links are also available through the site.

Apraxia Information ◎ ◎
http://laran.waisman.wisc.edu/fv/www/lib_apraxia.html

Visitors to this site will find synonyms to apraxia, suggested sources for additional resources, as well as links to chat forums, sites offering information about apraxia, and sites offering support.

Developmental Verbal Apraxia or Developmental Apraxia of Speech ◎ ◎ ◎
http://tayloredmktg.com/dyspraxia/das.html

This site contains an informative fact sheet on apraxia, including a description, its causes, main symptoms, related dysfunctions, behavioral problems, supportive therapy, and other speech therapies.

Mixed Receptive-Expressive Language Disorder

American Hyperlexia Association ◎ ◎
http://www.hyperlexia.org
"The American Hyperlexia Association is a nonprofit organization comprised of parents and relatives of children with hyperlexia, speech and language professionals, education professionals, and other concerned individuals with the common goal of identifying hyperlexia, promoting and facilitating effective teaching techniques both at home and at school, and educating the general public as to the existence of the syndrome called hyperlexia." This Web site includes links to pages describing hyperlexia and treatment options, as well as links to the mailing list, membership information, materials order list, organizations and therapist directories, other hyperlexia sites, and a guest book.

Hyperlexia and Language Disorders ◎ ◎ ◎
http://www.geocities.com/HotSprings/9402/index.html
The parent of a hyperlexic child hosts this page devoted to information on hyperlexia. Several articles presenting personal stories and education issues are available in both English and Spanish, and visitors can also access subscription information for a listserver. Many sites offering additional information resources are linked through this address. Site link categories include hyperlexia, language disorders, language skills, social skills, study skills, education issues, diet intervention, and commercial sites.

Hyperplexia Parent's Page ◎ ◎ ◎
http://www.geocities.com/Heartland/Meadows/9019/hyperlexia.html
This forum for parents with hyperlexic children offers articles, examples of story therapy, success stories, parents' letters, chat forums, pen pal resources for children, and links to professional associations. Articles and other resources are nontechnical and offer specific suggestions for dealing with hyperlexia issues in children.

9.7 **Delirium, Dementia, Amnestic, and Other Cognitive Disorders**

General Resources

Delirium, Dementia, and Amnestic Disorders and Other Cognitive Disorders ◎ ◎
http://www.chesco.com/~snowbaby/Cognitive.html#Deliriums

This site presents DSM-IV criteria taken from the site author's book, *DSM-IV Made Easy,* developed for use by mental health professionals, patients, relatives, and other lay people. Criteria and coding notes are available for different forms of deliriums, dementias, amnestic disorders, and mental disorders due to a general medical condition.

Institute of Gerontology ◎ ◎
http://www.iog.wayne.edu

Out of Wayne State University, this institute conducts research in, and provides education in the field of gerontology. There are summaries of the research programs at the Institute, including family and intergenerational relationships, health and healthcare (including psychological services), human development and expression, and independence and productivity (including cognitive training and aging). A faculty directory and bibliography, is provided, as well as colloquia and conference information.

AIDS/HIV Dementia

AIDS/HIV Support-Group.com ◎ ◎ ◎
http://www.support-group.com/cgi-bin/sg/get_links?aids_hiv

This Support-Group.com resource page provides links to support groups and organizations nationwide and internationally, governmental agencies and information sites, an AIDS/HIV bulletin board and USENET groups, and online journals. Professional organizations and resources are included as are sites related to AIDS/HIV prevention and alternative treatments.

BETA: AIDS Dementia Complex ◎ ◎
http://www.aegis.com/pubs/beta/1996/be963105.html

From the *Bulletin of Experimental Treatments for AIDS,* this informative document reviews the disorder, its causes, and symptoms in detail, and provides a useful psychiatric classification of the stages of disorder progression. HIV-related infections and their effect on patinet mental health is discussed, as well as diagnosis, theories of disease mechanisms, viral load, treatment, and prophylactic measures. Drug therapies are examined in detail, as well as current and future research topics.

HIV Insite Gateway to AIDS Knowledge ◎ ◎ ◎
http://HIVInSite.ucsf.edu/topics/mental_health

At HIV Insite, documents and abstracts on coping strategies, AIDS-related dementia complex (ADC), psychoactive pharmaceuticals, and the mind-body connection may be accessed. A powerful search engine may be used for browsing current news topics. Also included is HIV prevention and statistical information and a Spanish information section.

Opportunistic Infections: Neurological disorders ◎
http://www.hivpositive.com/f-Oi/OppInfections/4-Neuro/4-NeuroSubMenu.html

This site summarizes the possible neurological disorders resulting from HIV infection, and offers links to informative documents on the major effects of HIV on the central nervous system, the AIDS dementia complex, treatment efficacy, peripheral neuropath, confounding brain system disorders and HIV infection, as well as a list of references.

Project Inform: AIDS Dementia Complex Hotline Handout ◎ ◎
http://www.projinf.org/fs/dementia.html

This site provides detailed information on the symptoms of this newly classified dementia, its prevalence, diagnosis and assessment, as well as the mechanism behind AIDS-caused dementia. In addition, topics such as HIV infection, drug therapy, symptoms of various stages of AIDS-related dementia, and related issues are discussed. Contact and support information is also included.

Selected HIV/AIDS Bookmarks:
A Service of the Center for Mental Health Services ◎ ◎ ◎
Selected for their overall content and quality, the links made available provide the user with a variety of treatment, research, and prevention information. Top sites include the National Institutes of Health Guide to HIV/AIDS Information Services, AIDS Clinical Trial Information Service, and the Center for Disease Control and Prevention.

The Body: Depression, Anxiety, and Mental Health ◎ ◎ ◎
http://www.thebody.com/mental.html

Visitors to this address will find interactive questions and answers related to HIV, mental health, and spiritual support, as well as links to sites providing information on a variety of topics. These topics include coping with AIDS and HIV, stress, anxiety, depression, the mind-body connection, psychoactive drugs, relationships and sexuality, chemical dependency, death and mourning, issues for professionals, and resources for caregivers.

United Nations Programme on HIV/AIDS   ◎ ◎ ◎
http://www.unaids.org

HIV/AIDS information by subject or country, publications, press releases, and conference updates are all available at the site of the United Nations Programme on HIV/AIDS. This leading advocate for worldwide action against HIV/AIDS provides past and present issues of its newsletter in PDF and Word format, speech transcripts in English and French, information about its Africa Partnership, and a number of useful links on AIDS education, research, and treatment.

Alzheimer's Disease

Administration on Aging: General Resources   ◎ ◎
http://www.aoa.dhhs.gov/jpost/generalresources.html

This site lists links to resources on the Internet for geriatric issues such as Alzheimer's disease and other dementias, as well as general psychology and psychiatry. Resources include metasites (sites allowing users to search many sites from one location), Web sites, personal pages, articles, professional guidelines, organizations, discussion groups and listservers, research projects, and other related information.

Alzheimer Page   ◎ ◎
http://www.biostat.wustl.edu/alzheimer

Sustained by Washington University Alzheimer's Disease Research Center, this searchable database of information has links to questions and answers on more frequently discussed topics regarding this disease, a searchable archive of the mailing list, and a section on links to support groups, organizations, products, research, jobs, nursing homes, and personal Web sites related to Alzheimer's disease and other dementias.

Alzheimer Research Forum   ◎ ◎ ◎
http://www.alzforum.org

This Web site's information database consists of a professional and non-professional section. The non-professional section has links to Web sites on patient care, support groups, commercial products, news and general information about the disease, as well as associations and disease centers. The professional section contains a keyword searchable database, with links to research findings and treatment guides, online forums and tools, conference information, drug company directory, and the opportunity to receive and give information on specific Alzheimer research topics.

Alzheimer Web ◎ ◎ ◎

http://home.mira.net/~dhs/ad3.html

A directory of current Alzheimer's disease research endeavors, links to research laboratories, current papers via PubMed, and a listing of FAQs are included at this Web site, which focuses solely on Alzheimer's disease research. An up-to-date listing of cholinesterase inhibitors and other Alzheimer's drugs and a colorful depiction of the cholinergic pathways affected in the Alzheimer's brain can be viewed.

Alzheimer's Association ◎ ◎ ◎

http://www.alz.org

The Alzheimer's Association offers information and support on issues related to the disease. Patients and caregivers can access general facts about Alzheimer's disease, and detailed discussions of medical issues, diagnosis, expected lifestyle changes, treatment options, clinical trial participation, planning for the future, and contact information for special programs and support. Caregiver information and professional resources are also available. Resources for investigators include a summary of current research, lists of grant opportunities, lists of past grant awards, progress report forms, and information on the Reagan Institute. The Association also offers news, program, and conference calendars; publications; and information on advocacy activities at this site.

Alzheimer's Disease Education and Referral (ADEAR) Center ◎ ◎ ◎

http://www.alzheimers.org

This service of the National Institute on Aging offers information on Alzheimer's disease and related disorders. The site describes new features and the ADEAR information and referral telephone services. Fact sheets, research and technical reports, information on training programs, an online newsletter, public service announcements, and online lectures are available at the site. Other features include a bibliographic database of health education materials on Alzheimer's disease, a clinical trials database, a calendar of events, a site search engine, and links to related sites.

Alzheimer's Disease Information Directory ◎ ◎ ◎

http://www.zarcrom.com/users/yeartorem/index4.html

The Alzheimer's Disease Information Directory provides an overview of resources for Alzheimer's patients and their caregivers. Links are provided to Alzheimer's Association chapters, worldwide organizations, online discussions lists, and chats geared towards patients as well as caregivers. Information on related dementias, special sites for seniors, and comprehensive research and caregiver information are available. Pages from the Web site may be viewed in English, French, German, Italian, Portuguese, or Spanish via Alta Vista's translator.

Alzheimer's Disease Society

http://www.alzheimers.org.uk

Created to provide information about Alzheimer's disease and other dementias, this site has links to descriptive fact sheets on these disorders, their symptoms, and physical causes and consequences, treatment and prognosis. In addition, there are summaries of current research theories on these dementias. For caregivers, there is general support advice and related topics, as well as current news, information about the society itself, as well links to other related societies.

Alzheimers.com

http://www.alzheimers.com

General information on Alzheimer's disease including risk factors, prevention, and treatment are comprehensively covered at the Alzheimers.com Web site. Diagnostic tools, the 10 early warning signs of Alzheimer's disease, other similarly presenting dementias, and daily feature stories and research updates are included. Of great interest are the site's online pharmacy, with a variety of Alzheimer's treatment products available for direct delivery, and a coping section with plenty of information geared especially for caregivers.

American Association
for Geriatric Psychiatry (AAGP) ○ ○ ○ (some features fee-based)

http://www.aagpgpa.org

The AAGP Web site includes numerous links to various issues of interest for both professionals and interested laypersons. There are news reports, the AAGP bookstore, meeting information, consumer information, including brochures and a question/answer section, advocacy and public policy section, a link to the *American Journal for Geriatric Psychiatry*, a health professional bulletin, member meeting place, staff listing, and a link to the AAGP Education and Research Foundation.

American Health Assistance Foundation ○ ○

http://www.ahaf.org

This nonprofit organization is provided to promote research, education, and financial support to those involved in age-related degenerative diseases, such as Alzheimer's disease. There are links to information about the Alzheimer's disease research program and other related resources, including news updates and fact sheets, as well as support resources. There is general information presented on research updates, grants and upcoming events.

Baylor College of Medicine
Alzheimer's Disease Research Center ○ ○ ○

http://www.bcm.tmc.edu/neurol/struct/adrc/adrc1.html

As part of Baylor College of Medicine, this center conducts both clinical and scientific research on various aspects of the disease. Links to Alzheimer's related research projects provide overviews of the projects, which include psychosis, language, hemispheric asymmetry, cholinergic dysfunction, progressive disease studies, and more. A link to clinical drug trials for memory loss provides information on the various FDA-approved drugs for the disease, and information on a memory impairment project. In addition, there are fact files for diagnosis and medical evaluation, advances in diagnosis and treatment, genetic testing, and behavioral changes in the disease. There are links to educational opportunities, and other related links.

Geropsychology Central ○ ○ ○

http://www.premier.net/~gero/contents.html

This site provides information for seniors, professionals, and consumers interested in issues relating to gerontology and mental health. Included are links to related conferences, literature, journals, other gerontology related sites and organizations, geropsychology practice qualifications, a number of links for dementia resources, including Alzheimer's, and Parkinson's diseases, stroke, mental and quality of life assessment materials, and other mental health and geriatrics links to Web sites and research centers.

Institute for Brain Aging and Dementia ○ ○ ○

http://maryanne.bio.uci.edu

Located at the University of California, Irving, the Institute's research focuses on successful aging, preserving Alzheimer's patient abilities, beta-amaloid research, cell death, exercise and brain well-being, and other related areas. Brief summaries of these research areas are provided. In addition, information on the clinic, which has programs devoted to patient assessment and mental health, as well as their successful aging program is present. A list of the faculty and their research interests, and training opportunities is available.

LewyNet ○ ○ ○

http://www.ccc.nottingham.ac.uk/~mpzjlowe/lewy/lewyhome.html

This Web site provides information on Lewy bodies and associated dementias. Informative links include pathological and clinical descriptions of dementias, including figures and diagnostic criteria, consortium and conference information, links to fact files and Web sites on Alzheimer's and Parkinson's diseases, and information on relevant books.

Medical Glossary from Alzheimer's Outreach ◎ ◎ ◎
http://www.zarcrom.com/users/alzheimers/w-07.html

More than 50 medical terms related to Alzheimer's disease are available at this address, providing patients and caregivers with a valuable educational resource.

Memory and Dementia ◎ ◎
http://www.rcpsych.ac.uk/public/help/memory/memory.htm

This report offers a review of the problem of memory impairment, common signs, problems related to memory dysfunction, physical causes, and a review of types of dementias, such as Alzheimer's disease. Self-help advice, and support information are present.

Rush Alzheimer's Disease Center ◎ ◎
http://www.rush.edu/index.html

This Center's research projects focus on risk factors, symptoms and assessment, testing for the disease, examining the neurobiology of Alzheimer's, and devising treatments. There are links to the current clinical trials, which gives information on which drugs were tested, a link to educational grants, publications from the faculty, and the Rush Brain Bank, which aids research by providing the materials necessary for basic experiments; and processes, diagnoses, and stores brain specimens and other related materials. There are also a number of links for family support groups and information, and educational and training services available at the Center.

University Alzheimer Center ◎ ◎ ◎
http://www.ohioalzcenter.org

Affiliated with Case Western Reserve University, this Center conducts research on memory and aging issues. There are links to current studies being conducted at the center, consisting of brief summaries on topics such as apolipoprotien E, attention and Alzheimer's diseases, clinical and family studies regarding Alzheimer's and memory loss, life history studies and memory loss, visual spatial studies, and more. A list of publications by the Center's staff, as well as articles on research conducted at the Center are provided. A fact sheet on Alzheimer's disease, warning signs of Alzheimer's, medication updates, cell division and Alzheimer's, and exercise and Alzheimer's written by the staff and are present. General information about the Center, current news, and other related links are also present.

Washington University Alzheimer's Disease Research Center ◎ ◎
http://www.biostat.wustl.edu/adrc

Located in Washington University Medical Center in St. Louis, the Web site lists the overall research mission of the Center, including faculty and staff, and has basic information on the different cores of the Center (biostatistics, clinical psychometric, tissue resources, etc.). The biostatistics core has numerous links to various statistical and disease-related resources. There are links to the Center's *Horizon Newsletter*, informative links to certain projects, a list of relevant seminars, and a calendar of the center's daily events.

Amnestic Disorders

Amnestic Disorders ◎ ◎

http://www.psyweb.com/Mdisord/amnd.html

This brief introduction to amnestic disorders describes the cognitive impairment involved, lists the amnestic disorder types, and provides a link to summaries of nine psychotherapeutic alternatives, including Adlerian therapy, existential therapy, and transactional analysis. The bases, goals, and appropriateness of each theory to specific behaviors and conditions are explained.

Creutzfeldt-Jakob Disease (CJD)

Creutzfeldt-Jakob Disease ◎ ◎ ◎

http://wfh.org/CJD4Eng.html

Creutzfeldt-Jakob disease, its clinical presentation, causes, and transmission information are contained at this online CJD review. Concerns of the hemophilia community regarding CJD transmission are discussed, and prophylaxis of disease contraction through reduction of plasma pool sizes other methods is explored. An online glossary pertinent to CJD discussion is accessible.

Creutzfeldt-Jakob Disease Fact Sheet ◎ ◎ ◎

http://members.aol.com/crjakob/brochure.html

This site is very informative. Cruetzfeldt-Jakob Disease is defined, and discussions include pathology, susceptibility, diagnosis, prognosis, treatment, and research are well covered. For those wishing for continued research material, postal and Internet addresses for the Creutzfeldt-Jakob Disease Foundation, National Institute of Neurological Disorders and Stroke, and National Organization for Rare Disorders are provided.

Creutzfeldt-Jakob Disease Foundation, Inc. ◎ ◎ ◎

http://cjdfoundation.org/info.html

Creutzfeldt-Jakob Disease Foundation provides descriptions and fact sheets in an effort to educate the public and give awareness of the research needed to gain a better understanding of this Prion disease. There is also information on theories concerning the CJD agent, associated Internet resources, current news and statistics, postings of conferences/symposiums, and general information about the Creutzfeldt-Jakob Disease Foundation.

Neuropathology of Creutzfeldt-Jakob Disease ⊙ ⊙ ⊙
http://www.cjd.ed.ac.uk/path.htm

The characerization of Creutzfeldt-Jakob Disease is made at this Web location, where four neuropathological features are identified. Human prion disease histological investigation and abnormalties are described and illustrated, and classical and other changes associated with the condition are listed. Additional conditions associated with spongiform-like changes in the central nervous system are reviewed including Alzheimer's disease and frontal lobe dementia.

Delirium

Merck Manual of Diagnosis and Therapy: Delirium ⊙ ⊙ ⊙
http://www.merck.com/pubs/mmanual/section14/chapter171/171b.htm

The acute confusional state of delirium is fully reviewed at this page of the online *Merck Manual of Diagnosis and Therapy*. Factors such as coexisting brain disease or systemic illness affecting the brain are discussed, specifically in terms of metabolic, structural, and infectious causes. The rapidly fluctuating symptoms of the disorder, its diagnostic criteria, and the potential for reversibility of symptoms through rapid identification and proper management are summarized.

Huntington's Disease

Dementia in Huntington's Disease ⊙ ⊙
http://www.informatik.fh-luebeck.de/icd/icdchVF-F02.2.html

A clinical description and diagnostic guidelines for the dementia that occurs as part of the overall brain degeneration of Huntington's disease are offered at the site. Early symptom summaries may be accessed, and a list of differential diagnoses to be considered is presented. Four diagnostic criteria are explained, in addition to the accessible, requisite, general criteria for dementia that must be met. Development of additional extrapyramidal rigidity or spasticity with pyramidal signs is mentioned.

Pick's Disease

Pick's Disease of the Brain ◎ ◎
http://www.ncbi.nlm.nih.gov/htbin-post/Omim/dispmim?172700

Provided for professionals, this document provides clinical information and links to references on case studies, causes of the disease, diagnosis, heritability, neuropathology, and related disorders, such as Alzheimer's and Parkinson's disease. Included are links to medical databases.

Pick's Disease Support Group ◎ ◎
http://www.pdsg.org.uk

This support organization offers online access to the newsletter, which covers meeting and group information, disease information, personal stories, and scientific articles. In addition, there are links to contact resources, telephone and e-mail directories, articles written by the group's members on this disease, as well as related links.

Vascular Dementia

Vascular Dementia: Dementia Caused by Multiple Brain Strokes ◎ ◎
http://www.alzbrain.org/misc/vdementia.html

Dementia caused by multiple brain strokes is described at this site of Alzbrain.org, with seven related diseases and 10 facts about dementia from multiple brain strokes listed.

Prosopagnosia (Face Blindness)

Face Blind! Bill's Face Blindness (Prosopagnosia) Pages ◎ ◎
http://www.choisser.com/faceblind

An individual with face blindness (prosopagnosia) hosts this site, presenting an extensive discussion of face blindness in 13 chapters. Topics include physical causes, the importance of recognizing others, how most people recognize others, ways to recognize others without using the face, emotions, sexuality, suggested ways to cope, and other related subjects. Appendixes offer suggestions on finding medical articles related to the condition, diagnosis, and links to related sites.

9.8 **Dissociative Disorders**

General Resources

Colin A. Ross Institute: Diagnosing Dissociative Disorders ◎ ◎
http://www.rossinst.com/dddquest.htm
The full text and scoring rules for the Dissociative Disorders Interview Schedule, developed by the founder of the Ross Institute, is available for educational purposes at this site. This structured interview is used by professionals for systematic clinical assessment and research of dissociative disorders.

Dissociative Identity Disorder (DID)/
Trauma/ Memory Reference List ◎ ◎
http://www.sidran.org/refdid.html
This reference list composed in 1997 offers citations, sometimes accompanied by quotes or abstracts, related to dissociative identity disorder, trauma, false memory syndrome, amnesia, and related topics. Topics and resources include "Traumatic Amnesia In Holocaust Survivors," "Validity And Diagnosis Of DID," "Suggestibility and Hypnotic Pseudomemory," standard of care issues, and statistical references.

Healing Hopes, Inc. ◎ ◎
http://www.healinghopes.org
This nonprofit organization provides information and support resources for those interested or involved with dissociative identity disorders. There are links to fact sheets on anxiety, panic and anger management, depression, dissociation disorders and their treatment, eating disorders, self-injury and suicide prevention, stress, therapist information, support group issues and more. In addition, there are online forums, chat rooms, news, and related sites.

International Society for the Study of Dissociation (ISSD) ◎ ◎ ◎
http://www.issd.org
This nonprofit professional organization advocates research and professional training in the diagnosis, treatment and education of dissociative disorders, as well as serving to promote international communication among scientists and professionals working in this area. There are links to conference information, membership and society information, a link to the *Journal of Trauma and Dissociation,* the ISSD newsletter, education resources, including articles on related topics, and a list of dissociation disorder treatment guidelines. In addition, there is a set of professional and self-help links, and contact information.

National Alliance for the Mentally Ill (NAMI): Dissociative Disorders Helpline Fact Sheet ◎ ◎
http://www.nami.org/helpline/whatdiss.htm

Dissociative disorders are discussed at this site, including dissociative amnesia, dissociative fugue, dissociative identity disorder, and depersonalization disorder. Common treatments are also briefly discussed.

New England Society for the Study of Dissociation ◎ ◎
http://www.nessd.org

This Society, an affiliate of the nonprofit International Society for the Study of Dissociation (ISSD), serves professional members from Connecticut, Maine, Massachusetts, New Hampshire, Rhode Island, and Vermont. Quarterly meetings offer professional presentations, discussion groups, consultation clinics, networking opportunities, and the Society sponsors educational workshops on the treatment of dissociative disorders and other topics. This site provides visitors with a mission statement, membership information, a calendar of events, recent newsletter articles, a bulletin board, and links to related sites.

Snap.com: Dissociative Disorders ◎ ◎ ◎
http://uswest.snap.com/directory/category/0,16,-43444,00.html?st.sn.dir.alpha.cat_7

This address contains links to treatment centers, societies, information pages, support groups, therapy information, and self-help resources for dissociative disorders, including dissociative identity disorder, trauma and dissociation, and repressed memory. Resources explaining the signs and symptoms of these disorders are included at this site.

Synergy: The Institute for Dissociative Disorders ◎ ◎
http://ourworld.compuserve.com/homepages/Synergy_Institute

This nonprofit corporation's mission is to provide education and information to interested professionals and consumers. Book reviews are available, as well as a list of articles relating to dissociative disorders. Information on membership, and a long list of links to related sites are included.

Depersonalization Disorder

Merck Manual of Diagnosis and Therapy: Depersonalization Disorder ◎ ◎ ◎
http://www.merck.com/pubs/mmanual/section15/chapter188/188e.htm

This common psychiatric disturbance, characterized by distorted self-perception, is presented at this chapter of the online *Merck Manual of Diagnosis and Therapy*. The variable range of impairment; spontaneous resolution of symptoms; and a variety of successful psychotherapies, including psychodynamic, cognitive-behavioral, and hypnosis are discussed.

Dissociative Amnesia

Merck Manual of Diagnosis and Therapy: Dissociative Amnesia ❂ ❂ ❂
http://www.merck.com/pubs/mmanual/section15/chapter188/188b.htm

Lost information that is normally part of conscious awareness and further characteristics of dissociative amnesia are discussed here, including the trauma-related occurrences and the controversy surrounding accurate, later recollections. Diagnosis, based on physical and psychiatric exam, is provided, and supportive management goals are presented.

Dissociative Fugue

Merck Manual of Diagnosis and Therapy: Dissociative Fugue ❂ ❂ ❂
http://www.merck.com/pubs/mmanual/section15/chapter188/188c.htm

The loss of identity, formation of a new identity, and other characteristics of dissociative fugue, are found at this site of the online *Merck* reference. The disorder's relation to dissociative identity disorder, and the remarkable array of symptoms, causing much distress and disability, are described. Switching of personalities, amnesic barriers, and physical manifestations are presented. Evaluative and diagnostic procedures are listed, and variability of prognosis is explained. Successful treatment, with the aim of either achieving personality integration or cooperation among the personalities, is explained, and includes three separate phases of psychotherapy.

Dissociative Identity Disorder

Alliance for the Treatment of Trauma and Dissociation ❂
http://www.netreach.net/~alliance

This site describes the Alliance for the Treatment of Trauma and Dissociation, a professional practice of two psychotherapists offering services to practitioners, patients, and their families in the treatment of dissociative identity disorder. The disorder is discussed, as well as specific treatment services offered by the Alliance. Visitors can contact the Alliance by e-mail for further information or appointments.

Amongst Ourselves ◎ ◎ (free registration)
http://foxfiremad.com/amongst

This site contains links to information on dissociative identity disorder (DID), its causes, FAQs, symptoms, and lists a number of related links. In addition, interested parties can subscribe to the list, view the bulletin board, and join the chat room.

Dissociation.com: All About Multiple Personalities ◎ ◎
http://www.dissociation.com

Created by a professional and a person affected by dissociative disorder, this Web site offers a detailed theoretical description of dissociative disorder, including links to definitions of psychiatric terms, links to full text articles, course manuals and links to organizations, journals and other sites of interest. In addition, personal accounts of living with dissociative disorders are available, as well as a book list.

Sidran Foundation: Dissociative Identity Disorder ◎ ◎
http://www.sidran.org/didbr.html

The Sidran Foundation offers this report on dissociative identity disorder. Topics include related disorders, definition of dissociation, process of disorder development, behavioral symptoms, incidence, and diagnostic problems. Treatment information and offline support is available.

9.9 Eating Disorders

General Resources

Academy of Eating Disorders ◎ ◎ ◎
http://www.acadeatdis.org/mainpage.htm

This multidisciplinary professional organization focuses on anorexia nervosa, bulimia nervosa, binge eating disorder, and related disorders. Divisions of the Academy specialize in Academic Sciences, Human Services, Primary Medicine, Psychiatry, Psychology, Dietetics, Nursing, and Social Work. Visitors to the site can access membership information, annual conference details, facts on all eating disorders, and a bibliography of information sources. Specific topical discussions include the prevalence and consequences of eating disorders, courses and outcome of eating disorders, etiology, and treatment.

American Anorexia Bulimia Association ○ ○

http://www.aabainc.org

The American Anorexia Bulimia Association is a national nonprofit organization dedicated to the prevention and treatment of eating disorders. This site contains a number of links to informative pages on eating disorders, such as anorexia, bulimia, and binge eating. Information on symptoms, support, medical consequences, risk factors, a list of references about these disorders, as well as membership information is included.

Anorexia Nervosa and Bulimia Association ○ ○ ○

http://www.ams.queensu.ca/anab

Primarily a supportive organization for those affected by or interested in eating disorders, this Web site has extensive links to support groups, as well as lots of information on eating disorders in general, including an overview of the biology of eating disorders, treatment and diagnosis, as well as predisposing factors. There is a list of reference materials of interest, as well as online access to the Association's newsletter.

Anorexia Nervosa and Related Eating Disorders, Inc. ○ ○ ○

http://www.anred.com/toc.html

This comprehensive site offers links to fact sheets on eating disorder descriptions, statistics, warning signs and medical/psychological problems associated with these disorders, risk factors, causes, and treatment. Also, there are links to information about athletes, men, diabetes and eating disorders, less common eating disorders, such as bigarexia, night eating, Gourmand syndrome, Pica, and others. In addition, there are support resources and prevention information, a list of FAQs, personal stories, research projects, association information, reference lists, and other links of interest.

Center for Eating Disorders ○ ○ ○

http://www.eating-disorders.com

Located within Saint Joseph Medical Center, this Center provides complete treatment programs for eating disorders. Links include information about these types of disorders, online discussion forums, faculty and staff information, description of the Center, current news on relevant issues, such as body image, an events calendar, and other support information is available.

Concerned Counseling Eating Disorders ○ ○ ○

http://www.concernedcounseling.com/eatingdisorders/eatingdisordersindex.html

Supported by the Montecatini Residential Treatment Center for Women with Eating Disorders and Other Addictions, this site contains links to conference transcripts on various related topics, definitions and symptoms, warning signs, complications, treatment and recovery information, relapse issues, prevention, and support groups details. Research resources include information on clinical trials, causes, treatment, effects, and other related topics. Visitors can subscribe to the newsletter and access the referral network, online chat conference, and the concerned counseling journal.

Eating Disorders Awareness and Prevention (EDAP), Inc. ○ ○ ○

http://www.edap.org/frame337142.html

EDAP, a national nonprofit organization, increases awareness and prevention of eating disorders through community-based education and advocacy programs. Site visitors will find general information about the organization, news, notices of upcoming events, details of EDAP programs, eating disorder fact sheets, suggested reading lists, press releases for media use, links to related sites, and contact details.

Eating Disorders Site ○ ○ ○

http://closetoyou.org/eatingdisorders

Provided by the Close to You Family Network, this large database of provides comprehensive information on the various eating disorders and their assessment, diagnosis, treatment, self-tests, medical complications, nutrition-related resources, art therapy, a list of treatment centers, a reference list, current news in eating disorders, recovery and personal stories, and professional associations.

Harvard Eating Disorders Center ○ ○ ○

http://www.hedc.org

The Harvard Eating Disorders Center, a national nonprofit organization, conducts research and education activities in an effort to improve detection, treatment, and prevention of eating disorders. The site presents facts on eating disorders, suggestions on helping a child with an eating disorder and locating support resources, events calendars, program details, and information on providing support to the organization. Answers are available to common questions, helping visitors determine if they need professional help. Answers are also available concerning different forms of counseling, medication, and other forms of therapy.

International Association of
Eating Disorders Professionals (IAEDP) ○ ○

http://www.iaedp.com

The International Association of Eating Disorders Professionals offers a certification process for health professionals seeking specialized credentials in the treatment of patients with eating disorders. The Web site provides information regarding the Association, membership and certification information, and registration details for symposium events.

Mirror-Mirror: Eating Disorders Shared Awareness ◎ ◎ ◎

http://www.mirror-mirror.org/eatdis.htm

Visitors to this address will find resources on anorexia nervosa, bulimia nervosa, and compulsive overeating, including definitions, signs and symptoms, medical complications, dangerous methods of weight control, relapse prevention and warning signs, addictions, self-injury, and other topics. Specific resources are available for children, teenagers, college students, athletes, men, and older women. Additional site features include a chat forum, suggested readings, and links to national organizations, treatment centers, and other related sites. Content is written from a personal, nontechnical point of view.

New York State Psychiatric Institute's Eating Disorders Unit ◎ ◎

http://www.nyspi.cpmc.columbia.edu/nyspi/depts/psypharm/eating~1

The Eating Disorders Unit's Web page provides fundamental information for interested professionals and consumers on eating disorders, diagnostic criteria, treatment available for these disorders at the Institute, case examples and discussions, and information about the Unit itself.

Psychosomatics and Eating Disorders ◎ ◎

http://www.cyberpsych.org/pdg

The newsletter of the Psychosomatic Discussion Group is provided at this site. Links to articles on various topics such as anorexia nervosa, bowel disease and case studies, as well as links to abstracts and related papers are present. Academic course listings and links to discussion lists are also available.

Society for the Study of Ingestive Behavior ◎ ◎

http://www.jhu.edu/~ssib/ssib.html

This professional society's site includes links to current news and information on ingestive behavior topics, relevant journals, calendar of events, membership information, employment, access to the newsletter, awards, and grants, and links to related organizations and other sites. This site is searchable by keyword.

Anorexia Nervosa

Internet Mental Health: Anorexia Nervosa ◎ ◎ ◎

http://www.mentalhealth.com/dis/p20-et01.html

Information resources on anorexia nervosa at this site include American and European diagnostic criteria, an interactive online diagnostic tool, treatment information from the National Institute of Mental Health, research article citations found through PubMed, patient education booklets, general articles, and links to related sites.

National Association
of Anorexia Nervosa and Associated Disorders ◎ ◎ ◎
http://www.anad.org

This national nonprofit organization helps eating disorder victims and their families through hotline counseling, support groups, and referrals to healthcare professionals. The site offers information about the organization, eating disorder definitions, fact sheets, warning signs, therapy information, statistics and demographics, and suggestions on confronting someone with an eating disorder. Visitors will also find information on insurance discrimination and eating disorders, legislative alerts, and links to related useful sites.

Bulimia Nervosa

Internet Mental Health: Bulimia Nervosa ◎ ◎ ◎
http://www.mentalhealth.com/dis/p20-et02.html

Information resources on bulimia nervosa at this site include American and European diagnostic criteria, an interactive online diagnostic tool, treatment information from the National Institute of Mental Health, research article citations found through PubMed, patient education booklets, general articles, and links to related sites.

Cyclic Vomiting Syndrome

Bits and Pieces:
A Page for and By Adult Sufferers of Cyclic Vomiting Syndrome ◎ ◎
http://www.geocities.com/HotSprings/Falls/8150/index.html

This site provides information, discussion forums, and other resources for people interested in or affected by this disorder. At this site, there are links to professional articles, personal stories, news items, related literature resources, and links to interest.

Cyclic Vomiting Syndrome Association ◎ ◎
http://www.beaker.iupui.edu/cvsa/index.html

This organization's site provides basic information about the disorder, lists upcoming events and conferences, provides information about membership, and offers a list of related links to Web sites. In addition, there is a good amount of research information, as well as support resources.

Disease in Disguise: Cyclic Vomiting Syndrome ⊙ ⊙ ⊙
http://www.geocities.com/Heartland/Hills/4975/cvs_home.html

This Web site supplies information on the symptoms, incidence, diagnosis, treatment, causes, and presents brief case studies on this syndrome. Reference materials, links to related organizations, personal pages, and a Web ring are all found at the site.

Gourmand Syndrome

Lessons from Gourmand Syndrome ⊙ ⊙
http://www.sciencenews.org/sn_arc97/6_7_97/food.htm

Appearing as an article from *Science News Online,* information about this syndrome, its symptoms, neurological and psychological causes, behavioral consequences, and references are provided. In addition, personal accounts are available at this site.

Pica

Anorexia Nervosa and Related Eating Disorders, Inc. Pica Fact Sheet ⊙ ⊙
http://www.anred.com/pica.html

This fact sheet defines Pica, and provides general information on symptoms, causes, incidence, and consequences.

Rumination Disorder

HealthCentral.com: Rumination Disorder ⊙ ⊙
http://healthcentral.com/mhc/top/001539.cfm

The *General Health Encyclopedia* of Health Central offers several sections on rumination disorder, including its definition, symptoms, expectations, and potential complications. A link to associated medical conditions, such as hiatal hernia, may be found, and the importance of serum electrolyte and hematological workups is mentioned.

Screening Programs

National Mental Illness Screening Project:
National Eating Disorders Screening Program ○ ○ ○
http://www.nmisp.org/eat.htm

This site offers detailed information about the National Eating Disorders Screening Program, which includes an educational presentation on eating disorders, a written screening test, and the opportunity to meet privately with a health professional. The site presents general information and answers to questions about the screening program, a sample screening test, and links to program sponsors.

9.10 Elimination Disorders

Encopresis

Problems With Soiling and Bowel Control ○ ○
http://www.brooklane.org/whitepgs/children/chsoil.html

Reasons for soiling and the social and psychiatric difficulties that coexist with encopresis in children are discussed at this paper of the American Academy of Child and Adolescent Psychiatry. The importance of a complete physical exam is stressed, and a description of soiling not caused by an illness or disability is found. Combination treatment strategies are reviewed.

Treatment Guidelines for
Primary Nonretentive Encopresis and Stool Toileting Refusal ○ ○ ○
http://www.aafp.org/afp/990415ap/2171.html

American Family Physician presents this excellent online clinical guide to the treatment of primary encopresis, with the characteristics of the disorder and the necessary medical assessment introduced. A program of appropriate behavior management and an incentive/reward-based system, as well as other guidelines assimilated from the literature on toilet training and encopresis are provided. Identification of physical or behavioral pathology, a complete physical examination checklist, and a table outlining differential diagnoses to be considered are found. Several steps follow that emphasize practicality and ease of implementation of the guidelines. An illustrative case is provided, as well as a convenient, patient information handout.

Enuresis

Primary Nocturnal Enuresis: Current Concepts ◎ ◎ ◎
http://www.aafp.org/afp/990301ap/1205.html

Causative factors of primary nocturnal enuresis and the significant psychosocial impact associated with the condition are reviewed in this article, courtesy of *American Family Physician*. A comprehensive review of the literature includes the etiology of primary nocturnal enuresis, with complete summaries of genetic, maturational, and other potential causes; important assessment considerations; and suggestions for consistent, goal-oriented pharmacological and nonpharmcological interventions.

9.11 Factitious Disorders

Asher-Meadow Center for Education and Prevention of Munchausen Syndrome by Proxy ◎ ◎
http://www.bcpl.lib.md.us/~agravels

Resources at this site include links to current news articles and descriptive fact sheets about Munchausen Syndrome by Proxy, its symptoms, assessment and identification, a comprehensive FBI report on various aspects of this syndrome, and a bibliography. In addition, there are links and information about support groups and organizations, case studies, related Web sites, and access to an online newsletter.

Dr. Marc Feldman's Munchausen Syndrome, Factitious Disorder, and Munchausen by Proxy Page ◎ ◎ ◎
http://ourworld.compuserve.com/homepages/Marc_Feldman_2

Within this comprehensive site, there are links to articles, case reports, firsthand accounts, general information, and abstracts about various aspects of these psychiatric disorders.

Munchausen Syndrome by Proxy: by Keith T. Huynh ◎ ◎ ◎
http://www.medicine.uiowa.edu/pa/sresrch/Huynh/Huynh/sld001.htm

This site contains a slide presentation that provides comprehensive and descriptive information on this syndrome in an organized format. Topics presented include case study reports, definitions of the condition, history, epidemiology, causes, risk factors, incidence, diagnosis strategies, tools and assessment, clinical signs and evidence, prognosis and follow-up, as well as a worthwhile conclusion to the information and evidence presented.

9.12 **False Memory Syndrome**

False Memory Syndrome Facts ◎ ◎
http://www.fmsf.com

This site offers article citations (occasionally with quotes or abstracts), links and information resources related to false memory syndrome, presenting information mainly refuting the false memory syndrome theory. Resources are available under the categories of scientific analysis, clinical issues, legal issues, media, organizations, philosophy, and support.

False Memory Syndrome Foundation ◎ ◎
http://www.hiwaay.net

The False Memory Syndrome Foundation seeks reasons for the spread of this disorder, works for the prevention of new cases, and aids the primary and secondary victims of the Syndrome. Resources at the site include information on the Foundation, activities, bibliography, events, articles about this syndrome, an online newsletter, mailing lists, and links to related sites.

Recovered Memory Project ◎ ◎ ◎
http://www.brown.edu/Departments/Taubman_Center/Recovmem/Archive.html

This project's Web site is devoted to issues relating to recovered memory, including case files from legal proceedings, clinical and other scientific cases, and other corroborated recovered memory cases. There is access to articles, abstracts, data files, research summaries, peer-reviewed studies, and other publications relating to recovered memories. A large number of links to other resources is included in the research and scholarly resources section. The project is directed by Professor Ross Cheit of Brown University.

9.13 **Impulse-Control Disorders, Other**

Intermittent Explosive Disorder

Treating Intermittent Explosive Disorder with Neurofeedback ◎
http://www.brainwavetx.com/library/explosiv.html

This site presents a case study of a young male with intermittent explosive disorder, and his positive experience with neurofeedback. The article suggests that EEG biofeedback may help in reducing abuse of spouses, partners, and children.

Kleptomania

Kleptomania: Symptoms ○

http://mentalhelp.net/disorders/sx23.htm

Summarized criteria of kleptomania, taken from the *Diagnostic and Statistical Manual of Mental Disorders, 4th Ed.* is presented at this site of the Mentalhealth.Net online information source.

Pathological Gambling

CME Reviews: Pathological Gambling ○ ○ ○

http://www.cme-reviews.com/pathologicalgambling.html

CME Reviews offers online Continuing Medical Education courses for psychiatrists, neurologists, and primary care physicians. Professionals can read full-text articles on compulsive gambling, review educational objectives, and take a quiz at the end of the article. Titles include The Molecular Genetics of Pathological Gambling; Serotonergic and Nonadrenergic Function on Pathological Gambling; Pathological Gambling: A Negative State Model and Its Implications for Behavioral Treatments; Pharmacologic Approaches in the Treatment of Pathological Gambling; and Problem and Pathological Gambling: A Consumer Perspective.

Illinois Institute for
Addiction Recovery: About Pathological Gambling ○ ○

http://www.addictionrecov.org/aboutgam.htm

This site describes pathological gambling, including a discussion of differences between casual social gambling and pathological gambling, affected groups, and teen gambling. The site also discusses the Custer Three-Phase Model, including the winning, losing, and desperation phases. A link is available to information on diagnosis, prevention, and treatment of addiction in the workplace.

Mount Sinai Department of Psychiatry: Compulsive,
Impulsive, and Anxiety Disorders Program: Gambling ○

http://www.mssm.edu/psychiatry/gambling.html

This site provides a short description of pathological gambling, lists the department's research interests, and offers contact information. Cognitive-behavioral group therapy is currently offered by the department for this disorder.

**North American Training Institute
(NATI)—Compulsive Gambling** ❂ ❂ ❂ (free registration)

The North American Training Institute, a division of the Minnesota Council on Gambling, provides products and courses aimed towards the education and prevention of compulsive gambling, especially among senior citizens and teens at risk. A listing of educational books, audiovisual materials, and professional training programs offered by the organization are described. Current and back issues of *Wanna Bet* magazine are offered online especially for teens concerned about gambling. Also available from NATI are translated materials and information on state and national reports examining compulsive gambling problems and exploring long-term management strategies. Users who take an online survey can receive free informational packets. A brief registration for ordering materials is required.

Pyromania

Predictors of Violent Adult Behavior ❂ ❂ ❂

http://www.ozemail.com.au/~jsjp/violence.htm

A "predictive triad" of adult violent behavior, including persistent bedwetting, cruelty to animals, and firesetting, is described at this online review article. The classic analysis of a pyromaniac is discussed, and, out of the three triad characteristics, pyromania is described as being most widely associated with adult violent behavior. The distinctions between firesetters and nonfiresetters in attempting to seek internal solutions to their problems is explained, with firesetters more apt to seek external objects on which to project their emotions. The possible existence of physical unattractiveness, multiple medical problems, and social isolation often found in these individuals are discussed, and the importance of recognition of the triad in a person's background is emphasized.

Sexual Addiction

American Foundation for Addiction Research (AFAR) ❂ ❂

http://www.addictionresearch.com

This organization supports research and education on addictive disorders by providing funds for addiction research. In addition to organization information, there is a searchable database on sexual addiction, research project funding priorities, general facts about addiction, and donation information.

National Council on Sexual Addiction and Compulsivity (NCSAC) ❂ ❂

http://www.ncsac.org/main.html

This national nonprofit organization is devoted to the promotion of the awareness of sexual addiction and compulsivity in both public and professional areas. In addition to detailed member information, there are media contact resources, a suggested reading list, NCSAC position papers on sexual addictions, support groups, and general information about sexual addiction and compulsivity.

SexHelp.com: Dr. Carne's Online Resources ◎ ◎
http://www.sexhelp.com

This site provides information about sexual addiction, its causes and treatments, as well as interactive tests, articles by Dr. Carnes on sexual addiction and other topics. In addition, there is an online bulletin, a calendar of events, a suggested reading list, and links to sexual addiction databases, clinics and clinicians, and other support resources.

Trichotillomania

Trichotillomania Learning Center ◎ ◎ ◎
http://www.trich.org

This nonprofit organization provides informational resources on this compulsive disorder to interested persons. The site offers links to support groups, therapists, and other sites of interest, an events calendar, basic information on the disorder, membership information, and contact details.

9.14 Infancy, Childhood, or Adolescence Disorders, Other

Reactive Attachment Disorder

Association for Treatment and Training in the Attachment of Children ◎ ◎ ◎
http://www.attach.org

This coalition of parents and professionals exchanges information on attachment and bonding issues. Information on healthy attachment, membership details, events and training notices, a newsletter, recommended reading lists, book reviews, assessment instrument reviews, and clinical notes are found at this address. Details of the organization's structure, research reviews, links to related sites and contact details for non-Internet resources, and lists of suggested professional resources are also available.

Attachment Disorder Support Group ◎ ◎ ◎
http://www.syix.com/adsg

The Attachment Disorder Support Group provides education and support to parents facing the challenge of raising a child with reactive attachment disorder. A description of attachment disorder, symptoms, potential parenting mistakes in a child with this disorder, support resources, and links to related sites are listed at the address. Also provided are chat forums, articles, personal stories, answers to frequently asked questions (FAQs), information on choosing a therapist, directories of group homes, centers, and other resources, and lists of suggested books and other publications. Visitors can also search the site by keyword.

Selective Mutism

Selective Mutism Foundation ⚙ ⚙ ⚙

http://personal.mia.bellsouth.net/mia/g/a/garden/garden/home.htm

This foundation's site offers considerable information on the description, diagnosis, assessment, treatment, and other issues concerning selective mutism. Also available are current research studies, a bibliography, healthcare providers referral list, information about the Foundation and its members, and a number of links to related sites. Special education information can be accessed. Correspondence with Foundation directors is encouraged.

9.15 Learning Disorders

General Resources

Instant Access Treasure Chest:
The Foreign Language Teacher's Guide to Learning Disabilities ⚙ ⚙ ⚙

http://azstarnet.com/~ask/ed/ADD_Links.html

Links at this site provide visitors with access to valuable learning disability resources on the Internet. Sites are categorized by topic, including assistive technology, attention-deficit/hyperactivity disorder, auditory deficits, college policies for students with disabilities, commercial sites, conference handouts, dyslexia, foreign language and learning disabilities, general information, government resources, hyperlexia, learning styles, legal information, questions and answers, teaching students with disabilities, and visual deficits. Many sites are listed under each topic, making this site a valuable starting point for Internet information on learning disorders.

LD Online ⚙ ⚙ ⚙

http://www.ldonline.org

This interactive site offers a wealth of information on learning disabilities and attention-deficit/hyperactivity disorders, including assessment, behavior, legal information, and other related topics. Links to the online newsletter, the online store, various discussion forums and events calendars, and a large listing of resource guides are available. Personal stories and a searchable database are also present.

Learning Disabilities Association (LDA) ⊙ ⊙ ⊙
http://www.ldanatl.org

This national nonprofit organization is comprised of individuals with learning disabilities, their families, and professionals, and aims to enhance the education and general welfare of children and adults with learning disabilities. Information about LDA includes goals of the organization, a description of services offered, and membership details. Organizations and other sources for information are listed at the site, under topic categories including audio tapes, books on tape, culturally diverse national organizations, government agencies, links to other resources, other learning disabilities organizations, publications for professionals, recent publications, related organizations, toll-free resources for adults with learning disabilities, video tapes, and Web search tools. Information alerts and bulletins, notices of upcoming events, fact sheets, links to state chapters, contact details, and subscription information for LDA publications are all available at the address.

National Institute of Mental Health (NIMH): Learning Disabilities ⊙ ⊙ ⊙
http://www.nimh.nih.gov/publicat/learndis.htm

This online educational pamphlet describes different types of learning disabilities, the causes of these disabilities, diagnosis, education options, medication, and family coping strategies. The site also provides details on current research, government aid, and sources of information and support.

Unicorn Children's Foundation ⊙ ⊙ ⊙
http://www.saveachild.com

This nonprofit Foundation supports parents and professionals through research, treatment advocacy, and information exchange. A nationwide directory of professionals and involved parents, fact sheets, presentations, warning signs, chat forums for both parents and professionals, a list of accommodations for students with learning disorders, common questions and answers, news, event listings, and an online store are all available at this site. Visitors can also download forms, for both professional and caregiver use, helping in the diagnosis of communication and learning disorders.

Disorders of Written Expression (Dysgraphia)

Diagnosis and Intervention Strategies
for Disorders of Written Language ☺ ☺

http://www.udel.edu/bkirby/asperger/dysgraphia_mjkay.html

A detailed discussion of written language disorders, written by an Ed.D., is presented at this site. Topics include multiple brain mechanisms, physical and psychological requirements for written language, dysgraphia classification systems, assessment issues, intervention for written language disorders, and a discussion summary.

Mathematics Disorder (Dyscalculia Syndrome)

Dyscalculia International Consortium ☺

http://www.shianet.org/~reneenew/DIC.html

Resources on dyscalculia at this site include links to information related to diagnosis, research, prognosis, assistance, and education law. Educational math books are listed at the site, and can be ordered through links to Amazon.com.

Dyscalculia Syndrome: Master's Thesis by Renee M. Newman ☺ ☺ ☺

http://www.shianet.org/~reneenew/thesis.html

This site allows interested individuals to free access to this thesis devoted to the study of dyscalculia. Extensive coverage of various topics is present, including describing the disorder, personal accounts, statistical data, testing and diagnostic issues, treatment and therapeutic strategies, including educational and teaching advice, cognitive assessment, and other information. Tables, references, and related information are all included.

Nonverbal Learning Disorders

NLDline: Nonverbal Learning Disorders ☺ ☺

http://www.nldline.com/welcome.htm

Information at this site devoted to nonverbal learning disorders describes this disorder in detail, including specific types, and also offers a discussion of NLDline's purpose and a section devoted to useful information resources. These resources include suggested book and video lists, support resources, hotlines, links to related sites, and sources for audio tapes.

What is Nonverbal Learning Disorder Syndrome ◎ ◎

http://www.matrixparents.org/faqnonverbal.html

First appearing in *Hydrocephalus Association Newsletter*, this article describes the syndrome and its effects on various aspects of the patient life, including educational symptoms. Biological causes are discussed and therapeutic interventions are presented.

Reading Disorder (Dyslexia)

Bright Solutions for Dyslexia ◎ ◎ ◎

http://www.dys-add.com

Bright Solutions for Dyslexia is an organization offering seminars, inservices, training, and coordination of parent programs in techniques related to teaching dyslexics. Definitions of dyslexia from four sources—symptoms of dyslexia, research discussions, and testing and assessment tools are discussed at the site.

Davis Dyslexia Association International ◎ ◎ ◎

http://www.dyslexia.com

The Davis Dyslexia Association International offers workshops and training to teachers and professionals on helping individuals with dyslexia and other learning disabilities. A resource library at the site includes articles, questions and answers about dyslexia, book excerpts, and links to other information sources. Educational materials, professional resources, chat forums, a Davis Program provider directory, and workshop calendars are all found at the site. Resources are provided in English, Spanish, German, French, Dutch, and Italian.

Dyslexia—The Gift: Internet Circle of Friends ◎ ◎ ◎

http://www.dyslexia.com/links.htm

More than 200 sites related to dyslexia are linked through this address. Sites are indexed by topic or services offered, including information and other resources, education resources, autism and Asperger's syndrome information, resources, and support, general medical, psychological, and health resources, parenting resources and online communities, general education resources, home schooling resources, teacher magazines, ideas, and networks, gifted education resources, K–12 school resource sites, college and university sites, fundraising and foundation sites, virtual community and magazine sites, educational and curriculum materials, career information, online reference help with reading, writing, and spelling, the dyslexic viewpoint, learning centers and clinics, and international organizations and resources.

International Dyslexia Association ◎ ◎ ◎
http://www.interdys.org

This nonprofit Association is devoted to the study and treatment of dyslexia. Site resources include information about the organization, position papers, descriptions of branch services, membership details, conference and seminar calendars, an online bookstore, technology resources, legal and legislative information, research discussions, press releases, and a bulletin board for site visitors. The site also offers a detailed discussion of dyslexia, including information and links to Internet resources for adolescents, college students, parents, adults, educators, and other professionals.

Mathematics and Dyslexia ◎ ◎
http://www.ldonline.org/ld_indepth/math_skills/ida_math_fall98.html

The International Dyslexia Association provided this fact sheet outlining the problem of mathematical dyslexia. Related disorders, the symptoms and educational manifestations, intervention strategies, and references are included.

Sensory Integration Dysfunction

Sensory Integration Dysfunction ◎ ◎
http://www.comfortconnection.org/sensory_integration_dysfunction.htm

Supported by the Family Resource Center, this site provides links to home pages, fact sheets, support organizations, and an FAQ about sensory integration dysfunction. In addition, there are links to educational and school organization sites, related medical sites, and support groups.

9.16 Mental Retardation

American Association on Mental Retardation (AAMR) ◎ ◎
http://www.aamr.org

"AAMR promotes global development and dissemination of progressive policies, sound research, effective practices, and universal human rights for people with intellectual disabilities." Site resources include information about the AAMR, current news, bookstore, membership information, reference materials from the annual meeting, free access to the *American Journal on Mental Retardation* and *Mental Retardation*, a list of the divisions of the AAMR, and links to the discussion group and chat rooms.

Down's Syndrome WWW Page ◎ ◎ ◎

http://www.nas.com/downsyn

Created in part by members of the Down syndrome LISTSERV, this site provides a number of informative links for professionals and consumers. Included are links to worldwide organizations relevant to Down syndrome, support groups, a events and conferences calendar, education and inclusion information, family essays, healthcare guidelines, and a large number of online medical articles covering all aspects of the syndrome. There is online access to Disability Solutions, a publication providing information on mental disability, and links to medical essays and other informative Web sites on Down syndrome.

Mental Health Aspects of
Mental Retardation and Dual Diagnosis at The NADD ◎ ◎ ◎

http://www.thenadd.org/aboutdd.htm

NADD, an association for persons with developmental disabilities and mental health needs, provides this site on dual diagnosis: psychiatric disorders in persons with mental retardation. Topics that are discussed include a description of dual diagnosis and mental retardation, reasons for its prevalence, and available treatments.

The Arc of the United States ◎ ◎ ◎

http://www.thearc.org

This nonprofit organization is committed to the welfare of all children and adults with mental retardation and their families. The site offers contact details, information on government affairs, member, chapter, and communication services, publications, promotional products, fact sheets, and local and state home pages. A comprehensive list of links offers additional sources for information, parenting information and support, disability resource lists and directories, other national disability organizations, international disability organizations, assistive technology, software, and electronic information, health promotion and disability prevention resources, universities, disability service providers, federally funded projects on mental retardation, information on disability legislation, federal agencies, and organizational and grant resources.

9.17 **Mood Disorders**

General Resources

Depression and Related
Affective Disorders Association (DRADA) ⊙ ⊙

http://www.med.jhu.edu/drada

This site provides information about DRADA, links to research reports and other reference materials, book reviews, an online store for videos and books, support groups and other related organizations, as well as a link to clinical research studies seeking participants.

DSM-IV Criteria ⊙

http://members.aol.com/faery116/dsm.html

This site lists the DSM-IV criteria for major depressive episode, hypomanic episode, bipolar I disorder, bipolar II disorder, manic episode, major depressive disorder, mixed episode, dysthymic disorder, and cyclothymic disorder.

Mental Health Clinical Research Center ⊙ ⊙

http://www.mhcrc.unc.edu

This Center, located within the University of North Carolina at Chapel Hill, conducts research that examines the neurobiology and treatment of mood and psychotic disorders, as well as the psychopathology and physiology of stress. At this site, summaries of the major research focus issues, such as mood disorder neurobiology, pathophysiology of stress, neurobiology of psychotic disorders, and psychopharmacology are displayed. Overviews of the Center's core services programs, such as the behavioral and cognitive neuroscience core, and the clinical assessment and procedures core, are readily viewable. A link to clinical trials currently running at the University, news updates from the Center, and a faculty directory are located at this site.

Mood Disorders Association of British Columbia ⊙ ⊙

http://www.lynx.net/~mda

This association's Web site has links to general information about certain mood disorders, and offers an information request form and links to related sites.

Mood Disorders Clinic ⊙ ⊙

http://www.psychiatry.ubc.ca:80/mood/md_home.html

At this site there is information regarding depressive and bipolar disorders for both professionals and consumers. Information on assessment and diagnosis, symptoms lists, as well as information on the Canadian clinic itself is present.

National Depressive and Manic-Depressive Association ⊙ ⊙ ⊙
http://www.ndmda.org

The National Depressive and Manic-Depressive Association strives to educate patients, families, professionals, and the public concerning the nature of depressive and bipolar disorders as treatable medical disorders, foster self-help, eliminate discrimination, and improve access to care. The site contains extensive information on the Association and links to general information on depression and bipolar disorder and related issues. Links to support groups, patient assistance programs, education, advocacy, clinical trials, and reference materials are listed.

Bipolar Disorders

Bipolar Children and Teens Homepage ⊙ ⊙
http://members.aol.com/_ht_a/DrgnKpr1/BPCAT.html

Personal stories and links to useful Internet resources are included at this site devoted to bipolar disorder in children. General information for patients and parents, news, chat forums, service providers, professional associations, prevention resources, Internet directories, advocacy and policy information, medication information, support groups, and major organizations are found through this site.

Bipolar Disorder Diagnosis, Treatment, and Support ⊙ ⊙
http://www.ndmda.org/biover.htm

This fact sheet from the National Depressive and Manic-Depressive Association discusses major depressive disorder and bipolar disorder, including causes, general statistics, and symptoms of depression and mania.

Bipolar Disorder in Children and Adolescents ⊙ ⊙
http://www.klis.com/chandler/pamphlet/bipolar/content.htm

Visitors to this site will find a general description of bipolar disorder and associated disorders, including case studies. Other topics include prevalence (statistics), causes, diagnosis, comorbidity, mania in young children, the course and prognosis of bipolar disorder, factors making another episode more or less likely, and how bipolar disorder can adversely affect a person's life.

Bipolar Disorder in Children and Adolescents: Advice to Parents ⊙ ⊙
http://www.nami.org/youth/bipolar.htm

An article written by a professor of psychiatry at the University of Texas Medical Branch is available at this site. Detailed but nontechnical information about the disorder is available for parents, including symptoms in children and adolescents, evaluation, treatment, and medications. The article also offers specific issues in the education of children and teenagers about their disorder.

Bipolar Disorder Patient/Family Handout ⊚ ⊚ ⊚

http://www.psychguides.com/bphe.html

Resources at this site answer common questions about bipolar disorder, with topics including causes, diagnosis, genetics, symptoms, different patterns of the disease, treatment, medication and side effects, and psychotherapy. Contact information for support groups and suggestions for those diagnosed with the disorder, and a list of suggested readings are also found at the site.

Bipolar Disorders Portal ⊚ ⊚ ⊚

http://www.pendulum.org

Included in this Web site are various links to bipolar information, including diagnosis, treatment and medicine, support groups, books and other reference materials, alternative treatments, and a list of comorbid disorders. A number of bipolar-related links are also included.

Bipolar Information Network ⊚ ⊚

http://www.moodswing.org

This site was generated to provide online resources for the public interested in bipolar disorder. Links include an FAQ section, a bookstore, a list of advocacy groups, and links to related sites.

Bipolar Kids Homepage ⊚ ⊚

http://www.geocities.com/EnchantedForest/1068

This address serves as an Internet directory for patients, caregivers, doctors, and teachers searching for resources on bipolar disorders in children. General information sources, professional associations, articles, and resources on educational issues are found through the site. Parents will also find a questionnaire assisting physicians in diagnosing bipolar disorder and a mailing list for parents of bipolar children.

Internet Mental Health: Cyclothymic Disorder ⊚ ⊚ ⊚

http://www.mentalhealth.com/dis/p20-md03.html

Complete descriptions of cyclothymic disorders are found at this page of the Internet Mental Health database, with an outline of diagnostic criteria accompanied by links to differential diagnoses. Criteria for major depressive, manic, mixed, and hypomanic episodes are reviewed, and a link to the National Institute of Mental Health provides an overview of mood disorders, including courses of treatment and recovery. An online diagnosis to be used in conjunction with a full physical examination and diagnostic interview, is provided, and treatment information is offered.

Joy Ikelman's Information on Bipolar Disorder ◉ ◉

http://www.frii.com/~parrot/bip.html

As well as the author's own experiences with the disorder, there is information on treatment, self-education, assessment and classification of bipolar disorder information from professional organizations, suicide advice, news updates and links to related Web sites.

MEDLINEplus: Bipolar Disorder ◉ ◉ ◉

http://medlineplus.nlm.nih.gov/medlineplus/bipolardisorder.html

Resources from MEDLINEplus on bipolar disorder include links to information from the National Library of Medicine and National Institutes of Health, and other government and general resources. General information and overviews, research resources, information in Spanish, law and policy resources, news sites, organizations, information for teenagers, and treatment details are found through this address.

Mental Health InfoSource: Bipolar Disorders Information Center ◉ ◉ ◉

http://www.mhsource.com/bipolar/index.html

This site offers a general discussion of bipolar disorder, including diagnosis, treatment, and contact information for sources of help. Visitors can ask questions of experts, read archived questions and answers, and earn Continuing Medical Education credits while reading about current trends in the treatment of bipolar disorder. Chat forums, online support resources, treatment information, directories of support organizations, patient education articles, a site search engine, and links to related sites are all found through this address.

Moodswing.org:
Online Resources for People with Bipolar Disorder ◉ ◉

http://www.moodswing.org

Answers to frequently asked questions (FAQs), links to advocacy groups, an online bookstore through Amazon.com, and links to useful related sites are found at this address. Visitors can also search the site by keyword.

Psycom.net: Bipolar Disorder ◉ ◉ ◉

http://www.psycom.net/depression.central.bipolar.html

This site provides links to many resources on bipolar disorder, offering news of research advances, general information for patients, answers to frequently asked questions, suggested reading lists, practice guidelines, consensus statements, and support resources. Professionals can find links to sites offering specific discussions of diagnosis and treatment issues.

Resources for Parents of Kids with Bipolar Disorder ☺ ☺
http://www.bpso.org/BPKids.htm

The mother of a child diagnosed with bipolar disorder offers a list of suggested resources at this site. Materials include suggested books for children, books for parents, general books, articles from professional journals, books on therapy, organizations, Internet resources, audio tapes for children, videotapes, articles from popular media, and psychiatric hospitals for children. Links to online resources are provided when available.

Society for Manic Depression ☺ ☺
http://www.societymd.org

Online patient support forums, including a remission program, and a detailed description of bipolar disorder are available at this address. Topics include open communication with a psychiatrist, diagnosis, denial, manic and depressive states and medications. Some chat forums, allowing individual online communication with specialists, are available to those with a membership, which requires a fee.

Stanley Center for the Innovative Treatment of Bipolar Disorder ☺ ☺
http://www.wpic.pitt.edu/stanley

As part of the Stanley Foundation Bipolar Network, this research center's Web site includes informative links to current clinical trials, access to the Center's newsletter, affective disorders literature, information on genetics and bipolar disorder study, conference information, as well as an overview of the Center's background and goals.

World Wide Handbook on Child and Youth Psychiatry and Allied Disciplines: Bipolar Disorder ☺ ☺
http://Web.inter.nl.net/hcc/T.Compernolle/bipol.htm

An organizational and occupational psychiatrist has developed this handbook, and presents information on bipolar disorder in children at this site. Information includes an introduction to the disorder, symptoms, assessment, differential diagnosis, epidemiology, etiology, treatment, prevention, and prognosis. Reference citations and information about the author is available.

Depressive Disorders

Andrew's Depression Page ☺ ☺ ☺
http://www.blarg.net/~charlatn/depression/Depression.html

This site contains links to numerous online fact sheets and sites on various issues regarding depression. Topics included are treatment, suicide, online support resources, mood scales, general mental health, children and adolescents, general psychiatry links, a depression FAQ, and a collection of papers written by people with depression.

Asher Center for the Study and
Treatment of Depressive Disorders ⊚ ⊚

http://www.ashercenter.nwu.edu

As part of Northwestern University, this multidisciplinary center combines basic and applied research to address depressive disorders. Brief summaries of clinical research projects, as well as links to collaborating centers and departments are included. Faculty and staff information, as well as training opportunities, seminar information, and other links of interest are present.

Depression.com ⊚ ⊚ ⊚

http://depression.com

This online database of Internet resources on depression includes links to current news in depression, information on types of depression, therapies, anxiety, sleep, sex, suicide, weight and depression, support information for those living with a depressed person, information on the various drugs used in treatment, and a list of alternative therapies. Links to related sites are included.

Depression.com: Seasonal Affective Disorder ⊚ ⊚

http://www.depression.com/health_library/types/types_02_seasonal.html

This site describes different aspects of seasonal affective disorder, including case studies, the spectrum of the disorder, general statistics by geographic location, light therapy, simulated sunrise therapy, light therapy for nonseasonal depression, and general suggestions for those suffering from seasonal depression. Links are provided to information on several therapies.

Depression FAQ ⊚ ⊚

http://www.psych.helsinki.fi/~janne/asdfaq

This site defines depression and specific depressive disorders, including dysthymia, bipolar depression, seasonal affective disorder (SAD), postpartum depression, endogenous depression, and atypical depression. The causes and treatment of depression, including medications and electroconvulsive therapy (ECT) are discussed, and visitors can find links to related sites, a chat forum, and suggested readings.

Depression Resources List ⊚ ⊚ ⊚

http://www.execpc.com/~corbeau

This site contains numerous links to newsgroups, discussion forums, general mental health and specific disorder sites, support groups, and links to reference materials in five major areas: depression, bipolar disorder, suicide, panic, and depression treatment.

Depression: What You Need to Know ◎ ◎

http://www.vh.org/Patients/IHB/Psych/PatientEdMaterials/DepressionNIMH.html

This report summarizes the types of depressive disorders, supplying definitions for each, presents symptoms of depression and mania, suggests causes, discusses treatments, provides warnings about side effects, and offers information about behavioral therapy and self-help issues.

Dr. Ivan's Depression Central ◎ ◎ ◎

http://www.psycom.net/depression.central.html

This comprehensive site, devoted to information on the numerous types of depressive disorders and treatments for those suffering from depression and other mood disorders, contains a large number of links to articles, papers, and other informative sources of relevant topics, including support groups, research centers, and psychiatrists specializing in mood disorders. In addition, there are links to the diagnosis, classification, and treatment of depression and mood disorders, as well as to other important Web sites and newsgroups devoted to depression and other mental illnesses.

Dysthymic Disorder ◎ ◎

http://mentalhelp.net/disorders/sx14t.htm

This fact sheet describes Dysthymic Disorder, psychotherapy choices, drug treatment, and support issues.

Mentalhelp.net: All About Depression ◎ ◎ ◎

http://depression.mentalhelp.net

Depression information for consumers at this site includes details of symptoms, treatment, research (through PubMed), as well as links to online information resources, organizations, and online support. Visitors can also take an online quiz for a personal assessment of depression.

National Foundation for Depressive Illness (NAFDI), Inc. ◎ ◎

http://www.depression.org/index.html

Within this Web site there is information on the foundation's goals, descriptions of the symptoms, treatment and diagnosis of depressive illness, a list of the national board of directors and advisors, and online access to the NAFDI newsletter.

Post-Natal Depression ◎ ◎ ◎

http://www.rcpsych.ac.uk/public/help/pndep/dpn_frame.htm

In addition to describing the symptoms and frequency of occurrence, this article outlines the time course of onset, causes, especially endocrine factors, treatment options, related mental problems, prognosis, prevention information, and supportive organizations and literature.

Pregnancy and Depression ◎ ◎ ◎

http://www.angelfire.com/de2/depressionpregnancy/index.html

Resources on depression and pregnancy at this site include full-text professional journal articles, news stories, answers to readers' questions, discussion forums, and links to related sites. Similar resources are available on the treatment of depression during breastfeeding, pregnancy, childbirth, and mothering. Visitors will also find MEDLINE-based reference lists on pregnancy and breastfeeding, access to PubMed, MEDLINE, and MedExplorer for individual services, relevant sites listed by drug, and suggested reading lists.

Seasonal Affective Disorder (SAD): About Light, Depression, & Melatonin ◎ ◎

http://www.newtechpub.com/phantom/contrib/sad.htm

A professional therapist presents information at this site about seasonal affective disorder. Topics include light therapy, sadness, anxiety, irritability, violence, other symptoms, causes of the disorder, the history of light therapy, and the significance of winter holidays in coping with seasonal changes. Detailed discussions of light and melatonin, bright light therapy, and suggestions for avoiding seasonal depression are available at the site.

Seasonal Affective Disorder (SAD) Information Sheet ◎ ◎

http://www.outsidein.co.uk/bodyclock/sadinfo.htm

This Web site, created by Outside In, Ltd. provides information about seasonal affective disorder (SAD), including symptoms, treatment, products, mechanism of action, a symptom scoring table, and research abstracts.

Wing of Madness ◎ ◎ ◎

http://www.wingofmadness.com/index.htm

Described as one of the oldest depression pages available, this site offers a number of informative pages on all aspects of depression. There are a number of questions about depression and their answers, which include symptoms, treatments, online and offline support, reference materials, online articles and booklets, related newsgroups and support organizations, and more. There is a fact sheet on antidepressant advice, a book list, and a number of depression-related links.

Winter Depression Information ◎ ◎

http://www.psych.helsinki.fi/~janne/mood/sad.html

This article provides background information on winter depression, also termed seasonal affective disorder, as well as information about treatment products, and links to other Web sites related to the treatment of this disorder.

9.18 **Paranoia**

Aliens on Earth: Paranoia   ○ ○
http://www.ufomind.com/explore/psych/paranoid

Visitors to this address will find links to sites offering information on paranoia, conspiracy theories, and paranoid personality disorder. Links are categorized under topics, including general information, conspiracy claims, mental disorders, and flaws of logic and perception. A newsletter, search engine, and online bookstore are also available from the site. Many sites found through this address contain information unrelated to paranoid personality disorder.

Hopkins Technology: Paranoia   ○ ○
http://www.hoptechno.com/paranoia.htm

This site provides a patient education booklet on paranoia from the National Institute of Mental Health. The text defines paranoia and discusses specific mental conditions involving paranoia, including paranoid personality disorder, delusional disorder, and paranoid schizophrenia. Genetic contributions, biochemistry, and stress are discussed as possible causes of these disorders. Current treatments, including medications and psychotherapy, and outlook for paranoid patients are also discussed. The site lists references for additional information.

Useful Information on Paranoia   ○ ○
http://www.mhsource.com/hy/paranoia.html

This comprehensive fact sheet describes paranoia, presents case studies, provides information on paranoid symptoms, describes different types of paranoia, suggests causes, and offers information on treatment.

9.19 **Personality Disorders**

General Resources

Aggression and Transference in Severe Personality Disorders   ○ ○
http://www.mhsource.com/pt/p950216.html

This scientific article summarizes the association between aggressive behavior expression and personality disorders. Theories of aggression and how it relates to personality disorder, therapeutic procedures in dealing with the patients, symptoms, treatment assessment and reviews on recent literature dealing with this subject are included. References are listed.

Borderline Personality Disorder and More ◎ ◎
http://www.mental-health-matters.com/borderline.html

Links are available at this address to sites offering information and other resources related to antisocial, avoidant, borderline, conduct, and narcissistic personality disorders. Short descriptions are provided with each site link, and links are also available to book descriptions from Amazon.com, therapist and doctor directories, and hotlines.

Antisocial Personality Disorder

Internet Mental Health: Antisocial Personality Disorder ◎ ◎ ◎
http://www.mentalhealth.com/dis/p20-pe04.html

American and European diagnostic criteria, online interactive diagnostic tools, extensive treatment resources, research articles searches through PubMed, and patient education booklets are offered at this site. Links are also available to several additional sources for information. This site serves as a suitable source for general professional information on the disorder.

Psychopathology and
Antisocial Personality Disorder: A Journey into the Abyss ◎ ◎
http://www.flash.net/~sculwell/psychopathology.htm

This site discusses antisocial personality disorder, classification systems of psychopaths, and testing and assessment. Definitions of the primary psychopath, the secondary or neurotic psychopath, and the dyssocial psychopath are accompanied by discussions of comparative differences and the effects of studying a noninstitutionalized population. Information is technical, and presented for professional use.

Avoidant Personality Disorder

Avoidant Personality Disorder Homepage ◎ ◎
http://www.geocities.com/HotSprings/3764

This site is devoted to providing information on avoidant personality disorder. Included are a number of links to clinical descriptions, and diagnostic criteria for this and related disorders. Also included are three personal experience articles, a book list, and a list of relevant links.

PSYweb.com: Avoidant Personality Disorder   ☺

http://www.psyweb.com/Mdisord/avpd.html

A definition and DSM-IV criteria for avoidant personality disorder are available at this site, as well as links to descriptions of psychiatric therapies, including Adlerian, behavior, existential, gestalt, person-centered, psychoanalytic, rational-emotive, reality, and transactional analysis therapies.

Borderline Personality Disorder

Borderline Personality Disorder   ☺ ☺

http://www.palace.net/~llama/psych/bpd.html

This address offers a professional overview of several schools of thought concerning borderline personality disorder. Topics include Kernberg's Borderline Personality Organization, Gunderson's theories, the Diagnostic Interview for Borderlines, and the DSM-IV definition. The site also discusses possible causes of the disorder.

Borderline Personality Disorder (BPD) Central   ☺ ☺

http://www.bpdcentral.com

This comprehensive Web site is devoted to providing informative resources on BPD. Included are links to information and Web sites on the fundamentals of BPD, a list of professionals and therapists, BPD FAQs, a list of relevant books, self-help, abuse, and online resources, including support groups, mailing lists, and other related Web sites.

Borderline Personality Disorder Sanctuary   ☺ ☺ ☺

http://www.navicom.com/~patty

This site provides resources related to borderline personality disorder, including diagnosis and medication information, a forum for asking questions of professionals, articles, personal stories, suicide resources, a bulletin board, chat forums, and suggested reading lists. Profiles of site hosts are also found at the site. Visitors can also search MEDLINE and find information on non-Internet resources, professional directories, toll-free resources, contact details for mental health clinics, and listings of borderline personality disorder advocates at the site.

Internet Mental Health: Borderline Personality Disorder   ☺ ☺ ☺

http://www.mentalhealth.com/dis/p20-pe05.html

Information on borderline personality disorder at this site include American and European diagnostic criteria, an online interactive diagnostic tool, detailed treatment details, patient education booklets, and links to related sites. Visitors can also conduct searches for research articles on borderline personality disorder and specific subtopics through PubMed.

Dependent Personality Disorder

Dependent Personality Disorder: Treatment ◎ ◎
http://www.mentalhealth.com/fr20.html

This article focuses on the treatment of dependent personality disorder, including fundamental guidelines, psychosocial treatment, drug treatment, clinical signs of the disorder, behavior therapies, and hospitalization.

Histrionic Personality Disorder

Internet Mental Health: Histrionic Personality Disorder ◎ ◎ ◎
http://www.mentalhealth.com/dis/p20-pe06.html

The pervasive pattern of emotionality and attention-seeking typical of histrionic personality disorder is outlined, with eight characteristic behaviors noted. General information on personality disorders, numerous diagnostic differentials, and guidelines for diagnosis are found. Long-term psychotherapy and a flexible psychotherapeutic approach, emphasizing compassion and appropriate confrontation, is summarized. Online questions, to be answered by either professionals or patients, may assist with making an accurate psychiatric diagnosis.

Narcissistic Personality Disorder

Health Center.com: Personality Disorders—Narcissistic Behavior ◎
http://site.health-center.com/brain/personality/narcissistic.htm

A short discussion of narcissistic personality disorder is available at this address, including a description of major traits and suggested treatments.

Malignant Self-Love—Frequently Asked Questions Page ◎ ◎
http://www.geocities.com/Athens/Forum/6297/faq1.html

Information on narcissistic personality disorder is presented at this site in the form of answers to frequently asked questions (FAQs), related to narcissism and violence, parenting, personal relationships, exploitation, and many other topics. The site also offers information on publications authored by the host and book excerpts.

Paranoid Personality Disorder

Internet Mental Health: Paranoid Personality Disorder ◎ ◎ ◎
http://www.mentalhealth.com/dis/p20-pe01.html

Internet Mental Health provides the American and European descriptions of paranoid personality disorder, with links to an online diagnostic tool and an information booklet from the National Institute of Mental Health. Several characteristics and two principal diagnostic criteria are explained, including a pervasive distrust of others and the existence of the symptoms independent of any psychotic disorder. A treatment link offers information on the basic principles of both medical and psychosocial interventions, in addition to summaries of antianxiety medications, antipsychotic medications, and individual psychotherapy.

Mental Health Net: Paranoid Personality Disorder ◎ ◎
http://mentalhelp.net/disorders/sx37.htm

DSM-IV criteria for paranoid personality disorder are presented at this site, accompanied by links to symptoms and treatment information. Links are also available to related Internet resources, online support sources, organizations, and a directory of therapists. Book reviews and excerpts are also found at this address.

Schizoid Personality Disorder

Internet Mental Health: Schizoid Personality Disorder ◎ ◎ ◎
http://www.mentalhealth.com/dis/p20-pe02.html

Schizoid personality disorder, a pervasive pattern of detachment from social relationships, is presented at this Internet Mental Health Web location. Seven characteristics of the disorder, as outlined in the American description, are listed, in addition to nine symptoms and diagnostic guidelines found at the European description link. A unique online diagnostic tool may assist practitioners in making an accurate assessment. The basic principles of long-term psychosocial intervention and the advantages of group therapy are discussed.

9.20 **Pervasive Developmental Disorders**

General Resources

PDD Support Home Page ⊙ ⊙
http://www.geocities.com/HotSprings/9647

Designed to give the user as much information as possible concerning pervasive developmental disorder (PDD) general resources, this text-only site provides descriptions and connections to 16 links related to all aspects of pervasive developmental disorders. Selected links include "User to User," a correspondence site for communication with those in similar situations, "Dear Jim," a user-to-user advice page, a conferences/meetings link, publications list, and "Words of Wisdom."

Angelman's Syndrome (AS)

Angelman Syndrome (AS) Foundation, USA ⊙ ⊙ ⊙
http://chem-faculty.ucsd.edu/harvey/asfsite

This foundation was created to provide information and education, promote research, and serve as advocated for those interested in Angelman Syndrome. At this site, there are links to documents providing basic and specific information about the syndrome; diagnostic criteria and testing files; detailed information on the genetics of the syndrome, including clinical descriptions, differential diagnosis and molecular genetics; Foundation-based conferences, electronic forums, and other support; and advocacy links. Included are links to information and organizations in other countries, as well as other AS-related sites.

Angelman Syndrome Association ⊙ ⊙
http://www.australianholidays.com/asa/frames/asahome-f.htm

The Australian Angelman Association provides general information at its Web site pertaining to the diagnosis, research, and treatment of the rare, neuro-genetic disorder. The Angelman syndrome LISTSERV is provided for communication via e-mail as are past issues of the Association's newsletter.

Angelman Syndrome Information for Families & Professionals ⊙ ⊙ ⊙
http://www.asclepius.com/angel

This comprehensive site provides information and support resources for those interested in Angelman syndrome. Included are links to informative documents describing the symptoms of the syndrome, including physical and mental problems, issues regarding development, education, testing and genetic counseling, article references, detailed fact file on the genetics of the disorder and photographs of patients. Also included are links to conference information, a detailed summary of previous conference presentations and publications, and links to mailing lists for professionals and families interested by this syndrome.

International Angelman Syndrome Association (IASO) ○ ○
http://www.asclepius.com/iaso

The organization's mission and member countries are enumerated at this site along with information on joining the IASO electronic mailing list. The Web site's conference announcements are also available and may be viewed in English, French, Spanish, or German.

Asperger's Disorder

ASPEN of America, Inc. ○ ○ ○
http://www.asperger.org

This nonprofit organization promotes education and provides current information on social and communication disorders, such as Asperger's and nonverbal learning disorder. At this site, links to detailed fact sheets on Asperger's and nonverbal learning syndrome are available, as well as resources on related conditions. These fact sheets include links to FAQs, scientific articles, personal stories, research reports, and links to support organizations and other associations. Conference calendars and a reference list of books, videos and other materials is present, as well as membership information, the ASPEN newsletter, and contact information.

Asperger's Disorder Homepage ○ ○ ○
http://www.ummed.edu/pub/o/ozbayrak/asperger.html

A Web site providing information on the disorder, including its epidemiology, the biology, diagnostic criteria, treatment, bibliography, a list of clinicians that evaluate patients with the disorder, and the difference between this disorder and high functioning autism. Links to other Asperger's disorder related Web sites are included.

Asperger's Syndrome ○ ○ ○
http://www.autism-society.org/packages/aspergers.html

As the home page of the Autism Society of America, the Web site covers the general information concerning the recognition and treatment of this pervasive developmental disorder as well as effective strategies for working with individual's with the disorder. Educational packages, cassettes, videos, books, and links to related organizations are included. The Autism Society of America's periodical information list includes the *Journal of Autism and Developmental Disorders, Autism Research Review International,* and *European Child and Adolescent Psychiatry.*

Families of Adult's Afflicted With Asperger's Syndrome (FAAAS) ⊘ ⊘ ⊘
http://www.faaas.org

This informative and comprehensive site of the FAAAS strives to give support to family members of adults afflicted with Asperger's syndrome by promoting education and awareness of the neurological disorder and all its ramifications. Recommended educational materials, Asperger's syndrome specialists, adult evaluation centers, articles, and personal thoughts written by family members of affected individuals are included.

Autistic Disorders

Access:
Autistic Continuum Connections, Education, and Support Site ⊘ ⊘ ⊘
http://sr7.xoom.com/viah/

At this site, both general and support information related to autism is provided. An abundant amount of detailed information about autism and related disorders, language and communication disorders, and other related conditions is present, as well as summaries and articles of research on the causes, treatment, and psychology of autism. Support and research organizations links are offered, as well as resources for families and caregivers of autistic individuals. Resources on educating and mainstreaming affected children is available, as well as message boards, personal Web pages, and other online activities for autistic individuals and their families. Each topic includes links to related Web sites and support information. This is a very helpful site for those interested or affected by autism and related disorders.

Applied Behavior Analysis (ABA) Resources ⊘ ⊘ ⊘
http://members.tripod.com/RSaffran/aba.html

This personal Web page, created by the father of an autistic child, has a large number of links to organizations, articles, fact sheets, FAQs, and support resources. An informative section is presented on ABA research, including personal success stories, lists of support groups, specialized therapists and schools, treatment centers, legal and government resources, online discussion groups, and a great deal of information on ABA programs and how to start your own program. International autism resources and links to more detailed fact sheets on various aspects of ABA and autism are included.

Autism, Asperger's Syndrome, and Semantic-Pragmatic Disorder ⊘ ⊘ ⊘
http://www.jaymuggs.demon.co.uk/bishop.htm

From the *British Journal of Disorders of Communication,* this article abstract illustrates the confusion that surrounds the use of diagnostic terminology in the area where Neurology, Psychology, Psychiatry, and Speech Therapy converge. Rather than thinking in terms of rigid diagnostic categories, the author surmises that the core syndrome of autism may present as other milder forms of disorder (semantic-pragmatic disorder) and that the boundaries are not well-defined.

Autism Continuum Connections, Education, and Support Site: Verbal Dyspraxia/Apraxia ◎ ◎
http://access.autistics.org/information/ld/dvd.html

Newsgroups, suggested book lists, information resources, and sites from therapists are available through links at this address.

Autism Network International ◎ ◎ ◎
http://www.staff.uiuc.edu/~bordner/ani

This self-help and advocacy organization for autistic people describes its philosophies and goals as well as the services provided for all ANI members. Provided are an Internet discussion list, a pen-pal directory for autistic people, a growing reference library, and a speaker referral service for organizations wishing to engage autistic speakers. Autism as experienced by some individuals and as defined by some professionals is described. Articles and links to other autism Web sites are available.

Autism Research Foundation ◎ ◎
http://www.ladders.org/tarf

This organization promotes research of the neurobiological causes of autism and other childhood developmental disorders. At this site, the mission statement can be accessed, as well as an overview of current research projects at the Foundation, information on secretin, conference and employment resources, and brain donation information. Contact information is also included.

Autism Research Institute (ARI) ◎ ◎ ◎
http://www.autism.com/ari

The Autism Research Institute is devoted primarily to conducting research on the causes, prevention, and treatment of autism and to disseminating the results of such research. ARI's Web site provides its information request form for subscription to its newsletter, *Autism Research Review International (ARRI)* as well as ordering information for diagnostic checklists, and a parent/professional packet. Twenty-one newsletter excerpts and editorials are viewable from the Web site, providing many answers to autism controversies.

Autism Resources ◎ ◎ ◎
http://web.syr.edu/~jmwobus/autism

Visitors to this address will find links to autism resources on the Internet, answers to frequently asked questions (FAQs) on autism, advice to parents, book recommendations, a larger bibliography of autism publications, and information about the site creator (the parent of an autistic child).

Autism Society of America (ASA) ⊙ ⊙ ⊙

http://www.autism-society.org

The mission of the Autism Society of America is to promote lifelong access and opportunities for persons within the autism spectrum and their families, to be fully included, participating members of their communities through advocacy, public awareness, education, and research related to autism. This site contains a large amount of information and links pertaining to all aspects of autism. There are links to advocacy and government action alerts, the ASA and membership information, legislative action news, conference information, and a searchable directory of the Web site and mailing list. A link to research in autism, including articles from autism research professionals, and numerous links including reference materials, glossary, treatment and diagnosis, medical and insurance information, and links to other related organizations and sites are provided.

Autism-Resources.com ⊙ ⊙ ⊙

http://web.syr.edu/~jmwobus/autism

Offering information and links regarding the developmental disabilities autism and Asperger's syndrome, this comprehensive resource offers good advice to parents, autism FAQs, and a comprehensive bibliography of over 500 books on autism as well as a "top ten" publications list.

Autism/Pervasive Developmental Disorder ⊙ ⊙ ⊙

http://www.autism-pdd.net/autism.htm

The purpose of this site is to guide the visitor to the key issues associated with autism spectrum disorders. A growing awareness of the nature of autism and the multiple approaches to diagnosis, treatment, and care that are likely to be effective in meeting the needs of autistic individuals and their families are presented. The site is packed with valuable and unique information on such topics as job accommodation, college admissions, and respite care. Two online children's workbooks, and a parent's special guide to parent's rights and responsibilities regarding special education and related services are provided. Colorful, engaging books for children with autism and a large assortment of titles for parents and caregivers may be ordered.

Cambridge Center for Behavioral Studies: Links to Other Autism Sites ⊙ ⊙

http://www.behavior.org/autism/autism_links.html

Autism resources found through this site include support groups, information sources, professional associations, a directory of services, National Institute of Neurological Disorders and Stroke fact sheets, and clinical practice guidelines.

Center for the Study of Autism (CSA) ◎ ◎ ◎

http://www.autism.org

The Center for the Study of Autism provides information about autism to parents and professionals, and conducts research on the efficacy of various therapeutic interventions. The Web site includes an overview of autism in six different languages, subgroups and related disorders of autism, discussions of issues specific to autism, and interventions, such as music therapy and auditory integration training. Over 80 autism-related resource links can be accessed.

Future Horizons ◎ ◎ ◎

http://www.futurehorizons-autism.com

This world leader in the distribution of autism/PDD books, videos, and conferences provides an autism conference page listing, as well as publications and audiovisual materials available for online ordering. Browse the online library and find such titles as Behavioral Interventions, Asperger's syndrome, Little Rain Man, and Creating a "Win-Win" Individualized Education Program (IEP).

National Alliance for Autism Research (NAAR) ◎ ◎ ◎

http://babydoc.home.pipeline.com/naar/naar1.htm

The National Alliance for Autism Research is a nonprofit organization, dedicated to finding the causes, prevention, treatment, and, ultimately, the cure of the autism spectrum disorders. Promoting biomedical research in autism, the NAAR Web site details the facts about autism and the organization's mission. NAAR news, legislative updates, research funding information, conferences, and research articles can be found. An online store and e-mail notification of site updates are available.

On the Same Page Asperger/Autism Informational Index ◎ ◎ ◎

http://amug.org/~a203/table_contents.html

Plenty of interesting links are found in this large index of areas of interest to those concerned with autism/Asperger's syndrome. Included are the Asperger/Autism Rights section, the Asperger/Autism Bill of Rights with position statements, self-advocacy, and behavioral supports, a personal pleasure index, and a complete listing of links to relevant online journals. E-mail lists, bulletin boards, and much more make this page a good starting point for both professionals and lay people concerned with all aspects of Asperger's syndrome and autism.

Online Asperger's Syndrome Information and Support ◎ ◎ ◎

http://www.udel.edu/bkirby/asperger

This Web site has an extensive amount of information on Asperger's and related syndromes. There are links to fact sheets on the description of Asperger's, related research papers and research projects, diagnostic criteria, information about socialization and education, related disorders, support groups, clinicians, medical centers, newsletters, and a number of related links.

Society for the Autistically Handicapped ⊚ ⊚ ⊚
http://www.autismuk.com

The Society exists to bring an increased awareness of autism and expand patient's exposure to well-established and newly developed approaches in the diagnosis, assessment, education, and treatment of the disease. This site has many links describing autism, its treatment and diagnosis, including updated news on the latest research and treatment. There are large news and fact files, as well as informative links to topics such as sexuality, the culture and treatment of autism, and a list of worldwide conferences, workshops, and seminars relating to autism. There is also access to Europe's largest autism library, a message board, and related links. This site is a very informative resource for professionals and the public.

Support Groups by State ⊚
http://pddct.home.att.net/support.html

This Web site contains a concise listing of and contact information for support groups for autism in the mid-Atlantic states.

Syndrome of Hyperlexia versus
High Functioning Autism and Asperger's Syndrome ⊚ ⊚
http://www.hyperlexia.org/gordy001.html

This fact sheet, written by professionals from the Center for Speech and Language Disorders presents information on the symptoms of these disorders and the differences between them in order to aid in differential diagnosis.

University Students With Autism and Asperger's Syndrome ⊚ ⊚
http://www.users.dircon.co.uk/~cns/index.html

This site offers enlightening, first-person accounts from those with Asperger's and autism. FAQs, books, and the University Students With Autism and Asperger's Syndrome mailing list are available.

Childhood Disintegrative Disorder

Childhood Disintegrative Disorder ⊚ ⊚
http://anatomy.adam.com/ency/article/001535.htm

A synopsis of childhood disintegrative disorder is offered at this page of the adam.com Web reference. Alternative names for the disorder; causes, incidence, and risk factors; and links to symptoms and treatment information are provided.

Rett's Disorder

International Rett Syndrome Association ○ ○ ○
http://www.rettsyndrome.org

The International Rett Syndrome Association home page, available for translation into multiple languages, offers over 500 pages of information on breakthrough research, related news, patient education, and professional gatherings. Pages from the "Rettnet Digest" contain interesting posts and useful suggestions regarding communication and language, therapy, and special equipment, in addition to several other relevant topics. Personal stories of those afflicted with the disorder are found, and clinical information on Rett syndrome diagnosis, stages, and genetics is reviewed. A listing of upcoming scientific meetings, support groups and regional representatives, and a comprehensive listing of World Wide Web related resources can be found.

9.21 Schizophrenia and Other Psychotic Disorders

General Resources

Futurcom in Psychiatry ○ ○ ○ (free registration)
http://www.futur.com

Described as the first complete Web site dedicated to schizophrenia and other psychoses, both professionals and the public can access articles on schizophrenia and psychoses from a variety of scientific journals, information on major international conferences, learn about the treatment products available, and get online educational information on schizophrenia.

Schizophrenia Biological Research Center ○ ○
http://www.yale.edu/vayale

As part of Yale University's Department of Psychiatry, this center promotes progress in schizophrenia and other psychotic disorder treatment. The *Schizophrenia Newsletter* is available online, as well as faculty directories, clinical sites, and other related links within Yale and on the Internet.

Brief Psychotic Disorder

Brief Psychotic Disorder ⊙ ⊙ ⊙
http://www.mentalhealth.com/dis/p20-ps03.html

Brief psychotic disorder, formerly known as brief reactive psychosis, is detailed at this site of the Internet Mental Health database. An American description of the illness includes diagnostic symptoms, episode duration, and other disorder comparisons, as well as specifications regarding onset of symptoms in relation to marked life stressors. Associated features and differential diagnoses are included, in addition to the European version, termed "acute and transient psychotic disorder," which emphasizes acute stress, the absence of organic causes, and a rapidly changing and variable state. Internet links to psychotic disorder sites, psychotic disorder booklet connections, and instructions for accessing indexed literature on related, chosen subjects are available.

Delusional Disorder

Delusional Disorder ⊙ ⊙ ⊙
http://www.mentalhealth.com/dis/p20-ps02.html

Coverage of delusional disorder is found at this page of the Internet Mental Health database, where both American and European descriptions of the disorder may be accessed. Diagnostic criteria are outlined and subtypes to be assigned, based on predominant delusional theme, are recognized. Associated features and an extensive listing of differential diagnoses are included.

Delusional Disorder:
The Recognition and Management of Paranoia ⊙ ⊙ ⊙
http://www.psychiatrist.com/psychosis/commentary/current/c0106.htm

This professional article from the Department of Psychiatry and Human Behavior, Brown University School of Medicine, presents a detailed discussion of delusional disorder. Topics include a history of terms, phenomenology, epidemiology, etiology, subtypes (erotomanic, grandiose, jealous, persecutory, somatic, and unspecified), assessment principles, differential diagnosis, and treatment. A case study and references are also available.

Internet Mental Health: Delusional Disorder Research Topics ⊙ ⊙ ⊙
http://www.mentalhealth.com/dis-rs/frs-ps02.html

Articles related to delusional disorder research can be ordered through the Loansome Doc system at the National Library of Medicine. Users can search for articles categorized by topic. Some topics include classification, chemically induced delusion, complications, diagnosis, history, metabolism, prevention and control, rehabilitation, and many therapy topics.

Psychotic Disorder (NOS)

Psychotic Disorder Not Otherwise Specified ◎ ◎
http://www.psychcentral.com/disorders/sx83.htm

This Mental Health page of Psych Central summarizes the category of psychotic symptomatology for which no specific diagnostic criteria are met. Example disorders are listed, such as postpartum psychosis and persistent auditory hallucinations in the absence of any other features. A link to the criteria for brief psychotic disorder is accessible for differential diagnosis information.

Schizoaffective Disorder

Schizoaffective Disorder and Related Behaviors ◎ ◎ ◎
http://www.geocities.com/CollegePark/Classroom/6237

A registered nurse in the field of psychiatric nursing hosts this site, offering discussions of schizoaffective disorder, schizophrenia, mania, depression, and available treatments. A mental health resource directory, links to mental health sites, and links to mental health Internet reference sources, including general and professional articles, offer many valuable sources for additional information.

Schizophrenia

Expert Consensus Guidelines: Treatment of Schizophrenia ◎ ◎ ◎
http://www.psychguides.com

Full reprints of this expert consensus guidelines document, "Schizophrenia" from the *Journal of Clinical Psychiatry* can be downloaded in Adobe Acrobat PDF format from this site. A companion guide for patients and families is also available to download. Both guides offer a wealth of useful information on schizophrenia and its treatment.

Meador-Woodruff Laboratory ◎ ◎ ◎
http://www-personal.umich.edu/~jimmw

Located in the Department of Psychiatry at the University of Michigan Medical Center, this lab's primary research focus is on brain communication via chemical signaling and its pathology in mental illness, such as in schizophrenia. Specific information on the pathophysiology of schizophrenia experiments is provided, as well as summaries of recent experimental information and findings on various aspects of brain research and schizophrenia are available. A comprehensive description of schizophrenia is also present.

National Alliance for Research on Schizophrenia and Depression ⊙ ⊙ ⊙
http://www.mhsource.com/narsad.html

This organization appropriates funds for research into the causes, cures, treatments, and prevention of schizophrenia, depression, and bipolar disorders. Information on the organization, its newsletter and media news is included. Links to current events and announcements, educational materials, an information hotline and mailing list are provided. In addition, reading list, study participation, grant guidelines, and staff directory links are present.

Open the Doors: The World Psychiatric
Association Programme to Fight Stigma Due to Schizophrenia ⊙ ⊙ ⊙
http://www.openthedoors.com/index_2.htm

This international organization's Web site contains sections with resources for teens, families and friends, professionals and scientists, and information on the program itself. Information about the symptoms, physiological causes, societal problems related to schizophrenia, treatment, and the consequences of stigmatization are presented in a well-organized and comprehensive fashion. A large amount of information on support resources and links to related sites are provided.

Schizophrenia ⊙ ⊙ ⊙
http://www.vaxxine.com/schizophrenia

Provided by Magpie publishing, this Web site has links to information on schizophrenia and the problem of suicide, symptoms, medication, alternative treatment, rehabilitation, research and legal issues. A list of seminars and events, as well as companies and other contacts of interest are included. A database of schizophrenia information, provided by Janssen Pharmaceuticals, is accessible through the site. Links to *Schizophrenia Digest,* a magazine devoted to the disorder, as well as news updates, conference and meeting information, and success stories are provided.

Schizophrenia.com ⊙ ⊙
http://www.schizophrenia.com

This not-for-profit Web site contains an extensive number of links to articles and fact files on schizophrenia information, such as causes, diagnosis, treatment, support groups, success stories, assisted/involuntary treatment, and more. There are links to more comprehensive information for professionals, such as funding organizations, related journals, discussion forums, and current research. For consumers, there are a number of links to basic information about schizophrenia, as well as support groups, treatment, academic and pharmaceutical research, health insurance, and many other topics. A site search engine allows users to search the database of sites by keyword.

Schizophrenia—
Help Online Resource Center (Association for
the Psychotherapy of Schizophrenia, International) ◎ ◎
http://www.schizophrenia-help.com

This resource center is provided by the Association for the Psychotherapy of Schizophrenia and the Anne Sippi Foundation, and offers a discussion of the organization's philosophy, a newsletter of professional articles and archives, personal stories, and suggested reading. Links are available to the Anne Sippi Clinic and other related resources.

Schizophrenia Home Page:
Information for People Who Have Schizophrenia ◎ ◎ ◎
http://www.schizophrenia.com/newsletter/newpages/consumer.html

Information resources at this site devoted to schizophrenia include an introduction to neurobiologic disorders, personal stories, links to support resources and social centers, links to information on illegal drugs, and discussions and links to further information on causes, diagnosis, treatment, and medications. Links are also available to online education programs, employment resources for schizophrenics, clinical trials information for those wishing to participate, recommended reading lists, and additional information resources for consumers and patients.

Schizophrenia Therapy Online Resource Center ◎ ◎
http://www.schizophreniatherapy.com

The Anne Sippi Clinic offers a combination of medication and individual psychotherapy, in a residential setting, for the treatment of schizophrenia. This site offers a description of treatment facilities at the Clinic, articles from program directors, personal stories, and an informative online brochure for consumers.

Schizophrenia Treatment and Evaluation Program ◎ ◎
http://www.psychiatry.unc.edu/step/webtxt.htm#homepage.

This Web site offers basic information about schizophrenia, emergency psychiatric situations, and provides links to professional and support organizations.

Schizophreniform Disorder

Internet Mental Health: Schizophreniform Disorder ⊙ ⊙ ⊙
http://www.mentalhealth.com/dis/p20-ps04.html

Internet Mental Health's chapter on schizophreniform disorder offers both the complete American and European descriptions of the disorder, in addition to current research, online booklets, and accessible magazine articles. The diagnostic criteria; associated features of the disorder; and differential diagnosis, including schizophrenia and brief psychotic disorder, are found. By clicking on a chosen subject at the research page, visitors will gain access to ready-made MEDLINE literature searches.

Shared Psychotic Disorder

Shared Psychotic Disorder ⊙ ⊙ ⊙
http://www.mentalhealth.com/dis/p20-ps06.html

Formerly known as induced psychotic disorder, this Internet site offers visitors an overview of shared psychotic disorder, with both American and European descriptions found. The "folie a deux," shared by two or more people with close emotional links, is explained, and the likely schizophrenic illness of the dominant person is explained. The American reference of the disorder contains three diagnostic criteria, associated features, and a listing of five differential diagnoses. Internet links to psychotic disorder sites may be found.

9.22 Self-Injurious Behavior

Links to Self-Injury Sites ⊙
http://www.geocities.com/HotSprings/6446/selfinjury.html

Several sites related to self-injury can be accessed through this address. Support resources, personal stories, and organizations are included. Suggested books related to self-injury are also listed at the site.

Self-Injury ⊙ ⊙ ⊙
http://www.palace.net/~llama/psych/injury.html

An informative resource for consumers and professionals, this site contains links to information on the background of this behavioral disorder, its causes, demographics, associated diagnoses, support, self-help, personal stories, treatments, and other related links. In addition, there is a references list, and a number of links to online forums, mailing lists, and message boards related to self-injury. Also present are self-assessment tests and related links.

Self-Injury—Information and Resources ○ ○

http://cgi1.geocities.com/Wellesley/1520/selfharm.html

This United Kingdom based site includes links to informative pages about different aspects of self-injury; a comprehensive introduction to the disorder, including a personal experience story; methods to cope with the disorder; lessening the damage; myths; support groups; online resources; links to other self-injury sites; and an online forum.

9.23 Sexual and Gender Identity Disorders

Gender Identity Disorders

Gender Education and Advocacy: Gender Programs ○ ○

http://www.gender.org/resources/programs.html

Twenty-three clinics offering structured sex reassignment programs are listed at this site. The listing indicates clinics with resident surgeons, and provides detailed contact information.

Gender Web Project ○ ○

http://www.genderweb.org

In addition to providing links to forums and mailing lists related to gender identity issues, interested persons can access lists of scientific article abstracts, personal experiences, support groups, legal issues, and medical information, including fact sheets and links to sites on psychiatric information on gender identity topics. A list of related links is included.

Harry Benjamin International Gender Dysphoria Association, Inc. ○ ○

http://www.tc.umn.edu/nlhome/m201/colem001/hbigda

This professional Association is committed to the understanding and treatment of gender identity disorders, with members from the fields of Psychiatry, Endocrinology, Surgery, Psychology, Sociology, and Counseling. Site resources include general information about the Association, details of the Association's biennial conference, membership information, the full text of the Benjamin Standards of Care for Gender Identity Disorders (5th version), links to related sites, and contact details for those seeking more specific information.

Ingersoll Gender Centre:
Gender Dysphoria—A Sensitive Approach ◉ ◉ ◉

http://www.genderweb.org/medical/psych/dysphor.html

The Ingersoll Gender Centre hosts this site devoted to patient information about gender dysphoria. The Benjamin Standards of Care text with definitions is available at the site. Topical discussions include suggestions on seeking help, self-esteem and self-doubt, family and other relationships, employment, name changes and other documents, insurance, and dealing with emotional crisis after a sex change. Detailed information is available on hormones, surgical procedures, and the effects of these therapies on the body. Suggested reading and sources for support and products are also available.

International Foundation for Gender Education (IFGE) ◉ ◉

http://www.ifge.org

IFGE promotes "the self-definition and free expression of individual gender identity," providing information and referrals to the public. The site offers news, announcements, events notices, links and contact information for support groups and other organizations, links to related sites, commentary, membership details, and an online bookstore. Information resources at this site include general definitions and discussions of cross-dressing and transgenderism, legal and medical information, and links to activist groups and friendly businesses. Table of contents for current and archived issues of the organization's magazine, *Tapestry,* are also available at the site.

Psyweb.com: Sexual, Gender Identity Disorders ◉

http://www.psyweb.com/Mdisord/sexd.html

Information on sexual and gender identity disorders at this site includes a general definition and list of subtypes. General descriptions of Adlerian, behavioral, existential, gestalt, person-centered, psychoanalytic, rational-emotive, reality, and transactional analysis therapies are also available.

Transgender Resources ◉

http://www.drbanks.com/serious/transgender.html

Visitors to this address will find suggested books titles with links to Amazon.com for purchasing, as well as links to treatment centers and support groups.

Klinefelter's Syndrome

Understanding Klinefelter Syndrome: A Guide for XXY Males and Their Families ◎ ◎ ◎
http://www.nih.gov/health/chip/nichd/klinefelter

A description of the syndrome, including the genetic causes, as well as the physical and cognitive problems are discussed in this report from the National Institutes of Health. Issues such as diagnosis, social and personal problems, detection of the syndrome, education, legal advice, and treatment and consequences are discussed. Overviews of topics related to this syndrome and its effects in different stages of life are present, as well as support information.

Sexual Dysfunctions

Impotence Information Center ◎ ◎
http://www.medicdrug.com/impotence/impotence.html

Medic Drug's site on impotence offers links to fact sheets on the erectile process, impotence causes, treatment choices, implant types, premature ejaculation treatments, and related product information.

Impotence Partnerships ◎ ◎ ◎ (free registration)
http://www.impotencepartnerships.com

This site contains useful links to information for both consumers and professionals. For consumers, basic information on impotence, treatment, and patient stories are available. There are also a number of informative documents for partners of impotent patients, links to related Web sites and organizations, and an online "Ask the Doctor" section.

Merck Manual of Diagnosis and Therapy: Dyspareunia ◎ ◎ ◎
http://www.merck.com/pubs/mmanual/section18/chapter243/243d.htm

Painful coitus or attempted coitus is explained at this site of the online *Merck* publication, in addition to potential psychological factors involved. Inadequate stimulation, psychological inhibition of arousal, and other etiological features are discussed. Treatment of possible medical causes, such as cysts or abscesses, is summarized, and the prophylaxis of problems through patient education is emphasized.

Merck Manual
of Diagnosis and Therapy: Female Orgasmic Disorder ⊙ ⊙ ⊙
http://www.merck.com/pubs/mmanual/section18/chapter243/243c.htm

Orgasmic disorder, characterized as lifelong, acquired, general, or situational, is reviewed in this chapter of the online *Merck* reference. The etiological roles of relationship conflict, traumatic experiences, and fear of losing control are introduced. Counseling measures to remove obstacles to orgasm are discussed.

Merck Manual
of Diagnosis and Therapy: Sexual Arousal Disorder ⊙ ⊙ ⊙
http://www.merck.com/pubs/mmanual/section18/chapter243/243b.htm

Diminished capacity for sexual arousal, its etiology, and the distinction between decreased arousal and lessened desire is made at the site. Psychological and physical causes are reviewed, and an explanation of the importance of the history and physical exam is presented.

Merck Manual
of Diagnosis and Therapy: Sexual Dysfunctions ⊙ ⊙ ⊙
http://www.merck.com/pubs/mmanual/section15/chapter192/192b.htm

This general chapter on sexual dysfunctions presents information on proper sexual functioning, the sexual response cycle, and psychological factors involved in the etiology of lifelong and acquired dysfunction. Specific information regarding hypoactive sexual desire disorder, sexual aversion disorder, substance-induced disorder, male orgasmic dysfunction, and sexual dysfunction due to a physical disorder are differentiated.

9.24 Sleep Disorders

General Resources

About.com: Sleep Disorders ⊙ ⊙ ⊙
http://sleepdisorders.miningco.com/health/sleepdisorders

Links available at this site are listed by category, including bruxism, chronic fatigue syndrome, circadian rhythm, continuous positive airway pressure, delayed sleep-phase syndrome, dreams and nightmares, enuresis, fibromyalgia, herbal remedies, medication, restless legs syndrome, snoring, treatment centers, and many others. News, articles, newsletters, chat rooms, an online bookstore, and links to related About.com guides are also available from the site.

American Sleep Disorders Association (ASDA) ◎ ◎ ◎

http://www.asda.org

The professional section of the site provides links to information on membership, ASDA history and goals, directory of accredited centers, educational products, ASDA staff, accreditation information and policy, board certification, funding opportunities, position papers, professional education, free online access to publications from the National Center on Sleep Disorders (NCSDR), abstracts from the 1998 meeting, and the journal *Sleep Links* to other sleep-related sites are included. The patient and public area provides links to answers of common questions about sleep disorders, diagnoses and treatment, patient support groups, resources from NCSDR and other related links.

Basics of Sleep Behavior ◎ ◎ ◎

http://bisleep.medsch.ucla.edu/sleepsyllabus/sleephome.html

This online textbook, supported by the University of California, Los Angeles Medical School provides psychology students, clinicians and other interested persons with a comprehensive overview of sleep behavior. Descriptive and detailed chapters, with related images and tables, include the basic characteristics and phylogeny of sleep, types of sleep, brain processes in sleep and waking, chemical and neuronal mechanisms, pharmacology of sleep, dreams, regulation of and functions of sleep, sleep and other psychiatric disorders, and alertness. Links to definitions used within the textbook and a reference guide are also present.

Northside Hospital Sleep Medicine Institute ◎ ◎

http://nshsleep.com

This Institute is dedicated to the assessment and treatment of sleep disorders. A summary of various sleep disorders symptoms, as well as information of pediatric sleep disorders, the facilities, a staff directory, an online sleep disorders test, and links to related sites are provided.

Sleep Home Pages ◎ ◎

http://bisleep.medsch.ucla.edu

Bibliographic article lists, publications, funding opportunities, classifieds, links to related sites, training information, research chat forums, and other resources are available at this site. The site offers direct links to features of use to researchers, clinical professionals, and the public. Excessive daytime sleepiness, adolescent sleep, sleep and cognitive function, sleep and health, and the management of insomnia are discussed. Visitors can search the site by keyword, find contact information for site hosts, and find links to professional, scientific, and support organizations. Most resources are designed for use by investigators and clinicians.

Sleep Medicine   ◎ ◎ ◎

http://www.users.cloud9.net/~thorpy

This site houses a large number of links to online resources related to sleep disorders. Included are links to information about sleep discussion groups and FAQs, related Web sites, abstracts and text files, sleep disorder sites, clinical practice text files from the National Institutes of Health, professional associations, organizations and foundations, journals, medications, research sites, conferences, federal and state information, related products, and other mental health sites.

SleepNet   ◎ ◎ ◎

http://www.sleepnet.com

Resources at this address include a general site description, historical and background information on sleep disorders, trends in current research, public and professional chat forums, a weekly column, and disorder fact sheets. Links are provided to support groups, professional organizations, information on dreams, sleep deprivation information, research resources, news, and sleep laboratories.

Dyssomnias

About.com: Circadian Rhythm Abnormalities   ◎ ◎

http://sleepdisorders.about.com/health/sleepdisorders/msubcircadian.htm

Delayed sleep-phase syndrome (DSPS) may have its roots in individuals with an insufficient regulation of the sleep/wake cycle in response to environmental cues. This circadian rhythm disorder and others are described at the site, including additional sleep-phase syndrome conditions, jet lag, and information on the unique problems encountered by shift workers. The main symptoms of DSPS, such as sleep-onset insomnia, are outlined, and comprehensive information on causes, circadian rhythm abnormalities, and treatment is offered.

American Sleep Apnea Association   ◎ ◎

http://www.sleepapnea.org

This organization is dedicated to reducing injury, disability, and death from sleep apnea, and to enhance the well-being of those affected by this common disorder. General information and personal stories, publications, support groups, membership details, and links to related sleep medicine sites are found at this address. Visitors can e-mail questions to a doctor or lawyer, and request a general information packet from the organization.

Center for Narcolepsy ⊙ ⊙ ⊙

http://www-med.stanford.edu:80/school/Psychiatry/narcolepsy

Stamford University's School of Medicine includes this Center, whose Web site has information on symptoms, treatment options, drug information, and a comprehensive overview of the Center's research on the disorder. A publications list, with online access to one of the articles, a staff list, contact information, and a list of relevant links are included.

Evaluation and Management of Insomnia ⊙ ⊙ ⊙

http://www.hosppract.com/issues/1998/12/meyer.htm

This issue of *Hospital Practice* provides an online version of an article relaying the diverse causes of insomnia and its proper evaluation and treatment. Authored by a physician from the University of Colorado Health Sciences Center, the article provides information on the circadian rhythm of sleep; sleep cycles and associated brain wave patterns; and important, age-related changes in sleep patterns. The structure of sleep, depending on age, is illustrated via online graphs, and recommendations are made addressing the distressing complaints of insomnia in older patients. The etiology of insomnia, classifications of, and guidelines for evaluation and referral are presented. Management strategies described include behavior modification practices, exercise, and drug treatments. A table outlining the pharmacokinetic properties of these therapies is found, and differentiation is made between short/intermediate-acting and long-acting benzodiazepines.

Hypersomnia Mini Information Sheet ⊙ ⊙

http://www.ninds.nih.gov/patients/Disorder/hypersomnia/hypersomnia.HTM

The National Institute of Neurological Disorders and Stroke offers a listing of indexed journal articles as a source of in-depth information on hypersomnia. Information on obtaining suggested resources may be accessed, and contact information for related organizations is found.

Narcolepsy ⊙ ⊙

http://www.adam.com/ency/article/000802.htm

The etiology of narcolepsy is presented in this fact sheet, along with discussions of classic symptoms, supportive treatment procedures, prognosis, and consequences of the disorder.

Psychophysiological (Learned) Insomnia ⊙ ⊙

http://www.adam.com/ency/article/000805.htm

Related to insomnia, this article reviews the problems, causes and consequences of insomnia, including behavioral habits that contribute to sleep dysfunction. Treatment information and medical history questions are provided.

Parasomnias

Parasomnias ◎ ◎
http://sleepdisorders.about.com/health/sleepdisorders

Disruptive sleep events, such as sleepwalking, sleep terrors, and nocturnal seizures are summarized at this site of the About.com online resource. Definitions for hypnogogic hallucinations and sleep paralysis, rapid eye movement (REM) behavioral disorders, teeth grinding (bruxism), and sleeptalking (somniloquy) are presented, with each synopsis offering information on the symptom's relation to sleep disruption and the recommended medical intervention or behavior modification.

Parasomnias: Sleepwalking, Sleeptalking, Nightmares, Sleep Terrors, Sleepeating ◎ ◎
http://www.healthtouch.com/level1/leaflets/sleep/sleep006.htm

The information at the site, provided by the National Sleep Foundation, describes several sleep disorders of arousal and sleep-stage transition. Summaries of sleepwalking, sleeptalking, nightmares, sleep terrors, and sleep eating are found, along with each synopsis discussing possible causes and common concerns related to the disorder.

9.25 Somatoform Disorders

General Resources

American Psychological Association (APA): Common Body-Image Disorders ◎
http://www.apa.org/monitor/mar97/imageb.html

This site describes the full range of body image disorders, including benign discontentment, subclinical body disturbances, body image disturbances causing clinical mental disorders, eating disorders, and body dysmorphic disorder.

BehaveNet DSM-IV Somatoform Disorders ◎
http://www.behavenet.com/capsules/disorders/somatoformdis.htm

This site provides definitions of body dysmorphic disorder, conversion disorder, hypochondriasis, pain disorder, somatization disorder, undifferentiated somatoform disorder, and factitious disorder. Ordering information is available for the *American Psychiatric Association DSM-IV,* related publications, and books and other media through Amazon.com.

International Society of Psychosomatic Medicine, Obstetrics, and Gynecology ☺ ☺

http://www.ispog.org

The International Society of Psychosomatic Obstetrics and Gynaecology promotes the study and education of the psychobiological, psychosocial, ethical, and cross-cultural problems in the fields of obstetrics and gynecology. This site presents the objectives of the Society, as well as a newsletter and links to local chapters. Free online access to the abstracts of the *Journal of Psychosomatic Obstetrics and Gynecology* is available, as well as links to information on international meetings and congresses. Related links and a keyword search engine are available.

Snap.com: Somatoform Disorders ☺ ☺ ☺

http://uswest.snap.com/directory/category/0,16,uswest-51558,00.html

Sites listed at this address offer resources on somatoform disorders, including differential diagnosis, patient education, and Continuing Medical Education. More specific categories are available for detailed sites, including resources on body dysmorphic disorder, conversion disorder, hypochondriasis, Munchausen syndrome, and somatization disorder.

Somatoform Disorders Article ☺ ☺

http://www.uams.edu/department_of_psychiatry/syllabus/somatoform/somatoform.htm

This descriptive article provides an overview of the different somatoform disorders, including conversion, pain, hypochondriac behavior, and body dysmorphic disorders. Diagnostic criteria, symptoms, overviews of the specific disorders, and epidemiology and differential diagnosis are included in the discussion.

Somatoform Disorders Outline ☺

http://clem.mscd.edu/~hsp/syllabi/4320/somatoform.html

This site contains a concise outline of the characteristics and specific types of somatoform disorders, adapted from the *American Psychiatric Association DSM-IV,* 1994.

Body Dysmorphic Disorder

Body Dysmorphic Disorder (BDD): A Common But Underdiagnosed Clinical Entity ☺ ☺

http://www.mhsource.com/pt/p980111.html

First appearing in *Psychiatric Times,* this article describes BDD, its psychiatric history, symptoms, behavioral and social consequences, incidence, behavior therapies, and provides references.

HomeArts: Body Image-Body Dysmorphic Disorder Quiz ◉ ◉
http://www.homearts.com/depts/health/12bodqz1.htm

Body dysmorphic disorder is discussed at this consumer site. A description of the disorder and general discussion of prevalence is followed by a short questionnaire, designed to assess concerns about physical appearance. Users can complete the questionnaire and receive immediate results. Questionnaire results are accompanied by links to several related pages within the site.

Merck Manual of Diagnosis and Therapy: Body Dysmorphic Disorder ◉
http://www.merck.com/pubs/mmanual/section15/chapter186/186f.htm

This address offers a short discussion of body dysmorphic disorder, including a definition and overview of symptoms, diagnosis, and treatment. Links are available to information on related disorders within the Manual.

Muscle Dysmorphia ◉ ◉
http://anred.com/musdys.html

Basic information on muscle dysmorphia at this site includes a definition of this disorder, its symptoms, its effects, and treatment.

Something Fishy: Body Dysmorphic Disorder ◉ ◉
http://www.sfwed.org/bdd.htm

A thorough explanation of body dysmorphic disorder is available at this site. DSM-IV diagnostic criteria for the disorder are available, and links to several related sites are provided. Visitors can also find information on many eating disorders and related topics through this address.

Conversion Disorder

Merck Manual of Diagnosis and Therapy: Conversion Disorder ◉
http://www.merck.com/pubs/mmanual/section15/chapter186/186c.htm

A short discussion of conversion disorder at this address includes a definition and information on symptoms, diagnosis, and possible treatments. Links are available to information on related disorders within the Manual.

Hypochondriasis

Merck Manual of Diagnosis and Therapy: Hypochondriasis ○

http://www.merck.com/pubs/mmanual/section15/chapter186/186d.htm

Hypochondriasis is described briefly at this site, offering an overview of symptoms, diagnosis, prognosis, and treatment. Links are available to information on related disorders within the Manual.

Pain Disorder

Merck Manual of Diagnosis and Therapy: Pain Disorder ○

http://www.merck.com/pubs/mmanual/section15/chapter186/186e.htm

This site offers information on pain disorder, including a definition and descriptions of symptoms, signs, diagnosis, and suggested treatment. Links are available to information on related disorders within the Manual.

Somatization Disorder

Somatization Disorder: Symptoms ○ ○

http://bipolar.cmhc.com/disorders/sx94.htm

Pain, gastrointestinal, sexual, and pseudoneurological symptoms characteristic of somatization disorder are listed at the Web site, as well as additional criteria for making an appropriate diagnosis.

9.26 Substance-Related Disorders

General Resources

Addiction Research Foundation (ARF) ○ ○ ○

http://www.camh.net

Located in Ontario, the Addiction Research Foundation is now a component of the Centre for Addiction and Mental Health due to a recent merger. Drug and alcohol information at the site is provided by fact sheets and brochures, statistics, answers to frequently asked questions, public education materials, a list of staff publications, and links to sites providing additional information. Users can also access information on materials available at the ARF library, including a searchable library catalog, audiovisual subject lists, and a bibliography of library materials listed by subject. Professionals can access information on training courses and materials, and order publications from an online catalog. All resources are available in French and English.

Addiction Treatment Forum ◎ ◎ ◎

http://www.atforum.com

Devoted to issues surrounding addictions and their treatments, professionals and consumers can view online articles from Addiction Treatment Forum, obtain updates on treatment and medication news, get references to written information on addiction, and view current conference and events schedules. There are also a number of links to addiction related sites.

American Academy of Addiction Psychiatry ◎ ◎

http://www.aaap.org/index.html

Informational links on the Academy and membership, as well as the different committees and policy statements are provided. Links to previous, present, and future annual meetings, Accreditation Council for Graduate Medical Education (ACGME) information, as well as a Web store for reference tapes and other materials are present.

American Society of Addiction Medicine (ASAM) ◎ ◎ ◎

http://www.asam.org

The American Society of Addiction Medicine aims to educate physicians and improve the "treatment of individuals suffering from alcoholism and other addictions." Medical news items related to addiction treatment, clinical trials, practice guidelines, and other topics are available at the site. Publications offered at the site include practice guidelines, Chapter One of ASAM's *Principles of Addiction Medicine*, newsletters, patient placement criteria, and the table of contents and abstracts for the *Journal of Addictive Diseases*. General information about ASAM, activities of the AIDS and HIV Committee of ASAM, a physician directory, annual meeting details, membership information and directory, certification resources, discussion forums, news, resources on nicotine addiction, pain management information, contact information, state chapter details, and links to related sites are all found at this address.

Association for Medical Education and Research in Substance Abuse ◎ ◎

http://www.amersa.org

The Web site for this multidisciplinary organization of professionals interested in substance abuse has links to the mission statement, organization and membership information, conference information, an online discussion group, and a link to the table of contents for the journal, *Substance Abuse*.

Center for Education and Drug Abuse Research ◎ ◎

http://www.pitt.edu/~cedar

Funded by the National Institute on Drug Abuse, the Center is a collaborative effort of the University of Pittsburgh and St. Francis Medical Center. The Web site provides information on the mission, goals, experimental designs, research findings and faculty, research modules overviews, training, and education faculty list and overview. There is an informative link to an ancillary project, which includes the design and methods, literature review, and faculty involved in this study.

Center for Online Addiction ◎ ◎ ◎

http://www.netaddiction.com/index.html

The Center For Online Addiction provides resources on the psychology of cyberspace addiction. Risk factors involved, an online Internet addiction test, and treatment options for those addicted are available. A series of nationwide conferences and events as well as helpful links to online booklets, research, and resources on what makes certain Internet applications so time-consuming are offered. Additionally, a Virtual Clinic provides direct, online e-mail, chat room, or telephone counseling as necessary.

Center for Substance Abuse Prevention ◎

http://www.covesoft.com/csap.html

Funded by the federal government, this training service offers technical assistance to communities and professionals on program development, grantsmanship and fundraising, coalition building, multicultural communication, and more. A basic overview of the Center, as well as criteria for technical assistance services applications evaluations are provided.

Co-Dependents Anonymous ◎ ◎

http://www.codependents.org/siteindex.html

A large number of links, meeting information, organizational events and facts, recovery fact sheets, literature resources, and related links are provided at this site. Twelve-step programs, an FAQ section, employment opportunities, a directory, support information and documents, meeting reports, and international links are included.

Drug Abuse Research Center ◎ ◎

http://www.medsch.ucla.edu/som/npi/DARC

As part of University of California—Los Angeles, this research center is part of a larger drug abuse research consortium. A list of summaries for the over 30 current drug abuse research projects, as well as past projects are provided at this site. In addition, a list of the many publications, which can be ordered online, is available. Fellowship and other educational opportunities, ethnic issues projects, and research training information is obtainable. Links to other appropriate sites are present.

Drug Dependence Research Center ◎ ◎

http://itsa.ucsf.edu/~ddrc

This Web site serves as the home page to the Center, which is part of the Langley Porter Psychiatric Institute at the University of California, San Francisco. Comprehensive overviews of the Center's eight research projects, which focus on the pharmacology and psychology of drug abuse, as well as access to full-length research publications and posters are available. Contact information and links to other drug treatment centers, and related sites are provided.

Higher Education Center
for Alcohol and Other Drug Prevention ◎ ◎ ◎

http://www.edc.org/hec

Part of the U.S. Department of Education and supported by the Robert Wood Johnson Foundation, the Center's primary mission is to provide support to higher education institutions in their attempt to resolve alcohol and other drug abuse problems. There is free online access to many related publications, links to information on the learning opportunities, consultation services, and staff presentations. A number of links to other useful resources, as well as related databases, mailing lists, and other services are present.

National Center on Addiction and
Substance Abuse at Columbia University ◎ ◎ ◎

http://www.casacolumbia.org/information1455/information.htm

This national center provides the public with information on substance abuse and its impact on peoples' lives, prevention, treatment, and law enforcement. Full-text articles from the Center are available at the site, as well as news, information on research activities and training programs, links to federal resources, grants and funding resources, and resources for kids and teens, answers to frequently asked questions (FAQs), contact details, and a site search engine.

National Institute on Drug Abuse (NIDA) ◎ ◎ ◎

http://www.nida.nih.gov/NIDAHome1.html

As part of the National Institutes of Health (NIH), this organization supports international research, advocacy, and education on drug abuse and related issues. The site provides information on the mission and goals of the organization, current news, a list of descriptive fact sheets on commonly abused drugs and their treatment, links to publications, monographs, teaching materials, and reports on various aspects of substance abuse and addiction. Information on conferences, including summaries of previous meetings, relevant news articles, links to sites on the subdivisions of NIDA, funding and training opportunities and information, advocacy items, a clinical trial network, and links to the National Institutes of Health site and other professional organizations and centers related to substance abuse. This site also includes a search bar and employment listings.

New England Addiction Technology Transfer Center (ATTC) ⊚ ⊚ ⊚
http://center.butler.brown.edu/ATTC-NE

In an effort to exchange resources, promote culturally competent treatment services, and translate and disseminate research-based substance abuse information, the ATTC Web site provides online patient and professional education and resources. Useful links include upcoming conferences and training opportunities, multicultural and special population resources, an academia resource list, and the National ATTC Product Catalog. Connections to tobacco-related Web sites and prominent mental health organizations such as the Center for Mental Health Services and the Center for Disease Control can be found.

Prevline: Prevention Online from the National Clearinghouse for Alcohol and Drug Information (NCADI) ⊚ ⊚ ⊚
http://www.health.org

This excellent site, a service of the Substance Abuse and Mental Health Services Administration, offers valuable resources on drug use and abuse prevention for professionals and the general public. Search engines are available for locating information within the site or in 25 selected sites offering information on drug use and abuse. Links are provided to databases offering directories of prevention services, research summaries, conference reports, journal articles, and public education documents. Professional resources include monthly research briefs, a conference calendar, information on the latest research, funding and grants information, and links to important online forums. Publications on workplace issues are available for professionals and employers. Other resources include links to treatment organizations, information on funding opportunities, drug testing guidelines, a list of laboratories meeting minimum standards for urine drug testing, resources for runaways, and information on Addiction Technology Transfer Centers. The catalogs section lists available online publications from NCADI, presented by subject and audience. The online publications offer an abundance of resources for educators, family, and friends; health professionals and clinicians; scientists and researchers; teens/youth; and women. Spanish publications are also listed. Alcohol and drug fact sheets, media resources, and resources for children are also available from this comprehensive site.

Research Institute on Addictions ⊚ ⊚ ⊚
http://www.ria.org

Part of the New York State Office of Alcoholism and Substance Abuse Services, this institute's current research projects include alcohol abuse in minority teens, dual-diagnosed patients and drug coping skills, alcohol abuse and risk factors, teen alcohol use and high-risk sexual behavior, maternal substance abuse, schizophrenia and muscarinic receptors, woman's alcohol use, fetal alcohol syndrome and dopamine, as well as others. Links to clinical and scientific research findings provides online access to full-length articles and presentations from the Institute's faculty and staff. In addition, abstracts and summaries of related research studies performed at the Institute are available. A list of online documents at this site is given, as well as investigator and scientist directories.

Substance Abuse and Mental Health Services Administration ◎ ◎ ◎
http://www.samhsa.gov

The official Web site for the substance abuse and mental health agency for the U.S. Department of Health and Human Services. Links include professionals, programs and budget information databases, information on substance abuse and mental health issues, statistics, contracts, and updated news releases, as well as a search form for relevant documents. Links to other related centers are provided, as well as links to general information on substance abuse and mental health problems.

Substance Abuse/Addiction—
A Service of the Center for Mental Health Services (CMHS) ◎ ◎
http://www.mentalhealth.org/links/substanceabuse.htm

A variety of links to those in need of information/support for alcohol and drug abuse is provided at this CMHS Web page. Links include Mental Health Net and the National Clearinghouse for Alcohol and Drug Information (NCADI). Of particular interest is information on Web sites offering therapeutic options for addicts. Included are SMART Recovery, an abstinence-based alternative to Alcoholics Anonymous (AA), and the World Wide Web Rational Recovery Center, which presents an Internet Course on Rational Recovery, another 12-step alternative.

Virginia Addiction Technology Transfer Center ◎ ◎ ◎
http://views.vcu.edu/vattc

This Web site serves to provide information on the goals of the center, which is to provide current research on treatment for addiction. Links include addiction education programs, related conferences, access to technical publications on addiction and its treatment, current news and access to the newsletter, a calendar of local events, and a list of other addiction technology transfer centers. There are a large number of links, divided in categories such as substance abuse, drug and alcohol information, government professional organizations, research and addiction, treatment and prevention, and other informative Web sites.

Web of Addictions ◎ ◎ ◎
http://www.well.com/user/woa

This award-winning site provides information on drug and alcohol addictions. The drug information database has an extensive amount of fact sheets on the different drug issues, as well as technical information on the drugs themselves. Also included are links to meetings and conferences, contact information, support groups, and associations related to substance abuse.

Alcohol-Related Disorders

Al-Anon/Alateen Organization ⊙ ⊙ ⊙
http://www.al-anon.org

Al-Anon and Alateen are part of a worldwide organization providing a self-help recovery program for families and friends of alcoholics. Resources available at this official site include meeting information, the 12 steps, traditions, and concepts of the programs, information on Alateen, pamphlets, suggested readings and videotapes, an online newsletter, a calendar of events, and information on a television public service announcement developed by the organization. Professional resources include information on the organization, reasons people are referred to Al-Anon/Alateen, a description of group activities and how they help, and details of how Al-Anon/Alateen cooperates with professionals.

Alcoholism Index ⊙ ⊙ ⊙
http://www.alcoholismhelp.com/index

This searchable Web site has links to information under a number of topics regarding alcoholism, such as related organizations, drunk driving, relationships, health, information, support groups, treatment, personal pages, and more. Mental health information includes links to alcoholism and psychiatry, and related disorders, such as depression, suicide, denial, and bipolar disorder. This site contains a wealth of links to informative sites on alcoholism.

Alcoholism/Treatment ⊙ ⊙ ⊙
http://www.alcoholismtreatment.org

An excellent starting point for those exploring the possibility of alcoholism in themselves or loved ones, the site offers general information on the signs and symptoms of alcoholism. After a brief self-diagnosis, the user can gain access to treatment-oriented Web sites, including the Betty Ford Center, Hazleden Center link, as well as a 12-step overview Web site. Alcoholism experts can be directly e-mailed with questions.

Center for Alcohol and Addiction Studies ⊙ ⊙
http://center.butler.brown.edu/98report/activities.html

Devoted to the study of addiction and alcohol and located in Brown University, the Center's Web site provides information on training, research news, an online forum, a number of links to medical resources, as well as other links of interest. Also, the 1998 annual report is available online; topics include new grants and projects, research activities, medical education and clinical training, research training, a faculty directory and publications list, as well as other related information. This site is a comprehensive overview of the Center.

Internet Alcohol Recovery Center ○ ○
http://www.med.upenn.edu/~recovery

Provided by the University of Pennsylvania Health System, this online center provides information for both consumers and professionals. Consumer resources include treatment information, a reference list to substance abuse topics, help directories, and online forums. Professional resources include treatment information, a substance abuse reference list, alcohol-related news, and a comprehensive fact file on naltrexone for alcohol dependence treatment.

National Institute on Alcohol Abuse and Alcoholism (NIAAA) ○ ○ ○
http://www.niaaa.nih.gov

The National Institute on Alcohol Abuse and Alcoholism supports and conducts biomedical and behavioral research on the causes, consequences, treatment, and prevention of alcoholism and alcohol-related problems. Legislative activities, scientific review groups, and other activities of the Institute are described at the site, and users can also access a staff directory and employment announcements. The site provides professional online publications, press releases, conference and events calendars, research program information, links to other sites of interest, and answers to frequently asked questions. Users can also access fact sheets, MEDLINE, and ETOH, a database of alcohol-related research findings through this site.

Pittsburgh Adolescent Alcohol Research Center (PAARC) ○ ○ ○
http://www.pitt.edu/~paarc/paarc.html

This site dedicates itself to the accomplishments of the Center, including the generation of 167 publications, over 177 presentations, and the sponsorship of two scientific conferences. Also outlined is an overview of the Center's research training and major projects and studies conducted.

Psychoanalytic Perspective on the Problematic Use of Alcohol ○ ○
http://www.cyberpsych.org/alcohol/main.htm

This Web site's goal is the promotion of awareness of the psychoanalytic contributions to issues related to alcohol misuse. The psychoanalytic view of alcoholism is presented explaining many of the contributing factors leading to compulsive drinking.

Wernicke-Korsakoff Syndrome (Alcohol-Related Dementia) ◎ ◎
http://www.caregiver.org/factsheets/wks.html

In this fact sheet, the syndrome is defined, and the biological causes are discussed. Also, an overview of the related symptoms, diagnostic procedures, treatment options, and familial issues are mentioned. Caregiver information and references are provided. This site is offered by the Family Caregiver Alliance.

Amphetamine-Related Disorders

Internet Mental Health: Amphetamine Dependence ◎ ◎ ◎
http://www.mentalhealth.com/dis/p20-sb02.html

Amphetamine dependence leading to significant social and medical impairment is explained at the Internet Mental Health database, with connections to both American and European descriptions of the disorder. Withdrawal symptoms, greater use of the drug than intended, and other signs and diagnostic criteria are outlined. Six potentially present criteria are described at the European diagnostic page, and an online diagnostic quiz assists the practitioner in diagnosis. An introduction to management of amphetamine dependence outlines the basic principles of hospitalization, medications, and psychosocial intervention.

Caffeine-Related Disorders

Caffeine Dependence ◎ ◎
http://ndsn.org/SEPOCT94/CAFFEINE.html

A news review of a 1994 study from *JAMA* identifies "caffeine dependence syndrome" and reviews the criteria for this substance-abuse diagnosis. Questions are raised regarding the regulation of caffeine products.

Cannabis-Related Disorders

Internet Mental Health: Cannabis Dependence ◎ ◎ ◎
http://www.mentalhealth.com/dis/p20-sb03.html

Internet Mental Health provides visitors with an American and European description of cannabis dependence, its causes, six typical patterns of behavior, and associated features. An online diagnosis may assist the therapist or patient in assessment, and a treatment introduction, including medical and psychosocial principles, is found. Fact sheets on marijuana use are available, and a magazine article describing the long-term brain impairment associated with cannabis dependence is accessible.

Cocaine-Related Disorders

Cocaine Dependence ⊙ ⊙ ⊙
http://www.mentalhealth.com/dis/p20-sb04.html

Characteristics of cocaine abuse and the American criteria for dependence may be accessed from this page of the Internet Mental Health database. Cocaine tolerance, withdrawal symptoms, and continued usage despite recurrent related physical and psychological problems are explained, and 10 recognized associated features are listed. The European description of "cocaine dependence syndrome" is outlined, and an online diagnostic quiz is provided, which may be answered by either the patient or the therapist. An external link to treatment guidelines for patients with substance-abuse disorders may be accessed.

Codependence

NCC—The National Council on Codependence, Inc. ⊙ ⊙ ⊙
http://nccod.netgate.net/index.html

This organization's Web site contains the missions statement of the NCC, describes the general aspects of codependence as a disorder, and highlights upcoming events of interest to specialists in the field and lay people alike. Also available is information on the Codependents Anonymous support network, an educational material listing, and listing of 10 recovery links, including Codependency and Relationships, and the Self-Improvement Web Guide.

Dual Diagnosis

Dual Diagnosis Web Site ⊙
http://users.erols.com/ksciacca

This site is designed to provide information and resources for service providers, consumers, and family members seeking assistance and/or education in the field of dual diagnosis (the co-occurrence of mental illness with drug/alcohol addiction). Features include a glossary of terms defining various acronyms and terminology, clinical profiles of dual diagnosis, an education and upcoming training event section, and dual diagnosis literature, articles, chapters, and abstracts. A bulletin board is intended to furnish information regarding resources for dual diagnosis services, such as that pertaining to grants, legislation, and other pertinent resources. A 24-hour chat room and LISTSERV are available as is the Dual Diagnosis Directory of Programs and Services.

GAINS National Center for
People with Co-occurring Disorders in the Justice System ◎ ◎ ◎
http://www.prainc.com/gains/index.html

At the GAINS Center Web site, the organization's role as a national center for the collection and dissemination of information regarding mental health and substance abuse in those who come in contact with the justice system is described. The Center's primary goals, agenda, and functions are outlined, including information on the Center's technical services offered, publications produced, and the organization's sponsoring agencies and approaches. Programs to break the cycle of those who repeatedly enter the criminal justice system, such as the Jail Diversion Knowledge Development and Application Program, are discussed.

Hallucinogen-Related Disorders

Internet Mental Health: Hallucinogen Dependence ◎ ◎ ◎
http://www.mentalhealth.com/dis/p20-sb05.html

One of the unique features of the Internet Mental Health Web site is an online diagnostic tool, to assist the therapist with assessment or to give patients a better self-understanding of this condition. The American description of hallucinogen abuse and several associated features of dependence are reviewed. The European description, termed "hallucinogen dependence syndrome" and derived from the ICD-10 Classification of Mental and Behavioral Disorders is also found. Treatment recommendations may include antianxiety, antipsychotic, and antidepressant agents, as well as psychosocial interventions described at the site. A concise introduction to the Narcotics Anonymous program is offered.

Inhalant-Related Disorders

Inhalant Dependence ◎ ◎ ◎
http://www.mentalhealth.com/dis/p20-sb06.html

An online diagnosis, for use by either therapist or patient; introductions to both medical and psychosocial interventions; and complete descriptions of both the American and European diagnostic criteria for inhalant dependence are found, outlining the destructive patterns commonly occurring with abuse of this substance. Internet Mental Health's "Booklets" links contain further information on substance abuse, and connections to substance-related disorder sites are accessible.

Nicotine-Related Disorders

Internet Mental Health: Nicotine Dependence ☉ ☉ ☉
http://www.mentalhealth.com/dis/p20-sb07.html

The destructive pattern of nicotine use and symptoms of dependence are reviewed at this site of the Internet Mental Health Web pages. Associated features, such as sexual dysfunction, are listed, and an online diagnostic test, for use by either practitioners or patients, offers an aid to diagnosis. Practice guidelines for the treatment of nicotine dependence are accessible, and articles linking nicotine abuse with depression, as well as a higher mortality rate are found.

Practice Guideline for the Treatment of Patients With Nicotine Dependence ☉ ☉ ☉
http://www.psych.org/clin_res/pg_nicotine.html

The American Psychiatric Association (APA) presents a complete practice guideline for the treatment of nicotine dependence at this Internet location. These parameters of practice, developed by psychiatrists who are active in the clinical field, offer DSM-IV information on nicotine use disorders, specific features of diagnosis, and complete treatment principles and alternatives. Formulations and implementation of treatment strategies, clinical features influencing treatment, and future research directions are reviewed.

Opioid-Related Disorders

Internet Mental Health: Opioid Dependence ☉ ☉ ☉
http://www.mentalhealth.com/dis/p20-sb08.html

The Internet Mental Health database provides an excellent resource for general information and treatment guidance for opioid abuse. Visitors will find two clinical descriptions of opioid dependence, with diagnostic criteria completely outlined, in addition to external links on effective addiction management and practice guidelines for patients with substance-abuse disorders. Users may access topic-specific MEDLINE searches, and substance-related disorder booklets.

Recovery Organizations

Recovery Online ☉ ☉ ☉
http://www.recovery.alano.org

Recovery Online provides a comprehensive range of links to over 50 anonymous, self-help organizations ranging from the well-known Alcoholics Anonymous and Al-Anon

Family Groups to the less frequently encountered Depressed Anonymous, Phobics Anonymous, and Recovering Couples Anonymous. Eleven religious and secular anonymous group listings are included for help with alcoholism, homosexuality, survival of sexual abuse, and trauma. The variety also includes Schizophrenics Anonymous, Cleptomaniancs and Shoplifters, and Parents Anonymous. In addition to organizational listings, a listing of FAQs and a Recovery Message Board are available.

Recovery-Related Resources ◎ ◎ ◎

http://members.aol.com/powerless/recovtxt.htm

An enormous collection of recovery-related Internet links is organized at this site. Resources mentioned include Alcoholics Anonymous (AA) groups nationwide, a variety of anonymous organization listings, 12-step literature, and a state-by-state directory of AA meetings. Recovery chat room listings, message boards, and newsgroups are here as are recovery-related shopping sites.

Sedative-Related Disorders

Internet Mental Health: Sedative Dependence ◎ ◎ ◎

http://www.mentalhealth.com/dis/p20-sb10.html

The specifics of sedative abuse, with common withdrawal symptoms and other diagnostic features, are outlined at the American description page, accessible from the site. Seven associated problems, such as antisocial personality and learning disorders are listed, and a separate European description of "sedative or hypnotic dependence syndrome" is found. Information on barbiturate and benzodiazepine withdrawal, therapeutic communities and halfway houses, and psychosocial treatment principles is provided.

9.27 Suicide

American Association of Suicidology ◎ ◎ ◎

http://www.suicidology.org

This nonprofit organization is dedicated to the understanding and prevention of suicide. The Web site includes information regarding the Association, conference information, links to other relevant sites, internship information, and a directory for support groups and crisis centers. In addition, there are links to sources for books and other printed resources, links to legal and ethical issues, treatment, assessment and prediction, and certification/accreditation manuals.

American Foundation for Suicide Prevention ⊙ ⊙ ⊙

http://www.afsp.org

This foundation provides funds for the research, education and treatment programs for suicide prevention. The site has links to research updates, suicide facts, and survivor support. Other topics include assisted suicide, depression and suicide, neurobiology of, and youth suicide. Foundation information as well as current funding opportunities, research and treatment news is provided.

Doctor Assisted Suicide—
A Guide to WEB Sites and the Literature ⊙ ⊙ ⊙

http://Web.lwc.edu/administrative/library/suic.htm

The best and most informative sources on the subject are offered at this online guide to doctor-assisted suicide. Presented here are the multiple vantage points of the medical, legal, and religious communities, and provided is current coverage of the topic via recent publications, Web sites, and United States Supreme Court decisions. State statutes and proposed legislation are explored and provoke further discussion regarding the "right to die" debates.

Living With Suicide ⊙ ⊙

http://www.pbs.org/weblab/living/lws_0.html

A number of personal stories of experiences with suicide, a discussion group and links to suicide support groups, hotlines, associations, national directories of groups, and other related information are available at this site.

SA/VE—Suicide Awareness/Voices of Education ⊙ ⊙

http://www.save.org

This support organization's site provides answers to common questions on suicide, a list of symptoms and warning signs, personal stories, depression and suicide fact sheets, hospitalization information, resources on students and elderly depression, a book list, and a fact sheet on depression. Contact information and related links are included.

Suicide ⊙ ⊙ ⊙

http://www.metanoia.org/suicide

This Web site is a support page for those considering suicide, offering information on hotlines and links to additional Internet resources for aid and support. Suggested literature can be ordered from Amazon.com through the site. In addition, there is information on how to handle a person who is suicidal.

9.28 **Tic Disorders**

General Resources

Rush-Presbyterian—
St. Luke's Medical Center: Section of Movement Disorders ◎ ◎
http://www.rush.edu/patients/neuroscience/movement.html

This Center conducts research into the causes and treatment of movement disorders, treating patients with Parkinson's disease, Huntington disease, Tourette's disorder, other tic-related illnesses, dystonia, tremor, and myoclonus. Clinical features, causes, treatment, and current research projects associated with each disorder are described at the site.

Tics and Tourette's ◎ ◎ ◎
http://www.klis.com/chandler/pamphlet/tic/content.htm

This site presents a valuable patient and caregiver pamphlet on motor tics, vocal tics, complex tics, tic-related phenomena, and specific types of tic disorders. Discussions on the course, co-morbidity, prevalence, diagnosis, causes, and strategies, including non-medical and pharmacological interventions, are available.

Chronic Motor or Vocal Tic Disorder

BehaveNet Clinical Capsule:
DSM-IV—Chronic Motor or Vocal Tic Disorder ◎ ◎
http://behavenet.com/capsules/disorders/chrontic.htm

This BehaveNet Clinical Capsule, concisely defines the DSM-IV diagnosis of chronic motor or vocal tic disorder, in order to provide the reader with a rapid, basic understanding of the term and its relationship to other disorders. Provided are links to information on Tourette's disorder.

HealthCentral.com: Chronic Motor Tic Disorder ◎ ◎
http://planet-health.com/mhc/top/000745.cfm

HealthCentral's online encyclopedia presents an information sheet at the Web site relating to chronic motor tic disorder, with its definition, causes, symptoms, and treatments briefly reviewed. Links to fact sheets on transient tic disorder, facial tics, and other definitions and differential diagnoses are found.

Tourette's Disorder

Internet Mental Health: Guide to the Diagnosis and Treatment of Tourette's Syndrome ☺ ☺ ☺
http://www.mentalhealth.com/book/p40-gtor.html

This site presents an education booklet, providing physicians, psychologists, nurses, and other professionals with important information on Tourette's disorder. Topics include tic disorders, differential diagnosis, symptomatology, associated behaviors and cognitive difficulties, etiology, stimulant medications, epidemiology and genetics, nongenetic contributions, clinical assessment, and treatment. References, authors, and a link to the Tourette's Syndrome Association are listed at the site.

Tourette's Syndrome Association (TSA), Incorporated ☺ ☺ ☺
http://tsa.mgh.harvard.edu

Described as the only national organization dedicated to providing information on Tourette's Syndrome (TS), the Tourette's Syndrome Association's Web site includes links to public service announcements and a chat room. The site contains numerous general facts about TS, as well as scientific links, such as a publications list, research grant awards and TS diagnosis and treatment. Interested persons will find links to national chapters of the association, and international contacts. There are links to order TSA publications, and online access to selected relevant articles.

Tourette's Syndrome Resources ☺ ☺ ☺
http://members.tripod.com/~tourette13/links.html

Thirty-eight Internet resources related to Tourette's disorder are listed at this address. Specific site topics include disability, attention-deficit/hyperactivity disorder, neurology, patient advocacy, movement disorders, nervous system diseases, obsessive-compulsive disorder, psychology self-help, stuttering, and Ritalin. Resources specific to Tourette's disorder are provided through organizations and other Tourette's information sites.

Virtual Hospital: Medical Treatment of Tourette's Syndrome ☺ ☺
http://www.vh.org/Patients/IHB/Psych/Tourette/TSMed.html

This site offers an outline of medical treatments for Tourette's disorder, including suggested dose, side effects, and other notes. The medications information is accompanied by a list of sensory symptoms of Tourette's syndrome, biochemistry of the condition, environmental factors, and a list of possible reasons for poor attention in school.

Transient Tic Disorder

Transient Tic Disorder ◎ ◎

http://gohamptonroads.adam.com/ency/article/000747.htm

A simple definition and information on the causes, incidence, and risk factors associated with transient single or multiple motor tics are presented at this site of the adam.com online health information database. A symptom link stresses ruling out any physical causes of transient tics, and a treatment connection provides a list of actions to be taken if tics are recognized.

10. RARE DISORDERS

10.1 National Organization for Rare Disorders (NORD)

The National Organization for Rare Disorders (NORD) is a unique federation of voluntary health agencies, individuals, and medical professionals dedicated to the identification, treatment, and cure of rare "orphan" diseases. There are more than 6,000 of these serious health conditions, most of which are genetically caused. Each orphan disease affects fewer than 200,000 Americans, but combined, they affect more than 25 million people in the United States.

NORD came together during the late 1970s as an informal coalition of voluntary health agencies that were determined to solve the "orphan drug" dilemma. Each of the rare disease charities spent considerable effort raising funds to support research on "their" disease. However, as the cost of pharmaceutical development escalated, it became apparent that when academic scientists actually discovered a new treatment for a rare disorder, pharmaceutical companies did not want to make it commercially available. Thus, treatments for rare diseases became known as "drugs of limited commercial value," or "orphan drugs."

The "Orphan Drug Act" created financial incentives to entice pharmaceutical companies into developing orphan drugs. These incentives include seven years of exclusive marketing rights and a tax credit for the cost of clinical research. The FDA Office for Orphan Products Development also provides clinical research grants to academic scientists and small pharmaceutical companies for pivotal clinical trials.

After the law was enacted in 1983, NORD formalized its associations and incorporated as a nonprofit voluntary health agency serving the common needs of people with all rare diseases through programs of education, advocacy, research, and service. To this end, NORD became an international clearinghouse for information about rare disorders with a goal of creating understandable information for patients and families.

Education Programs

National Organization for Rare Disorders, Inc. (NORD): Rare Disease Database

During the struggle to pass the Orphan Drug Act, media attention highlighted the many problems people with rare diseases face in their daily lives. These patients contacted NORD and asked for assistance. Most importantly, orphan disease patients needed understandable information about their disease including the location of support groups (when they exist), and of clinical trials in which they might want to participate.

NORD's Rare Disease Database (RDB) can be accessed through NORD's Internet site, http://www.rarediseases.org. The database contains information on over 1,100 diseases written in layman's terminology, including: General Description (abstract), Synonyms, Symptoms, Causes (etiology), Affected Population (epidemiology), Related Disorders (for differential diagnosis), Standard Treatments, Investigational Treatments, Resources (contacts for further information), and References (bibliography). The database can be searched using the disease name, synonyms, or symptoms.

Several other databases can be accessed through the NORD home page at http://www.rarediseases.org, including:

Organization Database

This database lists approximately 1,200 disease-specific organizations and support groups, registries, clinics, Web sites, umbrella organizations, and service agencies. Information includes addresses, phone and fax numbers, Web addresses, publications, and services available through each agency. Most are American agencies, but Canadian and European rare disease organizations are also listed.

Orphan Drug Designation Database

The FDA has designated almost 1,000 pharmaceuticals as "orphan drugs." This database of approved and investigational orphan products lists officially designated orphan drugs, the indications for which they are approved, and ways in which to contact the manufacturers of these orphan drugs. The database is searchable by the name of the product, manufacturer, or the name of the disease.

Medical Equipment Exchange

Many patients do not have insurance with reimbursement benefits for durable medical equipment such as wheelchairs. This database contains ads placed by people who no longer need medical equipment and who are willing to sell, trade, or give the equipment away for free.

Other NORD Programs

Aside from its primary program of education and information, NORD acts as an advocate for programs and government services that benefit people with all rare diseases. NORD also supports biomedical research at academic institutions through clinical research grants. Donors can give for clinical research on all rare diseases, or restrict their gift to a specific rare disease.

NORD also provides services to rare disease patients and families including a Networking Program that links together the families of patients with the same diagnoses. At NORD's Annual Conference, families from throughout the United States come together to learn about the latest medical advancements in rare disease research, how to obtain services and benefits aimed at people with disabilities, coping mechanisms for patients and caregivers, etc. NORD also assists in locating free or low cost transportation for patients who must travel to distant medical facilities. Additionally, NORD administers several Medication Assistance Programs for pharmaceutical manufacturers, providing several free orphan drugs to uninsured and underinsured patients who cannot afford to purchase them.

NORD Is Here To Help

NORD's various programs and services have been created to serve the orphan disease community, patient organizations, and medical professionals who care for rare disease patients. Numerous surveys have shown that people with rare diseases go undiagnosed or misdiagnosed for extensive periods of time. Once diagnosed, they often have great difficulty locating information that they can understand and apply to their daily lives. Isolation and despair are common until they can obtain appropriate information. For some people, contacting others who have shared similar experiences is critically important. Most importantly, all people with rare diseases need hope that comes from knowledge that research is being pursued on their disease. If they wish to participate in a clinical research program, it is essential that patients can identify the location of clinical trials.

We invite you to contact NORD through the Web site www.rarediseases.org, by phone 203-746-6518 (or recorded Help-Line: 1-800-999-6673), or via mail at: NORD, P.O. Box 8923, New Fairfield, CT 06812.

Researching Rare Disorders

NORD rare disorder profiles are available at http://www.rarediseases.org. Clicking on the rare disorders database and entering a search term will return all related glossary entries. A summary of the rare disorder is provided, and a full report containing additional re-sources is available for a nominal sum.

PART TWO

GENERAL MEDICAL WEB RESOURCES

11. REFERENCE INFORMATION AND NEWS SOURCES

11.1 **Abstract, Citation, and Full-text Search Tools**

Doctor Felix's Free MEDLINE Page ◎ ◎
http://www.beaker.iupui.edu/drfelix/index.html

This site, a useful resource for those interested in performing MEDLINE searches for article citations, offers links to sites providing free MEDLINE access to visitors. More than thirty sites are profiled, with information on database coverage, frequency of updates, registration requirements, usage restrictions, document delivery information, and links to additional information on the site. Miscellaneous sources for full MEDLINE access trial periods are also listed.

Infomine: Scholarly Internet Resources ◎ ◎ ◎
http://infomine.ucr.edu/search/bioagsearch.phtml

Infomine offers searchable biological, agricultural, and medical resource collections. Web sites can be browsed by title of resource, subject and title, subject, and keyword. Recently added sites are stored in a separate section. The site also offers links to additional Internet medical resources.

Internet Grateful Med (IGM)
at the National Library of Medicine (NLM) ◎ ◎ ◎
http://igm.nlm.nih.gov

Internet Grateful Med (IGM) is one of the two NLM-sponsored free MEDLINE search systems. The default MEDLINE search includes articles published from 1966 to the present and includes PreMEDLINE. This version of IGM takes advantage of PubMed's ability to display related articles and links to the full text of participating online journals. Other searchable databases include AIDSLINE, AIDSDRUGS, AIDSTRIALS, BIOETHICSLINE, ChemID, DIRLINE, HealthSTAR, HISTLINE, HSRPROJ, OLDMEDLINE, POPLINE, SDILINE, SPACELINE, and TOXLINE. The site also offers a user's guide and specific information on new features of the site.

MEDLINE/PubMed at the National Library of Medicine (NLM) ◎ ◎ ◎
http://www.ncbi.nlm.nih.gov/PubMed

PubMed is a free MEDLINE search service providing access to 11 million citations with links to the full text of articles of participating journals. Probably the most heavily used and reputable free MEDLINE site, PubMed permits advanced searching by subject, author, journal title, and many other fields. It includes an easy-to-use "citation matcher" for completing and identifying references, and its PreMEDLINE database provides journal citations before they are indexed, making this version of MEDLINE more up-to-date than most.

11.2 **Daily Medical News Sites**

1st Headlines: Health ◉ ◉ ◉

http://www.1stheadlines.com/health1.htm

This medical news information site offers a keyword search engine for access to nationwide health news derived from seventy-one daily publications and reputable broadcast and online networks, including USA Today's Health section, Reuters Health, MSNBC, and drKoop.com. News coverage includes treatment discoveries, pharmacological updates, the latest in managed care, product recalls, and hundreds of other breaking news bulletins.

Doctor's Guide: Medical & Other News ◉ ◉ ◉

http://www.pslgroup.com/MEDNEWS.HTM

This site provides very current medical news and information for health professionals. Visitors can search the Doctor's Guide Medical News Database, and access medical news broadcast within the past week or the past month. News items organized by subject, firsthand conference communiqués, and journal club reviews are also available at this informative news site.

Health News from CNN ◉ ◉ ◉

http://www.cnn.com/HEALTH

Health News from CNN is produced in association with WebMD. Specific articles are available in featured topics, ethics matters, research, and home remedies, and an allergy report is also provided. National and international health news is presented, and users can access specific articles on AIDS, aging, alternative medicine, cancer, children's health, diet and fitness, men's health, and women's health. Visitors can also access patient questions and answers of doctors, chat forums, and special community resources available through WebMD. Information and articles are also offered by Mayo Clinic and AccentHealth.com.

Medical Breakthroughs ◉ ◉ ◉

http://www.ivanhoe.com/#reports

This site delivers daily News Flash Updates to your e-mail box. A fee of US$15 per quarter is required for receipt of bulletins on pending medical breakthroughs. Visitors can also search archived articles by keyword, read weekly general interest articles, find links to related sites, and watch videos related to current health issues. The site is sponsored by Ivanhoe Broadcast News, Inc., a medical news gathering organization providing stories to television stations nationwide.

Medical Tribune ○ ○ ○

http://www.medtrib.com

Daily medical news for health professionals is available at this site, and users can search archives for specific articles. The MD CyberGuide at the site describes and rates top medical Web sites, a valuable resource for physicians new to the Internet. Results of recent polls of physicians on many health topics and questions unrelated to health; clinical quizzes; a bulletin board; chat forums; and contact details are available at this informative site.

Reuters Health ○ ○ (some features fee-based)

http://www.reutershealth.com

Reuters provides an excellent site for breaking medical news, updated daily, as well as a subscription-based searchable database of the News Archives of Reuters News Service. Visitors can access MEDLINE from the site. Group subscribers have access to a database of drug information.

Science News Update ○ ○

http://www.ama-assn.org/sci-pubs/sci-news/1997/pres_rel.htm

This weekly online publication provides users with the Journal of the American Medical Association reports and a list of previous news releases. Visitors can also access site updates, search the site for specific articles, register for e-mail alerts of new issues, read classified advertisements, and find information on print subscriptions, reprints, and advertising rates.

This Week's Top Medical News Stories ○ ○ ○

http://www.newsfile.com/newsrx.htm

Conference coverage reports and summaries of recent research findings are available at this site from weekly online publications devoted to news such as HIV/AIDS, Alzheimer's disease, angiogenesis, blood products, cancer, gene therapy, genomics and genetics, CDC activities, hepatitis, immunotherapy, obesity, pain management, proteomics, transplants, tuberculosis and airborne diseases, vaccines, women's health, and world disease issues.

UniSci: Daily University Science News ○ ○

http://unisci.com

This site offers current articles related to all branches of science, including medicine. Many medical articles are available, and special archives offer additional medical resources. Users can access news from the past 10 days and perform searches for archived material.

USA Today: Health   ◎ ◎ ◎
http://www.usatoday.com/life/health/archive.htm

USA Today's feature stories and headline archives are directly accessible at this Web site where visitors can view some of the best in nationwide medical news coverage. Interesting articles include the safety of online pharmacies, news on unconventional remedies, and genetic research and discoveries. Visitors will also find the latest in groundbreaking medical and pharmacotherapuetic research.

Yahoo! Health Headlines   ◎ ◎ ◎
http://dailynews.yahoo.com/headlines/hl

Updated several times throughout the day, Health Headlines at Yahoo! offers full news coverage and Reuters News with top health headlines from around the globe. Earlier daily and archived stories may be accessed, and the site's powerful search engine allows viewers to browse, with full color, the latest in photographic coverage of news and events.

11.3 General Medical Supersites

American Medical Association (AMA)   ◎ ◎ ◎
http://www.ama-assn.org

The AMA develops and promotes standards in medical practice, research, and education; acts as advocate on behalf of patients and physicians; and provides discourse on matters important to public health in America. General information is available at the site about the organization; journals and newsletters; policy, advocacy activities, and ethics; education; and accreditation services. AMA news and consumer health information are also found at the site. Resources for physicians include membership details, information on AMA CPT/RBRVS Electronic Medical Systems, Y2K information and preparation suggestions, AMA Alliance information (a national organization of physicians' spouses), descriptions of additional AMA products and services, a discussion of legal issues for physicians, and information on AMA's global activities. Links are provided to AMA member special interest groups for physicians and students. Information for consumers includes medical news; detailed information on a wide range of conditions; general health topic discussions; family health resources for children, adolescents, men, and women; interactive health calculators; healthy recipes; and general safety tips. Specific pages are devoted to comprehensive resources related to HIV/AIDS, asthma, migraines, and women's health. Healthcare providers and patients will find this site an excellent source for accurate and useful health information.

BioSites ○ ○ ○

http://www.library.ucsf.edu/biosites

BioSites is a comprehensive catalog of selected Internet resources in the Biomedical Sciences. The sites were selected as part of a project by staff members of Resource Libraries within the Pacific Southwest Region of the National Network of Libraries of Medicine. Sites are organized by medical topic or specialty field, and users can also search the site by keyword. Featured Web sites are listed by title, but detailed descriptions are not provided.

CenterWatch ○ ○ ○

http://www.centerwatch.com/main.htm

This clinical trials listing service offers patient resources, including a listing of clinical trials by disease category, links to current NIH trials, listings of new FDA drug therapy approvals, and current research headlines. Background information on clinical research is also available to patients unfamiliar with the clinical trials process. Industry professional resources include research center profiles, industry provider profiles, industry news, and career and educational opportunities. Links to related sites of interest to patients and professionals are available at the site.

Health On the Net (HON) Foundation ○ ○ ○

http://www.hon.ch

The Health On the Net Foundation is a nonprofit organization advancing the development and application of new information technologies, notably in the fields of health and medicine. This site offers an engine that searches the Internet as well as the Foundation's database for medical sites, hospitals, and support communities. A media gallery contains a searchable database of medical images and videos from various sources. The site also features a list of online journals, articles and abstracts, and papers from conferences and various other medical sources. The HON MeSH tool allows you to browse Medical Subject Headings (MeSH), a hierarchical structure of medical concepts from the National Library of Medicine (NLM). Users can select a target group (healthcare providers, medical professionals, or patients and other individuals) to receive more tailored search results.

HealthGate.com ○ ○ ○

http://www.healthgate.com

HealthGate offers information resources and health-related articles for healthcare professionals and the general public. Health professional resources include links to research tools, including online journals, drug information, and medical search engines, Continuing Medical Education (CME) resources, news, and patient education materials. Resources for the general public and patients include articles on current health issues and advances, drug and vitamin information, symptoms and medical tests information, and several Webzines devoted to specific topics, including alternative medicine, fitness, nutrition, mental well-being, parenting, travel health, and sexuality. A joint effort of two medical publishers allows site access to full-text journal articles. Search engines allow users to search the site, MEDLINE, or a medical dictionary for information. The site provides users with a good starting point for medical information.

Medical Matrix ⊙ ⊙ ⊙ (free registration)
http://www.medmatrix.org

Medical Matrix offers a list of directories categorized into specialties, diseases, clinical practice resources, literature, education, healthcare and professional resources, medical computing, Internet and technology, and marketplace resources containing classifieds and employment opportunities. Additional features include a site search engine, access to MEDLINE, clinical searches, and links to symposia on the Web, medical textbook resources, patient education materials, Continuing Medical Education information, news, and online journals. Free registration is necessary to access the site.

MedNets ⊙ ⊙ ⊙
http://www.internets.com/mednets

This site houses a collection of proprietary search engines, searching only medical databases. Users can access search engines by medical specialty or disease topic. Other resources include links to the home pages of associations, journals, hospitals, companies, research, government sites, clinical practice guidelines, medical news, and consumer and patient information. The site also includes a set of medical databases and links to search engines provided on the Internet by medical schools.

Medscape ⊙ ⊙ ⊙ (free registration)
http://www.medscape.com

Medscape offers a searchable directory of specialty Web sites that provide information on a wide range of medical specialties. Registration is free, and users can customize the site's home page from a particular computer by choosing a medical specialty. Information in a personalized home page includes news items, conference summaries and schedules, treatment updates, practice guidelines, and patient resources, all pertaining to the chosen field of specialization. The site also includes clinical feature articles and links to special clinical resources.

Megasite Project: A Metasite Comparing Health Information Megasites and Search Engines ⊙ ⊙ ⊙
http://www.lib.umich.edu/megasite/toc.html

The Megasite Project, created by librarians at Northwestern University, the University of Michigan, and Pennsylvania State University, evaluates and provides links to 26 Internet sites providing health information. Criteria for evaluation and comparison include administration and quality control, content, and design. Users can access results of site evaluations, tips for successful site searches, lists of the best general and health information search engines reviewed, and site comparisons listed by evaluation criteria. A bibliography of articles on Web design and Internet resource evaluation is found at the address, as well as descriptions of other aspects of the project.

National Library of Medicine (NLM) ◉ ◉ ◉
http://www.nlm.nih.gov

The National Library of Medicine, the world's largest medical library, collects materials in all areas of biomedicine and healthcare, and works on biomedical aspects of technology; the humanities; and the physical, life, and social sciences. This site contains links to government medical databases, including MEDLINE and MEDLINE plus (for consumers); information on funding opportunities at the NLM and other federal agencies; and details of services, training, and outreach programs offered by NLM. Users can access NLM's catalog of resources (LocatorPlus), as well as NLM publications, including fact sheets, published reports, and staff publications. Also available are NLM announcements, news, exhibit information, and staff directories. NLM research programs discussed at the site include topics in Computational Molecular Biology, Medical Informatics, and other related subjects.

The Web site features 15 searchable databases, covering journal searches via MEDLINE, AIDS information via AIDSLINE, AIDSDRUGS, and AIDSTRIALS, bioethics via BIOETHICSLINE, and numerous other important topics. The "master search engine," nicknamed Internet Grateful Med (IGM), searches MEDLINE using the retrieval engine called PubMed. It is very user-friendly. There are 9 million citations among MEDLINE, PreMEDLINE, and other related databases.

Additionally, the NLM provides sources of health statistics, serials programs, and services maintained through a system called SERHOLD; medical images; international medical resources; and a searchable NLM staff directory.

WebMD ◉ ◉ ◉ (some features fee-based)
http://www.webmd.com

High-quality consumer health information and resources for healthcare professionals are available at this address. Consumer resources include information on conditions, treatments, and drugs; medical news and articles on specific topics; a medical encyclopedia; drug reference resources; a forum for asking health questions; online chat events with medical experts; transcripts of past chat events; message boards; and articles and expert advice on general health topics. Consumers can also join a "community" for more personalized information and forums. Physicians services are available for a fee of US$29.95 monthly (in a twelve-month contract), and includes access to medical news, online journals, and reference databases; online insurance verification and referrals; e-mail, voice mail, fax, and conference call capabilities; practice management tools; online trading; financial services; and other resources. The site includes a preview tour of the service for interested professionals.

11.4 **Government Information Databases**

CRISP: Computer Retrieval of Information on Scientific Projects ○ ○ ○

http://www-commons.cit.nih.gov/crisp

CRISP is a searchable database of federally-funded biomedical research projects conducted at universities, hospitals, and other research institutions. Users, including the public, can use CRISP to search for scientific concepts, emerging trends and techniques, or to identify specific projects and/or investigators. This site provides a direct gateway into the searchable database. The NIH funds the operation of CRISP.

Government Information Locator Service ○ ○ ○

http://www.access.gpo.gov/su_docs/gils/gils.html

Intended to pool access to government information through one search engine, this federal locator service enables a search by topic in which the search word or phrase is placed in quotation markets. Instructions for searching are located at the site.

Healthfinder ○ ○ ○

http://healthfinder.gov/moretools/libraries.htm

Healthfinder provides links to national medical libraries, such as the National Library of Medicine and the National Institutes of Health Library, and other medical or health sciences libraries on the Internet. Directories of libraries are also available to find local facilities. Visitors can use a site search engine to find specific health Web resources.

MEDLINEplus: Health Information Database ○ ○ ○

http://www.nlm.nih.gov/medlineplus/medlineplus.html

A comprehensive database of health and medical information, MEDLINEplus serves a different purpose from its sister service, MEDLINE, which is a bibliographic search engine to locate citations and abstracts in medical journals and reports. MEDLINEplus offers the ability to search by topic and obtain full information rather than citations. The search engine brings up extensive resources on every possible topic, giving complete information on all aspects of the topic. One can search body systems, disorders and diseases, treatments and therapies, diagnostic procedures, side effects, and numerous other important topics related to personal health and the field of medicine in general.

11.5 Government Organizations

Government Agencies and Offices

Administration for Children and Families (ACF) ⊙ ⊙ ⊙
http://www.acf.dhhs.gov

This site provides descriptions of, resources for, and links to ACF programs and services. These sites detail programs and services that relate to areas such as welfare and family assistance, child support, foster care and adoption, Head Start, and support for Native Americans, refugees, and the developmentally disabled. Updated news and information is provided as well.

Administration on Aging ⊙ ⊙ ⊙
http://www.aoa.dhhs.gov

This site provides resources for seniors, practitioners, and caregivers. Resources include news on aging, links to Web sites on aging, statistics about older people, consumer fact sheets, retirement and financial planning information, and help finding community assistance for seniors.

Agency for Toxic Substances and Disease Registry ⊙ ⊙ ⊙
http://www.atsdr.cdc.gov/atsdrhome.html

The mission of this agency is "to prevent exposure and adverse human health effects and diminished quality of life associated with exposure to hazardous substances from waste sites, unplanned releases, and other sources of pollution present in the environment." Toward this goal, the site posts national alerts and health advisories. It provides answers to frequently asked questions about hazardous substances and lists the minimal risk levels for each of them. The site has a HazDat database developed to provide access to information on the release of hazardous substances from Superfund sites or from emergency events and on the effects of hazardous substances on the health of human populations. A quarterly Hazardous Substances and Public Health Newsletter is available for viewing on the site, as are additional resources for kids, parents, and teachers.

Center for Nutrition Policy and Promotion (CNPP) ⊙ ⊙ ⊙
http://www.usda.gov/cnpp

The Center for Nutrition Policy and Promotion is "the focal point within USDA where scientific research is linked with the nutritional needs of the American public." It provides statistical information and resources for educators, and contains dietary guidelines for Americans, official USDA food plans, and means to request additional publications and information by mail or phone.

Department of Health and Human Services (HHS) Homepage

http://www.os.dhhs.gov

This site lists HHS agencies and provides links to the individual agency sites. It offers news, press releases, and information on accessing HHS records and contacting HHS officials. It also provides a search engine for all federal HHS agencies and access to HealthFinder.

Epidemiology Program Office

http://www.cdc.gov/epo/index.htm

Information and resources on public health surveillance is available here. Publications and software related to epidemiology are available for download. Updated news, events, and international bulletins are also featured at the site.

Federal Web Locator

http://www.infoctr.edu/fwl

This is a useful search engine for links to federal government sites and information on the World Wide Web. Users can search agency names and access a table of contents.

Food and Nutrition Service (FNS)

http://www.fns.usda.gov/fns

The Food and Nutrition Service (FNS) "reduces hunger and food insecurity in partnership with cooperating organizations by providing children and needy families access to food, a healthful diet and nutrition education in a manner that supports American agriculture and inspires public confidence." The site provides details of FNS nutrition assistance programs such as Food Stamps, WIC, and Child Nutrition. Research, in the form of published studies and reports, is also made available at the site.

Food & Drug Administration (FDA)

http://www.fda.gov

The FDA is one of the oldest consumer protection agencies in the United States, monitoring the manufacture, import, transport, storage, and sale of about $1 trillion worth of products each year. This comprehensive site provides information on the safety of foods, human and animal drugs, blood products, cosmetics, and medical devices. The site also contains details of field operations, current regulations, toxicology research, medical products reporting procedures, and answers to frequently asked questions. Users can search the site by keyword and find specific information targeted to consumers, industry, health professionals, patients, state and local officials, women, and children.

Food Safety and Inspection Service ☉ ☉ ☉

http://www.fsis.usda.gov

The Food Safety and Inspection Service (FSIS) is "the public health agency in the U.S. Department of Agriculture responsible for ensuring that the nation's commercial supply of meat, poultry, and egg products are safe, wholesome, and correctly labeled and packaged." This site offers a description of the FSIS and their activities, and provides news, consumer information, publications, and resources for educators.

Government Printing Office (GPO) Access ☉ ☉ ☉

http://www.access.gpo.gov/su_docs

Formed by the Government Printing Office to facilitate the transition of electronic documents, this site is the central location for accessing documents from all three branches of the federal government. It provides free access to the official government versions of some 140,000 titles in plain text or PDF format. GPO Access also contains links to governmental databases, including the Federal Register, the Code of Federal Regulations, and the Congressional Record.

Healthcare Financing Administration ☉ ☉ ☉

http://www.hcfa.gov

Information on Medicare, Medicaid, and Child Health insurance programs is provided here. Statistical data on enrollment in the various programs as well as analysis of recent trends in healthcare spending, employment, and pricing is also provided. The site offers consumer publications and program forms, which are available for download.

Indian Health Service (IHS) ☉ ☉

http://www.ihs.gov

Indian Health Service (IHS) is an agency "within the U. S. Department of Health and Human Services and is responsible for providing federal health services to American Indians and Alaska Natives." This site offers related news and press releases. It details management resources, medical programs, jobs, scholarships, office locations, and contact information.

National Bioethics Advisory Commission (NBAC) ☉ ☉

http://bioethics.gov/cgi-bin/bioeth_counter.pl

NBAC "provides advice and makes recommendations to the National Science and Technology Council and to other appropriate government entities regarding the appropriateness of departmental, agency, or other governmental programs, policies, assignments, missions, guidelines, and regulations as they relate to bioethical issues arising from research on human biology and behavior." It also advises on the applications, including the clinical applications, of that research. This site lists meeting dates, transcripts of meetings, reports, news, and links to related sites.

National Center for Chronic Disease Prevention and Health Promotion ◎ ◎ ◎

http://www.cdc.gov/nccdphp/nccdhome.htm

This site "defines chronic disease, lists major chronic diseases, and describes the cost burden of treating them as well as the cost-effectiveness of prevention." Risk behaviors that lead to chronic disease are discussed, and comprehensive and disease-specific approaches to prevention of chronic diseases are addressed. The site provides access to selected Center reports, newsletters, brochures, and CD-ROMs. Information on conferences, meetings, and news publications is provided along with links to related sites.

National Center for Environmental Health (NCEH) ◎ ◎ ◎

http://www.cdc.gov/nceh/ncehhome.htm

The NCEH "is working to prevent illness, disability, and death from interactions between people and the environment." Site links and information on programs and activities are provided, and access is available to publications and products including NCEH fact sheets, brochures, books, and articles. The site also offers current employment opportunities and information on training programs. Spanish and young adult versions of the NCEH site are also available.

National Center for Health Statistics (NCHS) ◎ ◎ ◎

http://www.cdc.gov/nchs/default.htm

The National Center for Health Statistics (NCHS) is the foremost federal government agency responsible for gathering, analyzing, and disseminating health statistics on the American population." To accomplish the mission of the Center, the NCHS Web site has a site-based search engine and collections of health related statistics organized alphabetically by topic. frequently asked questions are answered on various statistical topics. Useful resources at the site include contact information for obtaining copies of vital records, related catalogs, publications, and other information products.

National Center for Infectious Diseases ◎ ◎ ◎

http://www.cdc.gov/ncidod/index.htm

The mission of the National Center for Infectious Diseases "is to prevent illness, disability, and death caused by infectious diseases in the United States and around the world." The site contains an online bimonthly journal that tracks trends and analyzes new and reemerging infectious disease issues around the world. Resources include general information on infectious diseases, specific infectious disease discussions and descriptions, and links to organizations, associations, journals, newsletters, and other publications. One section of the site is devoted to resources related to travel health.

National Center for Toxicological Research (NCTR) ◎ ◎
http://www.fda.gov/nctr/index.html

The mission of NCTR "is to conduct peer-reviewed scientific research that supports and anticipates the FDA's current and future regulatory needs." This research is aimed at understanding critical biological events in the expression of toxicity and at developing methods to improve assessment of human exposure, susceptibility, and risk. The site details the accomplishments, current programs, and future goals of the NCTR.

National Guideline Clearinghouse (NGC) ◎ ◎ ◎
http://www.guidelines.gov/index.asp

The National Guideline Clearinghouse (NGC) is a database of evidence-based clinical practice guidelines and related documents produced by the Agency for Health Care Policy and Research (AHCPR), in partnership with the American Medical Association (AMA) and the American Association of Health Plans (AAHP). Users can search the database by keyword or browse by disease category.

National Institute for Occupational Safety and Health (NIOSH) ◎ ◎ ◎
http://www.cdc.gov/niosh/homepage.html

NIOSH "is part of the Centers for Disease Control and Prevention and is the only federal institute responsible for conducting research and making recommendations for the prevention of work-related illnesses and injuries." The site contains updated news, listings of special events and programs, and information on downloading or ordering related publications. It also provides access to databases such as a pocket guide to hazardous chemicals and a topic index of occupational safety and health information.

National Science Foundation, Directorate for Biological Sciences ◎ ◎ ◎
http://www.nsf.gov/bio/ibn/start.htm

The Division of Integrative Biology and Neuroscience (IBN) supports research aimed at understanding the living organism—plant, animal, microbe—as a unit of biological organization. Current scientific emphases include biotechnology, biomolecular materials, environmental biology, global change, biodiversity, molecular evolution, plant science, microbial biology, and computational biology (including modeling). Research projects generally include support for the education and training of future scientists.

IBN also supports doctoral dissertation research, research conferences, workshops, symposia, Undergraduate Mentoring in Environmental Biology (UMEB), and a variety of NSF-wide activities. This site describes in detail the activities and divisions of IBN, and offers a staff directory, award listings, and deadline dates for funding applications.

Office of National Drug Control Policy (ONDCP) ☉ ☉ ☉

http://www.whitehousedrugpolicy.gov

This site states the missions and goals of the ONDCP. It has a clearinghouse of drug policy information with a staff that will respond to the needs of the general public, providing statistical data, topical fact sheets, information packets and more. There is information on related science, medicine, and technology. There are also resources on prevention, education, and treatment programs. Information on the enforcement of the policies is provided for the national, state, and local levels.

Office of Naval Research—Human Systems Department ☉ ☉

http://www.onr.navy.mil/sci_tech/personnel/default.htm#biological

This site details Medical Science and Technology, and the Cognitive and Neural Science and Technology programs of the Human Systems Department. Procedures for submitting proposals are also outlined at the site.

Public Health Service (PHS) ☉ ☉

http://phs.os.dhhs.gov/phs/phs.html

Links to public health service agencies and program offices, and Health and Human Services vacancy announcements are available at this site. The site is linked to the Office of the Surgeon General, providing transcripts of speeches and reports, a biography of the current Surgeon General, and a history and summary of duties associated with the position.

Substance Abuse and Mental Health Services Administration ☉ ☉ ☉

http://www.samhsa.gov

The Substance Abuse and Mental Health Services Administration "is the federal agency charged with improving the quality and availability of prevention, treatment, and rehabilitation services in order to reduce illness, death, disability, and cost to society resulting from substance abuse and mental illnesses." The site provides substance abuse and mental health information, including details of programs for prevention and treatment in these areas, updated news and statistics, and notices of grant opportunities.

NIH Institutes and Centers

Center for Information Technology (CIT) ☉ ☉ ☉

http://www.cit.nih.gov/home.asp

The Center for Information Technology incorporates the power of modern computers into the biomedical programs and administrative procedures of the NIH by conducting computational biosciences research, developing computer systems, and providing computer facilities. The site provides information on activities and the organization of the Center, contact information, resources for Macintosh users, and links to many useful Information Technology sites. Users can search the site or the CIT Help Desk Knowledgebase for specific information.

Center for Scientific Review (CSR) ◎ ◎ ◎

http://www.drg.nih.gov

The Center for Scientific Review is the focal point at NIH for the conduct of initial peer review, which is the foundation of the NIH grant and award process. The Center carries out a peer review of the majority of research and research training applications submitted to the NIH. The Center also serves as the central receipt point for all such Public Health Service applications and makes referrals to scientific review groups for scientific and technical merit review of applications and to funding components for potential award. To this end, the Center develops and implements innovative, flexible ways to conduct referral and review for all aspects of science. The site contains contact information, transcripts of public commentary panel discussions, news and events listings, grant applications, peer review notes, and links to additional biomedical and government sites.

Centers for Disease Control and Prevention (CDC) ◎ ◎ ◎

http://www.cdc.gov

The mission of the Centers for Disease Control and Prevention is to promote health and quality of life by preventing and controlling disease, injury, and disability. The site provides users with links to 11 associated Centers, Institutes, and Offices; a Web page devoted to travelers' health; publications; software; and other products, data, and statistics; training and employment opportunities; and subscription registration forms for online CDC publications. Highlighted publications include *Emerging Infectious Disease Journal* and *Morbidity and Mortality Weekly Report,* both of which can be e-mailed on a regular basis by registering on this site. Links are available to additional CDC resources, and state and local agencies concerned with public health issues. CDC offers a comprehensive, alphabetical list of general and specific health topics at the site. Visitors can also search the site by keyword, and read spotlights on current research and information presented by the Web site.

Computer Database for Scientific Topics ◎ ◎ ◎

http://www-commons.cit.nih.gov/crisp

CRISP (Computer Retrieval of Information on Scientific Projects) is a comprehensive compilation of abstracts describing the federally-funded research projects of academic, healthcare, and research institutions. The database, maintained by the Office of Extramural Research at the National Institutes of Health, includes projects funded by many of the major government agencies, such as the National Institutes of Health (NIH), the Food and Drug Administration (FDA), and the Centers for Disease Control and Prevention (CDCP). Visitors to the site can use the CRISP search interface to identify emerging research trends and techniques, or locate specific projects and/or investigators. General information about the CRISP database and answers to frequently asked questions about CRISP are also available.

Fogarty International Center (FIC) ○ ○ ○
http://www.nih.gov/fic

The Fogarty International Center for Advanced Study in the Health Sciences leads NIH efforts to advance the health of the American public, and citizens of all nations, through international cooperation on global health threats. Resources at the site include Center publications, regional information on programs and contacts, research and training opportunities, a description of the Center's Multilateral Initiative on Malaria (MIM), details of the NIH Visiting Program for Foreign Scientists, and news and vacancy announcements.

Introduction to the National Institutes of Health (NIH) ○ ○ ○
http://www.nih.gov

NIH is one of eight health agencies of the Public Health Service which, in turn, is part of the U.S. Department of Health and Human Services. The NIH mission is to uncover new knowledge that will lead to better health for everyone. NIH works toward that mission by conducting research in its own laboratories; supporting the research of non-federal scientists in universities, medical schools, hospitals, and research institutions throughout the country and abroad; helping in the training of research investigators; and fostering communication of biomedical information. The site provides a Director's message about the agency, e-mail and telephone directories, visitor information, employment and summer internship program information, science education program details, and a history of NIH. A site search engine and links to the home pages of all NIH Institutes and Centers are available.

National Cancer Institute (NCI) ○ ○ ○
http://www.nci.nih.gov

The National Cancer Institute leads a national effort to reduce the burden of cancer morbidity and mortality, and ultimately to prevent the disease. Through basic and clinical biomedical research and training, the NCI conducts and supports programs to understand the causes of cancer; prevent, detect, diagnose, treat, and control cancer; and disseminate information to the practitioner, patient, and public. The site provides visitors with many informational resources related to cancer, including CancerTrials for clinical trials resources and CancerNet for information on cancer tailored to the needs of health professionals, patients, and the general public. Additional resources relate to funding opportunities, and events and research at NCI.

National Center for Biotechnology Information (NCBI) ◉ ◉ ◉

http://www.ncbi.nlm.nih.gov

A comprehensive site that provides a wide array of biotechnology resources to the user, the NCBI includes sources such as a genetic sequence database (GenBank); links to related sites, a newsletter, site and genetic sequence search engines; information on programs, activities, and research projects; seminar and exhibit schedules; and database services. Databases available through this site include PubMed (for free MEDLINE searching) and OMIM (Online Mendelian Inheritance in Man) for an extensive catalog of human genes and genetic disorders.

National Center for Complementary and Alternative Medicine (NCCAM) ◉ ◉ ◉

http://nccam.nih.gov

The National Center for Complementary and Alternative Medicine identifies and evaluates unconventional healthcare practices, supports, coordinates, and conducts research and research training on these practices, and disseminates information. The site describes specific program areas; answers common questions about alternative therapies; and offers news, research grants information, and a calendar of events. Information resources at the site include a citation index related to alternative medicine obtained from MEDLINE, a bibliography of publications; the NCCAM clearinghouse of information for the public, media, and healthcare professionals; and a link to the National Women's Health Information Center (NWHIC).

National Center for Research Resources (NCRR) ◉ ◉

http://www.ncrr.nih.gov

The National Center for Research Resources creates, develops, and provides a comprehensive range of human, animal, technological, and other resources to support biomedical research advances. The Center's areas of concentration are biomedical technology, clinical research, comparative medicine, and research infrastructure. The site offers more specific information on each of these research areas, grants information, news, current events, press releases, publications, research resources, and a search engine for locating information at the site.

National Eye Institute (NEI) ◉ ◉ ◉

http://www.nei.nih.gov:80

The National Eye Institute conducts and supports research, training, health information dissemination, and other programs with respect to blinding eye diseases, visual disorders, mechanisms of visual function, preservation of sight, and the special health problems and requirements of the visually impaired. Information at the site is tailored to the needs of researchers, health professionals, the general public and patients, educators, and the media. Resources include a clinical trials database, intramural research information, funding, grants, contract information, news and events calendar, publications, visitor information, a site search engine, and an overview of the NEI offices, divisions, branches, and laboratories.

National Heart, Lung, and Blood Institute (NHLBI) ☺ ☺ ☺

http://www.nhlbi.nih.gov

The National Heart, Lung, and Blood Institute provides leadership for a national research program in diseases of the heart, blood vessels, lungs, and blood, and in transfusion medicine through support of innovative basic, clinical, and population-based and health education research. The site provides health information, scientific resources, research funding information, news and press releases, details of committees, meetings and events, clinical guidelines, notices of studies seeking patient participation, links to laboratories at the NHLBI, and technology transfer resources. Highlights of the site include cholesterol, weight, and asthma management resources.

National Human Genome Research Institute (NHGRI) ☺ ☺ ☺

http://www.nhgri.nih.gov

The National Human Genome Research Institute supports the NIH component of the Human Genome Project, a worldwide research effort designed to analyze the structure of human DNA and determine the location of the estimated 50,000–100,000 human genes. The NHGRI Intramural Research Program develops and implements technology for understanding, diagnosing, and treating genetic diseases. The site provides information about NHGRI, the Human Genome Project, grants, intramural research, policy and public affairs, workshops and conferences, and news items. Resources include links to the Institute's Ethical, Legal, and Social Implications Program and the Center for Inherited Disease Research, genomic and genetic resources for investigators, a glossary of genetic terms, and a site search engine.

National Institute of Allergy and Infectious Diseases (NIAID) ☺ ☺ ☺

http://www.niaid.nih.gov

NIAID provides the major support for scientists conducting research aimed at developing better ways to diagnose, treat, and prevent the many infectious, immunologic, and allergic diseases that afflict people worldwide. This site provides NIAID news releases, contact information, calendar of events, links to related sites, a clinical trials database, grants and technology transfer information, and current research information (including meetings, publications, and research resources). Fact sheets for public use are available for different immunological disorders, allergies, asthma, and infectious diseases.

National Institute of
Arthritis and Musculoskeletal and Skin Diseases (NIAMS) ⊙ ⊙ ⊙

http://www.nih.gov/niams

The NIAMS conducts and supports a broad spectrum of research on normal structure and function of bones, muscles, and skin, as well as the numerous and disparate diseases that affect these tissues. NIAMS also conducts research training and epidemiologic studies, and disseminates information. The site provides details of research programs at the Institute and offers personnel and employment listings, news, and an events calendar. Health information at the site is provided in the form of fact sheets, brochures, health statistics, and other resources, and contact details are available for ordering materials. Scientific resources include bibliographies of publications, consensus conference reports, grants and contracts applications, grant program announcements, and links to scientific research databases. Information on current clinical studies and transcripts of NIAMS advisory council, congressional, and conference reports are also available at the site.

National Institute of
Child Health and Human Development (NICHD) ⊙ ⊙ ⊙

http://www.nichd.nih.gov

The NICHD conducts and supports laboratory, clinical, and epidemiological research on the reproductive, neurobiologic, developmental, and behavioral processes that determine and maintain the health of children, adults, families, and populations. Research in the areas of fertility, pregnancy, growth, development, and medical rehabilitation strives to ensure that every child is born healthy and wanted, and grows up free from disease and disability. The site provides general information about the Institute; funding and intramural research details; information about the Division of Epidemiology, Statistics, and Prevention Research; publications bibliography; fact sheets; reports; employment and fellowship listings; and research resources.

National Institute of Dental and Craniofacial Research (NIDCR) ⊙ ⊙ ⊙

http://www.nidr.nih.gov

The National Institute of Dental and Craniofacial Research provides leadership for a national research program designed to understand, treat, and ultimately prevent the infectious and inherited craniofacial-oral-dental diseases and disorders that compromise millions of human lives. General information about the Institute, news and health information, details of research activities, and NIDCR employment opportunities are all found at the site. A site search engine and staff directory are also available.

National Institute of
Diabetes and Digestive and Kidney Diseases (NIDDK) ◎ ◎ ◎
http://www.niddk.nih.gov

The National Institute of Diabetes and Digestive and Kidney Diseases conducts and supports basic and applied research, and provides leadership for a national program in diabetes, endocrinology, and metabolic diseases; digestive diseases and nutrition; and kidney, urologic, and hematologic diseases. NIDDK information at the site includes a mission statement, history, organization description, staff directory, and employment listing. Additional resources include news; a database for health information; clinical trials information, including a patient recruitment section; and information on extramural funding and intramural research at the Institute.

National Institute of Environmental Health Sciences (NIEHS) ◎ ◎ ◎
http://www.niehs.nih.gov

The National Institute of Environmental Health Sciences reduces the burden of human illness and dysfunction from environmental causes by defining how environmental exposures, genetic susceptibility, and age interact to affect an individual's health. News and Institute events, research information, grant and contract details, fact sheets, an Institute personnel directory, employment and training notices, teacher support, and an online resource for kids are all found at this site. Library resources include a book catalog, electronic journals, database searching, NIEHS publications, and reference resources. Visitors can use search engines at the site to find environmental health information and news, publications, available grants and contracts, and library resources.

National Institute of General Medical Sciences (NIGMS) ◎ ◎ ◎
http://www.nih.gov/nigms

The National Institute of General Medical supports basic biomedical research that is not targeted to specific diseases, but that increases the understanding of life processes, and lays the foundation for advances in disease diagnosis, treatment, and prevention. Among the most significant results of this research has been the development of recombinant DNA technology, which forms the basis for the biotechnology industry. The site provides information about NIGMS research and funding programs, information for visitors, news, publications list, reports, grant databases, a personnel and employment listing, and links to additional biomedical resources.

National Institute of Mental Health (NIMH) ◎ ◎ ◎
http://www.nimh.nih.gov

The National Institute of Mental Health provides national leadership dedicated to understanding, treating, and preventing mental illnesses through basic research on the brain and behavior, and through clinical, epidemiological, and services research. Resources available at the site include staff directories, information for visitors to the campus, employment opportunities, NIMH history, and publications from activities of the National Advisory Mental Health Council and Peer Review Committees. News, a calendar of events, information on clinical trials, funding opportunities, and intramural research are also provided. Pages tailored specifically for the public, health practitioners, or researchers contain mental disorder information, research fact sheets, statistics, science education materials, news, links to NIMH research sites, and patient education materials.

National Institute of Neurological Disorders and Stroke (NINDS) ⊙ ⊙ ⊙
http://www.ninds.nih.gov

The National Institute of Neurological Disorders and Stroke supports and conducts research and research training on the normal structure and function of the nervous system, and on the causes, prevention, diagnosis, and treatment of more than 600 nervous system disorders including stroke, epilepsy, multiple sclerosis, Parkinson's disease, head and spinal cord injury, Alzheimer's disease, and brain tumors. The site provides visitors with an organizational diagram, e-mail directory, links to advisory groups, the mission and history of NINDS, a site search engine, employment and training opportunities, and information on research at NINDS. Information is available for patients, clinicians, and scientists, including publications, details of current clinical trials, links to other health organizations, and research funding information.

National Institute of Nursing Research (NINR) ⊙ ⊙ ⊙
http://www.nih.gov/ninr

The National Institute of Nursing Research supports clinical and basic research to establish a scientific basis for the care of individuals across the life span, from management of patients during illness and recovery to the reduction of risks for disease and disability and the promotion of healthy lifestyles. NINR accomplishes its mission by supporting grants to universities and other research organizations as well as by conducting research intramurally at laboratories in Bethesda, Maryland. Visitors to this site can find the NINR mission statement and history, employment listings, news, conference details, publications, speech transcripts, answers to Frequently Asked Questions, information concerning legislative activities, research program and funding details, health information, highlights and outcomes of current nursing research, and links to additional Web resources.

National Institute on Aging (NIA) ⊙ ⊙ ⊙
http://www.nih.gov/nia

The National Institute on Aging leads a national program of research on the biomedical, social, and behavioral aspects of the aging process; the prevention of age-related diseases and disabilities; and the promotion of a better quality of life for all older Americans. The site presents recent announcements and upcoming events, employment opportunities, press releases, and media advisories of significant findings.

Research resources include news from the National Advisory Council on Aging, links to extramural aging research conducted throughout the United States, and funding and training information. Health professionals and the general public can access publications on health and aging topics, or order materials online.

National Institute on Alcohol Abuse and Alcoholism (NIAAA) ⊙ ⊙ ⊙
http://www.niaaa.nih.gov:80

The National Institute on Alcohol Abuse and Alcoholism conducts research focused on improving the treatment and prevention of alcoholism and alcohol-related problems to reduce the enormous health, social, and economic consequences of this disease. General resources at the site include an introduction to the Institute, extramural and intramural research information, an organizational flowchart, details of legislative activities, Advisory Council roster and minutes, information on scientific review groups associated with the Institute, a staff directory, and employment announcements. Institute publications, data tables, press releases, conferences and events calendars, answers to frequently asked questions on the subject of alcohol abuse and dependence, and links to related sites are also found at the site. The ETOH Database, an online bibliographic database containing over 100,000 records on alcohol abuse and alcoholism can be accessed from the site, as well as the National Library of Medicine's MEDLINE database.

National Institute on Deafness and Other Communication Disorders (NIDCD) ⊙ ⊙ ⊙
http://www.nih.gov/nidcd

The National Institute on Deafness and Other Communication Disorders conducts and supports biomedical research and research training in the normal and disordered processes of hearing, balance, smell, taste, voice, speech, and language. The Institute also conducts and supports research and research training related to disease prevention and health promotion; addresses special biomedical and behavioral problems associated with people who have communication impairments or disorders; and supports efforts to create devices that substitute for lost and impaired sensory and communication function. The site provides visitors with many fact sheets and other information resources on hearing and balance; smell and taste; voice, speech, and language; hearing aids; otosclerosis; vocal abuse and misuse; and vocal cord paralysis. Other resources include a directory of organizations related to hearing, balance, smell, taste, voice, speech, and language, a glossary of terms, an online newsletter, information for kids and teachers, clinical trials details, and a site search engine. Information on research funding and intramural research activities, news and events calendar, and general information about NIDCD is also available at this site.

National Institute on Drug Abuse (NIDA) ◎ ◎ ◎

http://www.nida.nih.gov/NIDAHome1.html

The National Institute on Drug Abuse leads the nation in bringing the power of science to bear on drug abuse and addiction through support and conduct of research across a broad range of disciplines, and rapid and effective dissemination of results of that research to improve drug abuse and addiction prevention, treatment, and policy. The site contains fact sheets on common drugs of abuse and prevention strategies, Institute announcements, media advisories, congressional testimonies, speech transcripts, online newsletters, scientific meeting dates and summaries, funding, training, legislation information, and links to related sites. Recent research reports and news related to drug addiction are highlighted at the site.

National Library of Medicine (NLM) ◎ ◎ ◎

http://www.nlm.nih.gov

The National Library of Medicine, the world's largest medical library, collects materials in all areas of biomedicine and healthcare; and works on biomedical aspects of technology; the humanities; and the physical, life, and social sciences. This site contains links to government medical databases, including MEDLINE and MEDLINE plus (for consumers), information on funding opportunities at the National Library of Medicine and other federal agencies, and details of services, training, and outreach programs offered by NLM. Users can access NLM's catalog of resources (LocatorPlus), as well as NLM publications, including fact sheets, published reports, and staff publications. Also available are NLM announcements, news, exhibit information, and staff directories. NLM research programs discussed at the site include topics in Computational Molecular Biology, Medical Informatics, and other related subjects.

The Web site features 15 searchable databases, covering journal searches via MED-LINE, AIDS information via AIDSLINE, AIDSDRUGS, AIDSTRIALS, bioethics via BIOETHICSLINE, and numerous other important topics. The "master search engine," nicknamed Internet Grateful Med (IGM), searches MEDLINE using the retrieval engine called PubMed. It is very user-friendly. There are 9 million citations in MEDLINE and PreMEDLINE and the other related databases.

Additionally, the NLM provides sources of health statistics, serials programs, and services maintained through a system called SERHOLD, medical images, international medical resources, and a searchable NLM staff directory.

Warren Grant Magnuson Clinical Center ◎ ◎ ◎

http://www.cc.nih.gov:80

The Warren Grant Magnuson Clinical Center is the clinical research facility of the National Institutes of Health, supporting clinical investigations conducted by the Institutes. The Clinical Center was designed to bring patient-care facilities close to research labs, allowing findings of basic and clinical scientists to move quickly from labs to the treatment of patients. The site provides visitors with news, events, details of current clinical research studies, patient recruitment resources, links to departmental Web sites, and information resources for NIH staff, patients, physicians, and scientists. Topics discussed in the Center's Medicine for the Public Lecture Series and resources in medical and scientific education offered by the Center are included at the site.

11.6 **Guides to Medical Journals on the Internet**

Amedeo   ◎ ◎ ◎   (free registration)
http://www.amedeo.com

Amedeo is a free medical literature service, allowing users to select topics and journals of interest. The service sends a weekly e-mail with an overview of new articles reflecting the specifications indicated by the user, and creates a personal home page with abstracts of relevant articles. The site allows registered users to access a Network Center, which facilitates literature exchange among users with similar interests. This service is supported through educational grants by numerous pharmaceutical companies.

BioMedNet:
The Internet Community for Biological and Medical Researchers   ◎ ◎ ◎
http://www.biomednet.com/library

Owned by publishing giant Reed Elsevier, this site contains a full text library of over 170 biomedical journals, most of which are available for a fee ranging from US$1–$20. Other features include a shopping mall for books, software, and biological supplies; an evaluated Medline system; a list of biomedical site links; a job exchange; and a science news journal. Free BioMedNet membership provides access to many of the site's features. Some publications, such as the Current Biology journals, offer free access to editorials, short articles, and letters. Prices and special offers can be found on each journal's home page under "Prices/Subscriptions." All visitors to the site can search the journals library and view abstracts without incurring charges.

Blackwell Science   ◎ ◎ ◎
http://www.blackwell-science.com/uk/journals.htm

This site offers online access to information regarding well over 200 Blackwell Science Publications. Journals are sorted alphabetically by title and are available in all major fields of science and medicine. Blackwell Science provides a good general overview regarding the content and aim of each of its journals. Tables of contents are available for current and back issues of each title. Access to abstracts and articles requires a fee.

Elsevier Science ⊙ ⊙ ⊙

http://www.elsevier.com

Covering the same Elsevier publications as Science Direct, this site's journal coverage is a bit more up-to-date, and it includes a table of contents search engine. The site also provides many links to journal-related information and subject categories for easy browsing of references in areas of interest. Information is also included on Elsevier's books, and an e-mail alerting service on subject-specific titles from Elsevier's books and journals is available free with registration.

EurekAlert ⊙ ⊙ ⊙

http://www.eurekalert.org

This site allows professionals and consumers to search the archives for the latest articles, news items, events, awards, and grants in science and medicine, including psychiatry. Current news from the Howard Hughes Medical Institute and the National Institutes of Health, as well as numerous links to institutions, journals, and other online resources are available.

Hardin Library Electronic Journal Showcase ⊙ ⊙ ⊙

http://www.lib.uiowa.edu/hardin/md/ej.html

The University of Iowa Hardin Library for the Health Sciences has compiled an index of free full-text journals on the Internet. Using this convenient listing, a user can go straight to a particular journal and retrieve the full text of an article, free-of-charge. Some journals are on a free-trial basis, and sample journal articles are provided for reference.

Highwire Press ⊙ ⊙ ⊙

http://highwire.stanford.edu

One of the largest producers of online versions of biomedical journals, Highwire Press's Web page presents an organized list (by alphabet or subject) of its biomedical journals, including detailed information regarding what is available at no charge for each title. For each journal, there is a link to its page, where tables of contents and abstracts are available. Full text of entire journals or back issues are available for a good number of titles.

Instructions to Authors in the Health Sciences ⊙ ⊙ ⊙

http://www.mco.edu:80/lib/instr/libinsta.html

Produced and maintained by the library staff of the Medical College of Ohio, this site contains a unique compilation of links to instructions for authors, for over 2,000 biomedical journals. All are links to the sites of the publishers who have editorial responsibilities for each title.

Karger ◎ ◎ ◎

http://www.karger.com

Karger provides online access to information on all of its publications. Journals are sorted by title and by subject area. Karger publishes hundreds of journals in an extensive variety of medical and related science fields. Table of contents and article abstracts are available free-of-charge. There is an extensive listing of back issues as well. A free sample issue of each publication is provided. However, a fee is assessed for access to articles.

MDConsult ◎ ◎ ◎ (fee-based)

http://www.mdconsult.com

MDConsult is a comprehensive online medical information service specifically designed for physicians. This is service is provided for a monthly fee of US$19.95, but a 10-day free trial is available. The service includes the ability to search 35 online medical reference books for information and 48 journals for full-text articles. Searches can also be performed for full text articles through MEDLINE and other databases. Members can also search patient education handouts, drug information, and practice guidelines. Additional resources include reviews of new developments from major journals, government agencies, and medical conferences, and a section devoted to what patients are reading in the popular press.

Medical Matrix ◎ ◎ ◎ (free registration)

http://www.medmatrix.org

Following a brief free registration, this site offers a wealth of information in all major medical fields, with continuous updating, rating, and annotating provided by an editorial board and contributors' group composed of physicians and librarians. Each link also includes a description of what can be accessed free-of-charge at that site. Most of the journal sites covered provide free access to table of contents and abstracts. However, some may assess a fee when accessing full text versions of journals. Links to other Web resources in a variety of specialty areas, diseases, and clinical practice subject are also provided, as well as a MEDLINE search engine, plus medical textbook and CME links.

MEDLINE Journal Links To Publishers ◎ ◎ ◎

http://www.ncbi.nlm.nih.gov/PubMed/fulltext.html

Through the National Library of Medicine, the MEDLINE service provides direct access to hundreds of medical journals in all fields, listed alphabetically by name, with direct links to their respective publishers. Upon accessing an individual publication, the reader can normally view the current issue table of contents and abstracts for the articles. In certain cases, the complete article texts are available without charge, but in other cases it is necessary to pay a fee and obtain an access password. Each page explains the available information and the conditions for access, since policies vary by publisher and journal.

PubList: Health and Medical Sciences ⊙ ⊙ ⊙

http://www.publist.com/indexes/health.html

This site contains an extensive list of links to medical journals, divided by subject areas. Useful information, such as frequency, publisher, and format is included for each publication, and a search engine can be used to identify titles of interest.

Science Direct ⊙ ⊙ ⊙

http://www.sciencedirect.com

A very useful site, Science Direct compiles an extensive list of links to online journal literature published by Elsevier Science in all major areas of scientific study, including clinical medicine. Access to full text is available by institutional subscription only; however, table of contents are provided free-of-charge for each journal. The site provides links to hundreds of journals categorized by subject and further subdivided by specialty. Journals are also listed alphabetically by title.

Springer-Verlag's LINK ⊙ ⊙ ⊙

http://link.springer.de

Covering the large list of journals published by Springer-Verlag, this site mostly contains abstracts, rather than full text. Full text is available for those titles for which individuals or institutions maintain print subscriptions. A bit slow to navigate, the site does cover a broad range of biomedical titles, all of which provide tables of contents from the most recent two to four years.

UnCover Web ⊙ ⊙ ⊙

http://uncweb.carl.org

This enormous database of medical and nonscientific journals' tables of contents permits searching by keyword, journal title, or author. Full articles can be faxed or e-mailed for a fee. For a modest price, the reveal service provides e-mailed tables of contents for specific journals as they are published and added to the database.

WebMedLit ⊙ ⊙ ⊙

http://webmedlit.silverplatter.com/index.html

WebMedLit provides access to the latest medical literature on the Web by indexing medical Web sites daily and presenting articles from each site organized by subject categories. All WebMedLit article links are from the original source document at the publisher's Web site, and most articles are available in full text.

Wiley Interscience ⊙ ⊙ ⊙

http://www3.interscience.wiley.com/index.html

This site is maintained by John Wiley and Sons, Inc. and provides links to all Wiley publications. Hundreds of titles are available online via direct link from the publisher. Journals are available in business, law, and all areas of science, including life and medical science. The Journal Finder option allows the user to search journals by title and subject. Free registration allows access to table of contents and abstracts abstracts published within the last 12 months. Full text access is available via registration to both individual and institutional subscribers of the print counterparts of the Wiley online journals.

11.7 **Health and Medical Hotlines**

Toll-Free Numbers for Health Information ⊙

http://nhic-nt.health.org/Scripts/Tollfree.cfm

A categorized list of toll-free health information hotlines is provided by this site. Each hotline provides educational materials for patients.

11.8 **Hospital Resources**

American Hospital Association ⊙ ⊙ ⊙

http://www.aha.org

Everything pertaining to hospitals is either available at this site or at a link from this site, including advocacy, health insurance, extensive hospital information, research and education, health statistics, and valuable links to the National Information Center for Health Services Administration as well as other organizations and resources.

Hospital Directory ⊙ ⊙ ⊙

http://www.doctordirectory.com/hospitals/directory

This useful site provides a listing of states and territories, each of which is a hot link to a further listing of cities in the state or territory. By clicking on a city, the database provides a listing of hospitals in that area, including name, address, and telephone numbers. The site offers other links for physicians pertaining to health plans, doctors, health news, insurance, and medical products.

HospitalWeb ⊙ ⊙ ⊙

http://neuro-www2.mgh.harvard.edu/hospitalwebworld.html

This site is a guide to global hospitals on the World Wide Web (not including the United States). It lists over 50 countries. Under each country, the names of a number of hospitals in that country are listed. By clicking on the hospital name, the user is taken to the hospital's Web site which provides further information.

11.9 Internet Newsgroups

General Medical Topic Newsgroups

Internet newsgroups are places where individuals can post messages on a common site for others to read. Many newsgroups are devoted to medical topics, and these groups are listed below. To access these groups you can either use a newsreader program (often part of an e-mail program), or search and browse using a popular Web site, http://www.deja.com.

Since newsgroups are mostly unmoderated, there is no editorial process or restrictions on postings. The information at these groups is therefore neither authoritative nor based on any set of standards.

sci.med	sci.med.nutrition	sci.med.vision
sci.engr.biomed	sci.med.occupational	alt.image.medical
sci.med.aids	sci.med.orthopedics	alt.med
sci.med.cardiology	sci.med.pathology	alt.med.allergy
sci.med.dentistry	sci.med.pharmacy	alt.med.cfs
sci.med.diseases.cancer	sci.med.physics	alt.med.ems
sci.med.diseases.hepatitis	sci.med.prostate.bph	alt.med.equipment
sci.med.diseases.lyme	sci.med.prostate.cancer	alt.med.fibromyalgia
sci.med.diseases.viral	sci.med.prostate.prostatitis	alt.med.outpat.clinic
sci.med.immunology	sci.med.psychobiology	alt.med.phys-assts
sci.med.informatics	sci.med.radiology	alt.med.urum-outcomes
sci.med.laboratory	sci.med.telemedicine	alt.med.veterinary
sci.med.nursing	sci.med.transcription	alt.med.vision.improve

11.10 Locating a Physician

American Medical Association (AMA): Physician Select Online Doctor Finder ⊙ ⊙ ⊙

http://www.ama-assn.org/aps/amahg.htm

The AMA is the primary "umbrella" professional association of physicians and medical students in the United States. The AMA Physician Select system provides information on virtually every licensed physician, including more than 650,000 physicians and doctors of osteopathy. According to the site, physician credentials have been certified for accuracy and authenticated by accrediting agencies, medical schools, residency programs, licensing and certifying boards, and other data sources. The user can search for physicians by name or by medical specialty.

HealthPages ○ ○ ○

http://www.thehealthpages.com

This search tool allows visitors to locate doctors in their area by specialty and location. Over 500,000 physicians and 120,000 dentists are listed. Doctors may update their profiles free-of-charge. Local provider choices are displayed to consumers in a comparative format. They can access charts that compare the training, office services, and fees of local physicians; the provider networks and quality measures of area managed care plans; the size, services, and fees of local hospitals; and more. Patients can post ratings and comments about their doctors.

Physicians' Practice ○ ○

http://www.physicianpractice.com

This site allows the user to search for doctors in many specialty areas. Searches are performed by specialty and zip code. Physicians must pay a fee to be listed but enjoy other benefits such as referrals, Internet presence, and a newsletter.

11.11 Medical Abbreviations and Acronyms

Ask MedBot ○ ○ ○

http://www.ncemi.org

The National Council for Emergency Medicine Informatics provides a searchable database for medical abbreviations and acronyms. Click on "Abbreviation Translator" and place the letters you wish to identify in the space and press "Enter." Single or multiple definitions will be printed on your screen.

Common Medical Abbreviations ○ ○

http://courses.smsu.edu/jas188f/690/medslpterm.html

Several hundred major medical abbreviations are defined in an alphabetical listing at this educational information site.

11.12 **Medical and Health Sciences Libraries**

Medical Libraries at
Universities, Hospitals, Foundations, and Research Centers ◎ ◎ ◎
http://www.lib.uiowa.edu/hardin-www/hslibs.html

This site includes an up-to-date listing of libraries that can be easily accessed through links produced by staff of the Hardin Library at the University of Iowa. Libraries are listed state by state enabling easy access to hundreds of library Web sites. There are also numerous foreign medical library links. These sites can be easily accessed from the central site established by the Hardin Library at the University of Iowa.

National Institutes of Health (NIH): Library Online ◎ ◎ ◎
http://libwww.ncrr.nih.gov

This site presents information about the NIH Library including a staff listing, current exhibits, hours, materials available to NIH personnel and the general public, current job vacancies, maps for visitors, and answers to frequently asked questions about the Library. Users can search the Library's catalog of books, journals, and other periodicals, access public and academic medical databases, and find seminar and tutorial information, as well as links to related sites.

National Library of Medicine (NLM) ◎ ◎ ◎
http://www.nlm.nih.gov

The National Library of Medicine, the world's largest medical library, collects materials in all areas of biomedicine and healthcare, and works on biomedical aspects of technology; the humanities; and the physical, life, and social sciences. This site contains links to government medical databases, including MEDLINE and MEDLINE plus (for consumers); information on funding opportunities at the NLM and other federal agencies; and details of services, training, and outreach programs offered by NLM. Users can access NLM's catalog of resources (LocatorPlus), as well as NLM publications, including fact sheets, published reports, and staff publications. Also available are NLM announcements, news, exhibit information, and staff directories. NLM research programs discussed at the site include topics in Computational Molecular Biology, Medical Informatics, and other related subjects.

The Web site features 15 searchable databases, covering journal searches via MEDLINE, AIDS information via AIDSLINE, AIDSDRUGS, and AIDSTRIALS, bioethics via BIOETHICSLINE, and numerous other important topics. The "master search engine," nicknamed Internet Grateful Med (IGM), searches MEDLINE using the retrieval engine called PubMed. It is very user-friendly. There are 9 million citations in MEDLINE, PreMEDLINE, and other related databases.

Additionally, the NLM provides sources of health statistics, serials programs and services maintained through a system called SERHOLD, medical images, international medical resources, and a searchable NLM staff directory.

National Network of Libraries of Medicine (NN/LM) ◎ ◎ ◎
http://www.nnlm.nlm.nih.gov

Composed of 8 regional libraries, the NN/LM also provides access to numerous health science libraries in each region, located at universities, hospitals, and institutes. The Web site enables the user to link directly to each of the libraries in any regional of the United States. These libraries have access to the NLM's SERHOLD system database of machine-readable holdings for biomedical serial titles. There are approximately 89,000 serial titles that are accessible through SERHOLD-participating libraries.

11.13 Medical Conferences and Meetings

Cell Press Online: Meetings and Conferences ◎ ◎ ◎
http://jobs.cell.com/events

Focused on mostly research-oriented meetings, this is a comprehensive listing of forthcoming conferences, with searching capabilities, by research area, location, and keywords. A unique feature of this site is its e-mail alerting service.

Doctor's Guide: Medical Conferences & Meetings ◎ ◎ ◎
http://www.pslgroup.com/medconf.htm

This is a very extensive list of several hundred conferences and meetings, including Continuing Medical Education (CME) programs worldwide, organized by date, meeting site, and subject. Location and other details are provided.

Health On the Net (HON) Foundation ◎ ◎ ◎
http://www.hon.ch/cgi-bin/conferences

This site provides a limited listing of conferences and meetings in medical specialty areas, and they are not categorized or indexed by fields. Information is chronological by month.

Medical Conferences.com ◎ ◎ ◎
http://www.medicalconferences.com

This site covers a broad range of medical conference listings, including meetings related to many different areas of healthcare including pharmaceuticals and hospital supplies, as well as the clinical medical specialties. An easy-to-use search mechanism provides access to the numerous listings, each of which links to details concerning each conference. The site claims to be updated daily, providing details on over 7,000 forthcoming conferences.

MediConf Online ○ ○ ○ (some features fee-based)
http://www.mediconf.com/online.html

This well-organized site lists conferences by medical subject, chronology, and geographic location, mostly covering meetings to be held in the next month or two. The listings include research conferences, seminars, annual meetings of professional societies, medical technology trade shows, and opportunities for CME credits. What is provided free on the Internet is only a small percentage of the complete fee-based database, which includes more than 60,000 listings of meetings to be held through 2014, and is available through the information vendors, Ovid or Dialog.

MedMeetings ○ ○ ○
http://www.medmeetings.com

This site claims to be "an interactive guide to medical meetings worldwide." The site is a service of International Medical News Group (IMNG), which publishes six major independent newspapers for physicians. The database includes information on thousands of medical meetings and conventions. Searches can be performed by disease, specialty group, date, location, availability of CME credit, and other criteria.

Medscape: Conference Summaries & Schedules ○ ○ ○
http://www.medscape.com

This service enables members to attend important meetings, catch up on missed meetings, or review sessions later by way of "comprehensive next-day summaries by world-renowned faculty in the form of in-depth online coverage." Medscape also provides access to both free and fee-based continuing medical education courses online. Schedules for upcoming conferences in specialty areas are provided.

Physician's Guide to the Internet ○ ○ ○
http://www.physiciansguide.com/meetings.html

Dates and locations for major national medical meetings are listed alphabetically by association at this site. There are also some hyperlinks to association pages and contact persons.

Princeton Medicon: The Medical Conference Resource ○ ○ ○
http://www.medicon.com.au

This comprehensive site contains details regarding worldwide major medical conferences of interest to medical specialists and primary care professionals. It is also periodically published in printed form. Access to lists of meetings is provided through a useful search engine that permits searching by specialty, year, and geographic region.

11.14 **Medical Data and Statistics**

Centers for Disease Control and Prevention (CDC) Biostatistics/Statistics ⊙ ⊙ ⊙
http://www.cdc.gov/niosh/biostat.html

This address provides visitors with links to sources of national statistics. Resources include federal, county and city data, as well as statistics related to labor, current population, public health, economics, trade, and business. Sources for mathematics and software information are also found through this site.

Health Sciences Library System (HSLS): Health Statistics ⊙ ⊙ ⊙
http://www.hsls.pitt.edu/intres/guides/statcbw.html

The University of Pittsburgh's Falk Library of the Health Sciences developed this site to provide information on obtaining statistical health data from Internet and library sources. Resources include details on obtaining statistical data from United States population databases, government agencies collecting statistics, organizations and associations collecting statistics, and other Web sites providing statistical information. The site explains specific Internet and library tools for locating health statistics, and offers a glossary of terms used in statistics.

National Center for Health Statistics (NCHS) ⊙ ⊙ ⊙
http://www.cdc.gov/nchs/default.htm

The NCHS, located within the Centers for Disease Control and Prevention of the U.S. Department of Health and Human Services, provides an extensive array of health and medical statistics for the medical, research, and consumer communities. This site provides express links to numerous surveys and statistical sources at the NCHS.

University of Michigan Documents Center: Statistical Resources on the Web: Health ⊙ ⊙ ⊙
http://www.lib.umich.edu/libhome/Documents.center/sthealth.html

Online sources for health statistics are cataloged at this site, including comprehensive health statistics resources and sources for statistics by topic. Topics include abortion, accidents, births, deaths, disability, disease experimentation, hazardous substances, healthcare, health insurance, HMOs, hospitals, life tables, mental health, noise, nursing homes, nutrition, pregnancy, prescription drugs, risk behaviors, substance abuse, surgery, transplants, and vital statistics. Users can also access an alphabetical directory of sites in the database and a search engine for locating more specific resources.

World Health Organization (WHO) Statistical Information System ⊘ ⊘ ⊘

http://www.who.int/whosis

The Statistical Information System of WHO (WHOSIS) is intended to provide access to both statistical and epidemiological data and information from this international agency in electronic form. The site provides health statistics, disease information, mortality statistics, AIDS/HIV data, immunization coverage and incidence of communicable diseases, links to statistics from other countries, as well as links to the Centers for Disease Control and Prevention in the United States. This site is the premier resource for statistics on diseases worldwide. See also the WHO main site: http://www.who.int for some additional disease-related statistics.

11.15 Medical Dictionaries, Encyclopedias, and Glossaries

Bio Tech's Life Science Dictionary ⊘ ⊘ ⊘

http://biotech.icmb.utexas.edu/search/dict-search.html#H

This free online dictionary designed for the public and professionals contains terms that deal with biochemistry, biotechnology, botany, cell biology and genetics. The dictionary also contains some terms relating to ecology, limnology, pharmacology, toxicology and medicine. The search engine allows the user to search by a specific term or by a term contained within a definition.

Diagnostic Procedures Handbook ⊘ ⊘ ⊘

http://www.bewell.com/dph/html/chapter/A.asp

This alphabetical listing of procedures, courtesy of Healthgate's supersite, provided an easy to access listing of diagnostic procedure information. Individual entries contain procedure synonyms, indications, contraindications, patient preparation, and special considerations and instructions. The techniques are fully described and related procedure links may be included.

Disease Finder from Healthanswers.com ⊘ ⊘ ⊘

http://www.healthanswers.com/adam/index_new/index.asp?topic=Disease

A wide range of diseases are listed in this alphabetical directory of information for patients and consumers. Visitors can search by keyword or browse the directory for information. Details include alternative names, definitions, causes, incidences, risk factors, prevention, symptoms, signs and tests, treatment, prognosis, and complications. Any helpful diagrams or representative photographs related to the condition are also provided.

Diseases and Conditions from Yahoo! Health ◎ ◎ ◎

http://dir.yahoo.com/Health/Diseases_and_Conditions

Consumers will find an alphabetical list of health topics at this address. Each entry provides a definition or information on alternative names, causes, incidence, and risk factors, prevention, symptoms, signs and tests, treatment, and prognosis. Information is included on medical terms, diseases, medical conditions, vaccines, and other related topics.

Diseases and Conditions Index from MedicineNet.com ◎ ◎ ◎

http://www.medicinenet.com/Script/Main/AlphaIdx.asp?li=MNI&d=51&p=A_DT

Medicinenet.com offers this comprehensive, user-friendly index to common and not so common diseases and conditions for reliable consumer information. Individual entries contain related terms as well as mini forums that offer concise encyclopedic articles on each disease, related news and updates, and ask the expert sections in which physicians answer common patient inquiries. Individual entries may also contain links to fact sheets on related topics of interest.

Glossary of Insurance—Related Terms at drkoop.com ◎ ◎

http://www.drkoop.com/hcr/insurance/glossary.asp

This site provides descriptions of both terms and phrases relating to health insurance. Terms are listed alphabetically.

HealthGate.com: Medical Tests ◎ ◎ ◎

http://www.bewell.com/tests/index.asp

This page of the Healthgate supersite offers consumers information on over 400 diagnostic tests. Educational facts and descriptions are accessible by entering keywords or phrases or by scrolling through an alphabetical listing of topics. This complete guide to medical testing contains concise information for each test entry including category of test, material studied, estimated cost and time necessary for testing, predicted reliability rating, as well as purpose, risks, and required patient preparation.

HealthGate.com: Symptoms, Illness, and Surgery ◎ ◎ ◎

http://www.bewell.com/sym/index.asp

As a service of Healthgate's supersite, this easy to use reference provides consumers with an excellent resource for a more complete understanding of disease diagnosis and treatment. By entering keywords or phrases or by browsing through an alphabetical listing of topics, visitors can obtain general information, signs and symptoms, causes, increased risk factors, and what to expect with respect to diagnostic and appropriate health care. Possible complications, prognosis, and general treatment measures are discussed for each entry listing.

Injury Finder from Healthanswers.com ⊚ ⊚ ⊚

http://www.healthanswers.com/adam/index_new/index.asp?topic=Injury

Patients can access an alphabetical directory of common injuries at this address. Information available includes a definition and important considerations about the injury, causes, symptoms, prevention, and suggested first aid.

List and Glossary of Medical Terms ⊚ ⊚

http://allserv.rug.ac.be/%7Ervdstich/eugloss/welcome.html

This site offers a multilingual glossary of technical and popular medical terms.

MedDictionary.com ⊚ ⊚

http://www.meddictionary.com

MedDictionary.com is an online bookstore specializing in medical, nursing, and other health-related dictionaries. Additional products include software and terminology guides. Users can order all products online.

Medical Dictionary from MedicineNet.com ⊚ ⊚ ⊚

http://www.medicinenet.com/Script/Main/AlphaIdx.asp?li=MNI&d=51&p=A_DICT

This valuable addition to the physician's electronic library contains all-inclusive entries that are revised on an ongoing basis for a considerable and ever-changing repertoire of classical and more modern medical terminology. The dictionary is unique in that it contains mini-encyclopedic entries for concise general information as well as definitions. With this easy to access reference tool, entries come complete with standard medical terms, related scientific terms, abbreviations, acronyms, jargon, institutions, projects, symptoms, syndromes, eponyms, and medical history.

Medical Spell-Check Offered by Spellex Development ⊚ ⊚ ⊚

http://www.spellex.com/speller.htm

Spellex Medical and Spellex Pharmaceutical online spelling verification allows visitors to check the spelling of medical terms. The search returns possible correct spellings if the word entered was not found.

Merck Manual of Diagnosis and Therapy ⊚ ⊚ ⊚

http://www.merck.com/pubs/mmanual

This online version of the 17th edition of the *Merck Manual* (1999) contains general medical text describing disorders and diseases that affect all organ systems. The site also provides links to the *Merck Manual of Geriatrics* and the *Merck Manual of Medical Information—Home Edition*. All manuals are searchable and use of the services is free-of-charge.

National Organization for Rare Disorders, Inc. (NORD) ☺ ☺ ☺ (some features fee-based)
http://www.rarediseases.org

The National Organization for Rare Disorders, Inc. (NORD) is a federation of more than 140 nonprofit organizations serving people with rare disorders and disabilities. The site provides access to current news items, conference details, an online newsletter, a rare disease database providing useful information for patients, an organizational database providing links to support and research organizations dedicated to rare disorders, and information specific to NORD. Users must pay a fee for full access to disease information.

Online Medical Dictionary from CancerWeb ☺ ☺ ☺
http://www.graylab.ac.uk/omd/index.html

This site offers a comprehensive medical dictionary online for clinical, medical student, and patient audiences, although a great many of the entries are very technical. It is a convenient source for a quick definition of an unfamiliar term.

Phys. Fitness Encyclopedia ☺ ☺
http://www.phys.com/fitness/welcome/welcome2.html

This online encyclopedia includes exercise guides for working each part of the body. The encyclopedia also describes sports and activities, detailing the physical benefits, necessary equipment, related terms, and additional resources. It also provides tips for preparing, playing, and training for the activities.

Procedures and Tests Index from MedicineNet.com ☺ ☺ ☺
http://www.medicinenet.com/Script/Main/AlphaIdx.asp?li=MNI&d=133&p=A_PROC

MedicineNet.com offers this comprehensive, user-friendly index to common and not so common diagnostic tests and treatment procedures. Each diagnostic and treatment mini-forum contains a main article for general information, outlining the purpose and safety of the procedure, related diseases and treatments, articles written by physicians on related topics of interest, and interesting related consumer health facts.

Test Finder from Healthanswers.com ☺ ☺ ☺
http://www.healthanswers.com/adam/index_new/index.asp?topic=Test

Common medical tests are listed alphabetically at this address, providing patients and consumers with a definition of the test a descriptions of how the test is performed, patient preparation for the test, how the test will feel, risks, reasons the test is performed, normal values, the meaning of abnormal results, cost of the test, and special considerations.

Tests and Procedures, University of Michigan Health System ◉ ◉
http://www.med.umich.edu/1libr/tests/testa00.htm

An alphabetical directory of medical test and procedures is found at this address. Clear, non-technical explanations of each test are offered to interested consumers. Visitors will also find discussions of health topics and other UMHS resources through this site.

Vitamin Glossary A–Z ◉ ◉ ◉
http://www.intelihealth.com/IH/ihtIH/WSIHW000/408/408.html

The InteliHealth site provides a link to descriptions of vitamins and minerals. The glossary is divided into three main groups: fat soluble vitamins, water soluble vitamins, and minerals. Each description includes the following areas: Good to Know, Recommendations, Benefits, Food Sources, Day's Supply In, and Watch Out.

11.16 Medical Legislation

American Medical Association (AMA) ◉ ◉
http://www.ama-assn.org/ama/basic/category/0,1060,165,00.html

The purpose of this site is to encourage physicians around the country to get involved in the AMA's grassroots lobbying efforts. It covers information on legislation relevant to the medical profession, the AMA's Congressional agenda, and educational programs available through the AMA on political activism for physicians. The Web site is updated regularly with the latest news on medical issues in the government.

American Medical Group Association (AMGA) Public Policy and Political Affairs ◉ ◉
http://www.amga.org/gov/pos.htm

The AMGA Web site contains position papers concerning major issues in the medical profession currently debated in Congress, and information on ordering publications providing news, legal resources, and compliance information to healthcare professionals. One section is devoted to suggestions on communicating with Congressional representatives on policy issues.

American Medical Student Association (AMSA) Legislative Affairs ◉ ◉ ◉
http://www.amsa.org/lad/index.html

The AMSA is an organization that attempts to improve healthcare and medical education. Its Legislative Affairs section of the Web site contains news of legislation that affects medical education, educational information on how to be a health policy activist, information on internship and fellowship opportunities in the field of health policy, and legislative links.

American Medical Women's Association (AMWA) ◎ ◎

http://www.amwa-doc.org/index.html

The AMWA promotes issues related to women's health and professional development for female physicians. The site's advocacy and actions sections contain articles on news and legislation that is relevant to these issues and gives advice on how to get involved.

Hugnet Legislation ◎ ◎

http://www.hugnet.com

The Hugnet site has information on current legislation that concerns the medical community and those interested in healthcare. It encourages visitors to contact members of Congress to voice their opinions on this legislation.

Public Citizen ◎ ◎ ◎

http://www.citizen.org

Public Citizen, a group founded by Ralph Nader, is an organization dedicated to political activism in issues concerning public health and safety. Within the site, there is information on legislation and activities related to the group's purpose of "protecting health, safety, and democracy." An extensive list of links to specific subjects include medically-related topics, such as "Healthcare Legislation," "HMO Accountability," and "Medical Malpractice Reform."

Thomas—U.S. Congress on the Internet ◎ ◎ ◎

http://thomas.loc.gov

Within Thomas, one can find information on bills, laws, reports, or any current U.S. federal legislation. The site's engine can be used to find current congressional bills by keyword or bill number.

U.S. House of Representatives Internet Office of the Law Revision Counsel ◎ ◎ ◎

http://uscode.house.gov/fast.htm

The Office of the Law Revision Counsel of the U.S. House of Representatives prepares and publishes the United States Code pursuant to section 285b of title 2 of the Code. The Code is a consolidation and codification by subject matter of the general and permanent laws of the United States. U.S. Code can be searched by keyword or other classification criteria, and titles and chapters of the Code can be downloaded from the site. Classification tables listing sections of the U.S. Code affected by recently enacted laws are also available.

11.17 **Medical Search Engines and Directories**

Achoo Healthcare Online ⊙ ⊙ ⊙
http://www.achoo.com

This site offers a directory of Web sites in three main categories: Human Health and Disease, Business of Health, and Organizations and Sources. The site has extensive subcategories and short descriptions for each site. Daily health news of interest to patients, the public, or medical professionals is available at the site, as well as links to journals, databases, employment directories, and discussion groups.

All The Web ⊙ ⊙ ⊙
http://www.alltheweb.com

This comprehensive site provides a variety of search engines including Fast Search. Fast Search allows users to search the Internet in 25 language catalogs and covers over 200 million high quality Web pages in very high speed. Visitors can copy the code needed to add Fast Search to their Web sites. Additionally at this site are search engines to search pictures and sounds.

Argus Clearinghouse ⊙ ⊙ ⊙
http://www.clearinghouse.net

The Argus Clearinghouse provides a central access point for value-added topical guides which identify, describe and evaluate Internet-based information resources. Its mission is to facilitate intellectual access to information resources on the Internet. Users can search for Web resources at this site using a directory or search engine. Many general categories are available including "Health & Medicine" and "Science & Mathematics." Subcategories under "Health & Medicine" include disabilities, diseases and disorders, fitness and nutrition, general health, medical specialties, medicine and medical services and sexuality and reproduction. Information about each site includes the compiler name or organization, detailed ratings, related keywords and the date the site was last checked by Argus Clearinghouse.

BigHub ⊙ ⊙ ⊙
http://www.thebighub.com

Formerly known as iSleuth.com, the BigHub allows users to search multiple engines including Yahoo, AltaVista, Infoseek, Excite, WebCrawler, Lycos, HotBot and Goto, Web directories and news databases simultaneously, and receive one summary of results. The BigHub provides advanced search options in relevant specialty topics including Health, Science and Reference resources. Users can also access news, weather, financial information, and more.

CliniWeb International ☺ ☺ ☺

http://www.ohsu.edu/cliniweb

CliniWeb, a service of Oregon Health Sciences University, is a searchable index and table of contents to clinical resources available on the World Wide Web. Information found at the site is of particular interest to healthcare professional students and practitioners. Search terms can be entered in five different languages: English, German, French, Spanish, and Portuguese. The site offers links to sites for additional search resources, and is linked directly to MEDLINE.

Daily Diffs ☺ ☺ ☺

http://www.dailydiffs.com

This site catalogs and provides updates on useful sites in many categories, including Health and Medicine. This section provides current news items related to fitness and wellness, diseases and disorders, risks, prevention, current treatments, and many specific topics covered in detail. Users can also search for resources by keyword.

Doctor's Guide ☺ ☺ ☺

http://www.docguide.com

The Doctor's Guide to the Internet is provided by P\S\L Consulting Group, Inc. and its purpose is to provide a comfortable environment for physicians to search the Internet and World Wide Web. The site contains a professional edition for healthcare professionals and a section directed at patients. Information of medical and professional interest includes medical news and alerts, new drugs or indications, medical conferences, a Congress Resource Center, a medical bookstore, and Internet medical resources. Patient resources are organized by specific diseases or condition. Users can search the World Wide Web through Excite, InfoSeek, McKinley, and Alta Vista search engines or can search the Doctor's Guide Medical News and Conference database.

Dogpile ☺ ☺ ☺

http://www.dogpile.com

Dogpile is a metasearch service that integrates several medium and large Web search and index guides into a single service. Visitors can complete a dogpile or geographic search (provides information about cities in the United States) or browse sites listed by categories such as "Health and Science" and their multiple subcategories. In addition this site offers yellow pages search, stock quotes, usenet articles, weather forecasts, job opportunities, shopping, and more.

drkoop.com ☺ ☺

http://www.drkoop.com

drkoop.com is an Internet-based consumer healthcare network. Included is a site search engine, reviews of Internet sites and multiple health-related topics and conditions to browse. In addition there are health-related news stories, a variety of resources such as information on drugs, books online, insurance, a physician locator, chat rooms, message boards, and much more.

Federal Web Locator ☉ ☉ ☉
http://www.infoctr.edu/fwl

The Federal Web Locator is a service provided by the Center for Information Law and Policy and is intended to be the one stop shopping point for federal government information on the World Wide Web. Links to relevant sites are available in the following categories: legislative, judicial and executive branches, independent and quasi-official agencies, federal boards, commissions, committees and nongovernmental federally related sites. Additionally users can access a variety of search engines including Aliweb, Alpha Legal Directory, Alta Vista, Cyber411, EINET Galaxy, Excite, Google, Inference Find, InfoSeek, Law Crawler-Legal Search Information, Lycos, McKinley, Metacrawler, OpenText Index, SavvySearch, Snap, WebCrawler, World Access Inernet Navigator, and Yahoo.

Galaxy ☉ ☉ ☉
http://galaxy.einet.net

This site houses a searchable directory of quality Web sites. Subcategories under medicine include diseases and disorders, health law, health occupations, history, human biology, medical informatics, operative surgery, philosophy, political issues, reference and therapeutics. There are also several site search options available.

Galen II ☉ ☉ ☉
http://galen.library.ucsf.edu

Galen II is the digital library of the University of California San Francisco. The site includes UCSF and UC resources and services, links to the AMA Directory, Drug Info Fulltext, Harrison's Online (requires a password), Merck Manual, Consumer Health, and a searchable database of additional resources and publications including electronic journals. Visitors can search the Galen II database or the World Wide Web using a variety of search engines.

Global Health Network ☉ ☉ ☉
http://www.pitt.edu/HOME/GHNet/GHNet.html

The Global Health Network offers national and international resources with information on agencies, organizations, academic programs, workshops, and conventions. The site maintains an online newsletter and offers links to related health networks. The site is also available in Japanese, Portuguese, Spanish, German, Chinese, Turkish, and Taiwanese.

Hardin Meta Directory of Internet Health Services ◉ ◉ ◉

http://www.lib.uiowa.edu/hardin/md/index.html

The purpose of the Hardin Meta Directory is to provide easy access to comprehensive resource lists in health-related subjects. It includes subject listings in large "one stop-shopping" sites such as MedWeb and Yahoo, and also independent discipline-specific lists. Sites are categorized by specific diseases and the number of links found at each site and only those that are well maintained are included. Additionally there is a list of free, full-text general medical journals available online.

Health A to Z ◉ ◉ ◉

http://www.healthatoz.com

This site offers visitors many useful resources for locating specific health information. A site search engine locates professionally reviewed health and medical information from other Internet resources including news headlines and updates, additional general health information, and a forum for asking questions of experts. Fact pages are dedicated to many specific health topics including diseases, alternative medicine, vaccines, nutrition, and fitness.

Health On the Net (HON) Foundation: MedHunt ◉ ◉

http://www.hon.ch/MedHunt

Health on the Net Foundation (HON) is a nonprofit organization and international initiative with a mission to help individuals and health care providers realize the potential benefits of the World Wide Web. This site provides several widely used medical search engines including MedHunt, Honselect, and Medline. Users can access databases containing information on newsgroups, LISTSERVs, medical images and movies, upcoming and past healthcare-related conferences, and daily news stories on health-related topics.

Health Sciences Information Service ◉ ◉ ◉

http://www.lib.berkeley.edu/HSIS/other2.html

The Health Sciences Information Service at University of California, Berkeley offers links to Internet medical and health resources. Electronic journals, books, indexes, and databases on the Internet are cataloged. The Service offers links to sites providing general medical information, institutes, and organizations on the Web, current news related to health and medicine, clinical sites, and sites related to Medical Informatics.

Health Web ◉ ◉ ◉

http://www.healthweb.org

HealthWeb provides links to specific, evaluated information resources on the World Wide Web, selected by librarians and information professionals at leading academic medical centers in the Midwest. Members, mainly universities or research centers, provide information that is sorted by alphabetical order and can be searched by keyword. Each member provides information on affiliated libraries as well as subject areas.

Indiana University Ruth Lilly Medical Library ◎ ◎ ◎

http://www.medlib.iupui.edu

Although portions of this site are restricted, many WWW medical resources can be accessed through links, including other libraries, government libraries and information sources, national agencies, associations, and numerous other vital resources.

InfoMine ◎ ◎

http://infomine.ucr.edu/search/bioagsearch.phtml

Provided by the University of California, InfoMine provides access to all types of Internet resources in the biological, agricultural, and medical sciences. Visitors can browse sites by subject, title, or keyword, or complete a search using InfoMine's search engine or a variety of Internet search and metasearch engines, virtual libraries and subject indexes, and mailing lists and newsgroups. Other features include access to BioAgMed and general references, online journals, the *Merck Manual* and educational resources.

MDchoice.com ◎ ◎

http://www.mdchoice.com

MDchoice.com is a privately held company founded by academic physicians with the goal of making access to health and medical information on the Internet as efficient and reliable as possible. The site features an UltraWeb search with all content selected by board-certified physicians. In addition, users have access to MEDLINE, drug information, health news, and a variety of clinical calculators. Also offered are several interactive educational exercises, online journals and text books, and employment opportunities.

Med Engine ◎ ◎ ◎

http://fastsearch.com/med/index.html

The Med Engine provides a general search engine called InferenceFind and several others including Microsoft's Multiple Search Engines, All-At-Once General Search, The Med Engine's I-Explorer, and Internet Sleuth. InferenceFind is unique in that it searches several search engines on the Internet, merges the results, removes redundancies and groups the results into understandable clusters. Additionally there are links to drug information, publications, physician directories, illnesses and diseases, educational sources, audio medicine, news, medical libraries and dictionaries, medical support, medical-legal issues, consumer information, associations and institutes, legislative action, hospital information, medical employment, government agencies, and more.

Med411.com ⊙ ⊙ ⊙

http://www.Med411.com

This medical search engine contains a collection of Web sites in the following categories: ancillary medical fields, associations, hospitals, import/export, insurance companies, journals/publications, medical equipment, medical legal, medical specialty, medical supplies, nursing, osteopathy, pharmaceuticals, and schools. Users can browse for sites by category or search for sites by keyword. A reference section titled "research" is available with links to medical associations, medical reference sites, medical libraries, medical dictionaries, sites that offer medical support, U.S. federal government sites and agencies and a search engine for the site of the Food and Drug Administration. Medical professionals may submit URLs of sites they are associated with to Med411.com online.

MedExplorer ⊙ ⊙ ⊙

http://www.medexplorer.com

MedExplorer is a comprehensive, searchable medical and health directory. Short descriptions of each site are provided. The site also lists related newsgroups and has information on conferences and employment.

MedFinder ⊙ ⊙ ⊙

http://www.netmedicine.com/medfinder.htm

MedFinder is an indexed database of WWW medical content. The database is searchable by type of Web page, with choices including information for patients, news articles, brief reviews, in-depth reviews or chapters, case presentations, simulations, practice guidelines, original research, and links directories. Searches can also be performed by topic, and specific criteria can be selected to further limit sites returned. Criteria can limit searches to pages containing peer-reviewed content, CME credits, audio or video resources, simulations, photos/animations, EKGs, radiographs, ultrasound/echo, nuclear images, CT scans, MRIs, and other images.

Medical Matrix ⊙ ⊙ (free registration)

http://www.medmatrix.org

Medical Matrix offers peer-reviewed, annotated, updated clinical medicine resources, and assigns ranks to Internet resources based on their utility for point-of-care clinical application. Visitors can access several search engines including Medical Matrix, MEDLINE and others or access sites through categories such as medical specialties, diseases, clinical practice, literature, education, healthcare and professionals, medical computing and Internet and technology, and marketplace. Additional information available includes online journals and textbooks, news, CME, prescription assistance resources, symposia on the Web, and classifieds. Access to site requires free registration.

Medical World Search ◎ ◎ ◎

http://www.mwsearch.com

This search engine indexes Web pages from selected medical Web sites. A directory of sites is not available. Users can chose to search indexed sites, selected general search engines, or MEDLINE. The search engine utilizes a medical thesaurus to increase the amount of returns from one query.

MedicineNet ◎ ◎ ◎

http://medicinenet.com/Script/Main/hp.asp

MedicineNet is a network of doctors producing health information for public use. The site offers an alphabetically arranged directory that provides information about diseases, treatments, procedures, tests, and drugs. The site also provides a comprehensive medical dictionary with thousands of terms and disorders along with prefixes and association designations. Other features include news, treatment updates, and health facts.

MedMark ◎ ◎ ◎

http://www.medmark.org

This comprehensive site provides users with a searchable directory of medical resources by specialty, free MEDLINE links, and other Internet resources. A search engine is available for locating additional medical and general sites.

Medscape ◎ ◎ ◎

http://www.medscape.com

Medscape provides several databases from which users can search the Web. These include articles, news, information for patients, MEDLINE, AIDSline, Toxline, drug information, dictionary, book store, Dow Jones Library, and medical images. There is a wealth of additional information provided including articles, case reports, conference schedules and summaries, continuing medical education resources, job listings, journals, news, patient information, practice guidelines, treatment updates, links to medical specialty sites, and more. Requires free online registration.

MedSurf ◎ ◎ ◎

http://www.medsurf.com/cgi-bin/OpenPage.cgi?Home.txt;Home

MedSurf offers links and a keyword search tool to find links to health and medical resources. The "Healthy Surfing" section provides news about the latest medical technologies and breakthroughs, while "Medicine Bag" guides physicians and healthcare providers to news and in-depth information on new timesaving technologies, advanced treatment alternatives, aging research, and upcoming educational forums.

MedWeb ◎ ◎

http://www.medweb.emory.edu/Medweb

Offered by Emory University, this site provides a searchable database of Web sites providing medical and health information. Searching is possible by entering keywords or by browsing subject categories.

Metacrawler ◎ ◎

http://www.metacrawler.com/

At the Metacrawler site users can search for Web resources through a directory or search engine. In addition, search engines are provided for newsgroups, audio, and shopping.

MMRL: Multimedia Medical Reference Library Medical Student Study Center ◎ ◎ ◎

http://www.med-library.com/medlibrary

The Multimedia Medical Reference Library, developed by medical students and professionals at Tufts University School of Medicine, is a searchable database of reviewed medical Web sites. Visitors can find links to sites offering audio resources, clinical trials information, online journals, medical equipment auctions, medical reference libraries, medical services, software, products, and links to medical schools and professional organizations. Each site is listed with a short description.

NetMed.com ◎ ◎ ◎

http://www.netmed.com/intro.html

NetMed.com provides users with links to useful sites grouped by medical condition. A relatively detailed description is given for most sites.

Online Medical Resources ◎ ◎

http://www.doctorbbs.com/searchall.htm

This site invites the user to search 20 different sites or online publications related to health and medicine. Links to MEDLINE and other general medical sites are also available.

Stanford MedWorld MedBot ◎ ◎ ◎

http://www-med.stanford.edu/medworld/medbot

Offered by Stanford University, this site allows users to search medical and health resources on the Web using major general and medical search engines. More specific searches can be performed on index and reference, education and learning, news and information, and medical images, and multimedia resources topics. Users can specify engines to employ in the search.

University of Iowa Libraries ☼ ☼ ☼

http://www.lib.uiowa.edu/index.html

This site includes links to OASIS, Healthnet, and other electronic resources available to University of Iowa students, faculty, and staff. Links are available to home pages for the Main Library and to each of the branch libraries.

Virtual Medical Center ☼ ☼ ☼

http://www-sci.lib.uci.edu/~martindale/Medical.html

This site, hosted by the University of California and written by Jim Martindale, provides users with links to a wealth of useful information, including travel warnings and immunization details, reference resources on a wide range of scientific subjects, and pathology and virology educational resources. Co-contributors include the UCI Science Library, the Department of Defense, the National Institutes of Health, and the National Science Foundation.

Yahoo! ☼ ☼ ☼

http://www.yahoo.com

Yahoo offers visitors the opportunity to search the Web and browse sites listed in multiple categories including health and science. Within each category are more specific subcategories that indicate the number of entries available. Most sites are suggested by users. Additionally Yahoo offers a wealth of services such as free e-mail, shopping, people search, news, travel, weather, stock reports, and more.

11.18 Pharmaceutical Information

Doctor's Guide: New Drugs and Indications ☼ ☼ ☼

http://www.pslgroup.com/NEWDRUGS.HTM

Doctor's Guide provides an ongoing source of new drug information, including FDA approvals and drug indications. Drug stories are presented in order of article datelines, with the most current stories listed first. Information for drug releases for the past 12 months is provided.

drkoop.com Drug Interactions Search ☼ ☼

http://www.drkoop.com/drugstore/pharmacy/interactions.asp

Users can enter several drug names into a search tool, checking for drug interactions.

Drug InfoNet ☼ ☼ ☼

http://www.druginfonet.com/phrminfo.htm

Information and links to areas on the Web concerning healthcare and pharmaceutical-related topics are available. The drug information is available by brand name, generic name, manufacturer, and therapeutic class. Visitors can ask questions of experts, and access disease information, pharmaceutical manufacturer information, healthcare news, and other resources.

Food and Drug Administration (FDA): Center for Drug Evaluation and Research ◎ ◎ ◎

http://www.fda.gov/cder/drug/default.htm

The Center for Drug Evaluation and Research broadcasts valuable information on prescription, consumer, and over-the-counter drugs at this address. Resources include alphabetical lists of new and generic drug approvals, new drugs approved for cancer indications, a searchable Orange Book listing all FDA approved prescription drugs, a National Drug Code directory, new over-the-counter labeling notices, patient information on over-the counter drugs, and alerts of new over-the-counter indications. Links are available to many resources related to drug safety and side effects, public health alerts and warnings, and pages offering information on major drugs. Reports and publications, special projects and programs, and cancer clinical trials information are also found through this address.

Food & Drug Administration (FDA) ◎ ◎ ◎

http://www.fda.gov

The FDA site provides extensive information on all aspects of drug research, regulations, approvals, trials, adverse reactions, enforcement, conferences, clinical alerts, reports, and drug news. The FDA Web Site Index is the first place to go to research a topic. There are several hundred subjects listed. One of these many sections covers FDA-related acronyms and abbreviations, which itself is a very useful tool in understanding much of the material at this site. For many researchers and physicians, however, information about FDA drug approvals is of central concern. A separate service, not included within the FDA, offers a concise summary of such approvals by medical specialty and condition for each year up to the present. This information can be accessed at the following Web site: www.centerwatch.com/drugs/DRUGLIST.HTM.

Medications Index from MedicineNet.com ◎ ◎ ◎

http://www.medicinenet.com/Script/Main/AlphaIdx.asp?li=MNI&d=51&p=A_PHARM

This all-inclusive pharmacological database from Medicinenet.com includes a mini forum for each prescription and nonprescription medication, containing a brief main article pertaining to the medication, related medications, related news and updates, diseases associated with the medication, and a listing of articles pertinent to the pharmacological agent's usage.

MedWatch—The FDA Medical Products Reporting Program

http://www.fda.gov/medwatch

The FDA Medical Products Reporting Program, MedWatch, is designed to educate health professionals about the importance of being aware of, monitoring for, and reporting adverse events and problems to the FDA and/or the manufacturer, and to disseminate new safety information rapidly within the medical community thereby improving patient care. To these ends, the site includes an adverse event reporting form and instructions, as well as safety information for health professionals, including "Dear Health Professional" letters and notifications related to drug safety. It also includes relevant, full-text continuing education articles and reports regarding drug and medical device safety issues.

Pharmaceutical Information Network ○ ○ ○

http://pharminfo.com

PharmInfoNet is a source of information on diseases, disorders, drug treatments, and research. In addition, there are links to more than one hundred pharmaceutical companies, both domestic and international. Organized by specialty areas, the site is a well-organized compilation of resources for physicians, researchers, medical students, and the public. The site is organized into information on disorders, archived articles, drugs used in the treatment of disorders, and other information sources, including newsgroups, e-mail lists, and related Web sites. An extensive Medical Sciences Bulletin Section and Pharmacotherapy Department provide articles on dozens of developments in research and drug therapies. Finally, the site provides a lengthy listing of drugs for treating disorders, with links to more extensive information sources.

Pharmaceutical Research and Manufacturers of America ○ ○ ○

http://www.phrma.org

This association Web site includes a "New Medicines in Development" database; a publications section containing reports relating to the pharmaceutical industry; various links for facts and figures on pharmaceutical research and innovation; and an issues and policies section covering many current topics of interest to pharmaceutical companies, such as genetics research and healthcare liability reform.

RxList—The Internet Drug Index ○ ○ ○

http://www.rxlist.com

This site allows users to search for drug information by name, imprint code, or keyword (action, interaction, etc.) The top 200 prescribed drugs for 1998, 1997, 1996, and 1995 are listed alphabetically or by rank. Patient monographs are available for a wide range of drugs, and one section is devoted to alternative medicine information and answers to frequently asked questions. The site also provides statistics related to site visits, and a forum for drug-specific discussions.

Virtual Library Pharmacy ⊙ ⊙ ⊙

http://www.pharmacy.org

This is truly a library of pharmacy information for professionals in all medical areas. The site provides information on pharmacy schools, companies, journals and books, Internet databases relating to pharmaceutical topics, conferences, hospital sites, government sites, pharmacy LISTSERVs, and news groups. Hundreds of site links are provided for the above areas.

World Standard Drug Database ⊙ ⊙

http://209.235.64.5:8888/cgi-bin/drugcgic.exe/START

Information on pharmaceutical products at this address includes ingredients, dosage, routes of administration, indications, contraindications, prescriber cautions, patient cautions, toxicity, side effects, liver disease cautions, renal failure procedures, pregnancy and lactation warnings, pharmacological actions, and diagnostic procedures. Visitors can search for relevant information by drug, ingredient, indications, contraindications, or side effects.

11.19 Physician Directories

Introduction

In order to obtain background information on practicing physicians in the United States, and to verify certification in various specialties, several important Web sites can be consulted, as listed below.

American Board of Medical Specialties (ABMS) ⊙ ⊙ ⊙

http://www.certifieddoctor.com/verify.html

This is a very useful verification service containing all physicians certified by an ABMS member board. It permits the public to verify credentials and certification status of any physician free-of-charge, searching by name, city, state, and specialty within the 24 member board specialty areas. The user enters the name of the physician and information is immediately available.

Healthgrades.com ⊙ ⊙ ⊙

http://www.healthgrades.com

This resource specializes in health care ratings, providing hospital ratings by procedure or diagnosis, physician ratings by specialty and geographic area, and ratings of health plans. Directories of hospitals, physicians, health plans, mammography facilities, and fertility clinics are also available. Visitors can access tips on choosing a hospital, physician, or health plan, as well as a glossary of terms and health news articles. Online health stores offer books, videos, magazines, greeting cards, flowers and gifts, pharmaceutical products, nutritional products, and insurance quotes. This service will soon include long-term care facilities, dentists, ambulatory surgery centers, and chiropractors in the ratings process.

Medi-Net Physician Background Information Service ✪ ✪ ✪

http://www.askmedi.com

Medi-Net describes itself as "an information delivery service that provides background information on every physician licensed to practice in the United States," providing name of medical school and year of graduation, residency training record, ABMS certifications, states where certified, and records of sanctions or disciplinary actions. There is a fee for reports.

12. PROFESSIONAL TOPICS AND CLINICAL PRACTICE

12.1 Anatomy and Surgery

Anatomy of the Human Body ⊙ ⊙ ⊙

http://rpisun1.mda.uth.tmc.edu/mmlearn/anatomy.html

This site offers images of the brain, elbow, arm, hand, knee, and foot. There are also sections that show slices of the ankle, foot, head, and neck in detail with nerves, muscles, and blood vessels identified.

Atlas of The Body ⊙ ⊙ ⊙

http://www.ama-assn.org/insight/gen_hlth/atlas/atlas.htm

The Atlas of the Body is a site offered by the American Medical Association that provides detailed information and labeled illustrations of the various systems and organs of the human body. The site also provides descriptions of disorders that affect these systems and organs.

Martindale's Health Science Guide, The "Virtual" Medical Center—Anatomy and Histology Center ⊙ ⊙

http://www-sci.lib.uci.edu/HSG/MedicalAnatomy.html

This site offers links to examinations, tutorials, and associations. It lists numerous atlases and sites with anatomical images, including some on embryology and developmental anatomy. Anatomy is just one of the many medical areas covered by the Virtual Medical Center, which also provides links to general medical dictionaries, glossaries, and encyclopedias, plus sites containing information on metabolic pathways and genetic maps.

Online Atlas Of Surgery ⊙ ⊙ ⊙

http://www.bgsm.edu/surg-sci/atlas/atlas.html

This site provides descriptions of specific surgical techniques, anatomy, instrumentation, positioning, room setup, and dissection. Also provided are indications leading to surgery and possible problems that may develop as a result of the surgery.

Online Surgery ⊙ ⊙ ⊙

http://www.onlinesurgery.com

Online Surgery gives the public an opportunity to view general and cosmetic surgical procedures online. Patients can fill out an application to finance an elective procedure and to be considered for a free procedure. Surgeries are viewed using RealPlayer.

Vesalius ⚙ ⚙ ⚙
http://www.vesalius.com

This site is a resource of medical illustrations with the purpose of providing educational material for surgeons and other medical professionals. Clinical Folios provide users with short educational narratives on surgical anatomy and procedures designed for online reference and study. There is an archive of images that demonstrate surgical techniques and other resources, including story boards, procedure descriptions using illustrations, photographs, x-rays, scans, animations and text, and short interactive programs or videos.

Virtual Body ⚙ ⚙ ⚙
http://www.medtropolis.com/vbody

This creative, informative site provides the viewer with labeled medical illustrations of various parts of the body. The human anatomy and body functions are presented in detail with interactive options that help the viewer learn the material.

Whole Brain Atlas, Harvard University ⚙ ⚙ ⚙
http://www.med.harvard.edu/AANLIB/home.html

This site, administered by the Harvard Medical School, shows imaging of the brain using magnetic resonance imaging (MRI), roentgen-ray computed tomography (CT), and nuclear medicine technologies. Structures within the images are labeled. Normal brain images are provided, as well as images of brains subjected to cerebrovascular disease, neoplastic disease, degenerative disease, and inflammatory or infectious disease. The entire atlas is available free-of-charge online or can be ordered on CD-ROM for a fee.

12.2 Biomedical Ethics

American Society of Bioethics and Humanities (ASBH) ⚙ ⚙ ⚙
http://www.asbh.org

The American Society of Bioethics and Humanities is an organization that promotes scholarship, research, teaching, policy development, and professional development in the field of bioethics. The site offers information on the Society, the annual meeting, position papers, awards, and links.

American Society of Law, Medicine, and Ethics (ASLME) ⚙ ⚙ ⚙
http://www.aslme.org

This site offers information on the American Society of Law, Medicine, and Ethics; *The Journal of Law Medicine and Ethics;* and *The American Journal of Law and*

Medicine. There is also information on research projects, a news section that gives information on recent developments in Law, Medicine, and Ethics, and information on future and past conferences held by the Society.

Bioethics Discussion Pages ◎ ◎ ◎
http://www-hsc.usc.edu/~mbernste/#Welcome

This page is a forum for people to discuss and share their views on selected topics in the field of biomedical ethics. There are also polls and articles on ethical issues.

Bioethics.net ◎ ◎ ◎
http://www.med.upenn.edu/bioethics/index.shtml

Produced by the Center for Bioethics of the University of Pennsylvania, Bioethics.net contains a host of resources relating to biomedical ethics. Included are sections on cloning and genetics, emergency room bioethics, surveys for pay, and assisted suicide. There is also a virtual library with links to Internet resources. A beginner's site (Bioethics for Beginners) contains material that is meant to educate the general public and people interested in the field about bioethics, its meaning, and its applications. At this beginner's site, there are resources for students and educators, and a list of different biomedical ethics associations.

Careers in Bioethics ◎ ◎
http://www.ethics.ubc.ca/brynw/jobs.html

This site has information on jobs that are being offered throughout the world in the field of Bioethics. Information on postdoctorals and fellowships is also available.

Center for Medical Ethics and Mediation ◎ ◎ ◎
http://www.wh.com/cmem

This site contains resources that help enable the Center to provide information on education, research, consultations, and mediations for healthcare professionals and organizations. These resources include information on workshops and seminars; requests for the Center to send a mediator to help with a dispute or conflict; profiles of the Center's mediators; and related links.

Health Priorities Group, Inc. ◎ ◎ ◎
http://www.bioethics-inc.com

The Health Priorities Group is made up of professionals in the field of Ethics, Medicine, Law, Nursing, and Theology. It offers training and support of corporate and hospital ethics committees, clinical case review, and help in health policy development for private and government institutions. The Web site has sections on services, publications, and reports on ethics issues.

Human Genome Project: Ethical, Legal, and Social Issues (ELSI) ◉ ◉

http://www.ornl.gov/TechResources/Human_Genome/resource/elsi.html

This site attempts to disseminate information on the Human Genome Project and the ethical, legal, and social issues surrounding the availability of genetic information. Available on this site are updates, publications, description of research in progress, and basic information on the Human Genome Project.

International Bioethics Committee ◉ ◉

http://www.unesco.org/ibc

Includes information on various ethical issues, including a section on the Human Genome Project. The site also has information on the International Bioethics Committee and its proceedings.

Medical Ethics—Where Do You Draw the Line? ◉ ◉

http://www.learner.org/exhibits/medicalethics

This site deals with issues by presenting real-life scenarios and letting the viewer take part in ethical decisions. There are also links to related resources and an ethics forum.

Midwest Bioethics Center ◉ ◉ ◉

http://www.midbio.org

This community-based Center is dedicated to the integration of ethical considerations in all health care decisions. Visitors to this address will find information about the organization, including a staff listing, membership details, and consortia information. Current events, publications, a discussion group, and advance directive pamphlets are also found at the site. Resources on community-state partnerships include policy, briefs, press releases, staff listings, a call for proposals, directories of grant seekers and recipients, and answers to questions. The Center's Compassion Sabbath program is also profiled at the site, offering information on conferences for clergy and other programs, lists of participants, answers to frequently asked questions, and links to related sites.

National Bioethics Advisory Commission (NBAC) ◉ ◉ ◉

http://bioethics.gov/cgi-bin/bioeth_counter.pl

In addition to providing information on current research trends in the biotech industry, NBAC explores the ethical implications of technological advances. The site acts a forum for the ethical concerns of the public regarding a rapidly advancing technology. NBAC's policy is outlined at the site.

National Reference Center for Bioethics Literature ⊙ ⊙ ⊙
http://www.georgetown.edu/research/nrcbl

Linked to the Kennedy Institute of Ethics of Georgetown University, this Center holds the world's largest collections of literature on Biomedical Ethics. Serving as a resource for both the public and scholarly researchers, the library lists its resources on this Web site. The site also provides access to free searching of the world's literature in this area using BIOETHICSLINE or the Ethics and Human Genetics Database. Other relevant links are provided in the areas of Educational and Teaching Resources and other bibliographies and Internet links on bioethics.

Physicians Committee for Responsible Medicine (PCRM) ⊙ ⊙
http://www.pcrm.org

PCRM is dedicated to preventative medicine, higher ethical standards of research, and access to managed care. The organization provides extensive material on ethics and research as well as prevention and nutrition. The site also offers news and events about numerous PCRM activities, details on clinical research projects, and summaries of texts produced by the organization.

The Hastings Center ⊙ ⊙ ⊙
http://www.thehastingscenter.org

The Hastings Center is a major center for the study of Biomedical Ethics. Their Web site provides information about the center as well as detailed explanations of current research activities. General listings of resources found at the Center, including an online library catalog, can also be accessed.

University of Buffalo
Center for Clinical Ethics and Humanities in Health Care ⊙ ⊙ ⊙
http://wings.buffalo.edu/faculty/research/bioethics/nav.html

Information about the Center, news and events notices, a library of bioethics and medical humanities documents, and the Ethics Committee Core Curriculum are available at this address. Links are presented to Internet resources on featured topics, including bioethics education, hospice and palliative care, advance directives, philosophy of mind, medical record privacy, genetics and ethics, and other relevant sites.

12.3 **Biotechnology**

Bio Online ⊘ ⊘ ⊘
http://www.bio.com

Bio Online is a comprehensive Web site for the life sciences and the biotechnology industry. This site provides general information, current news, an industry guide, academic and government links, and an extensive career center. It is an excellent resource for seeking information on the biotech industry and related sciences.

Biofind.com ⊘ ⊘ ⊘
http://www.biofind.com

Biofind.com provides insight into the biotechnology industry and is a resource for general information, news, and developments in emerging technologies. The site also contains a job search database, chat room, the "Biotech Rumor Mill" for anonymous public discussion of current events in the field, and links to other biotech Web sites. A subscription service is also available for a fee, which provides daily e-mail updates on jobs, candidates, business opportunities, innovations, press releases, or company "rumors" posted at the site.

Bioresearch Online ⊘ ⊘ ⊘
http://www.bioresearchonline.com/content/homepage

Bioresearch Online is a virtual community, forum, and marketplace for biotechnology professionals. Users have access to the latest headlines, product information, new and industry analyses, as well as career information. There are also specific pages devoted to pharmaceutical research and laboratory science.

Biotechnology: An Information Resource ⊘ ⊘ ⊘
http://www.nal.usda.gov/bic

Dedicated to providing current information in all areas of biotechnology, this site is a subsidiary of the National Agricultural Library and the U.S. Department of Agriculture. The site catalogs press releases and offers an exhaustive listing of links to other Web-based resources from around the world, and is an excellent source for information, especially in the area of Agricultural Biotechnology.

Biotechnology Industry Organization ⊘ ⊘ ⊘
http://www.bio.org/welcome.html

This industry-sponsored Web site provides weekly news updates on developing technology and world news. The site also offers general information, links to corporate Web sites, an online library, and a number of other educational resources. Although corporate sponsored, the site does not focus solely on product promotion, but has a genuine educational quality. Those seeking to learn more about this growing industry will find this site to be a valuable resources.

BioWorld Online ⚙ ⚙ ⚙

http://www.bioworld.com

BioWorld Online tracks the growth of the biotechnology market. In addition to providing stock and financial information, the site provides access to current industry headlines, job search resources, forums, and news worldwide.

CorpTech Database ⚙ ⚙ ⚙

http://www.corptech.com

This comprehensive database provides details on companies involved in high-tech industries, including biotechnology and pharmaceutical companies. Basic information such as each company's description, address, annual sales, and CEO name is available free; however, more in-depth financial and business data is only accessible to fee-paying subscribers. Searches for products or names of company officers are also available, again with some amount of information provided at no cost.

Enzyme Nomenclature Database ⚙ ⚙

http://www.expasy.ch/enzyme

Enzyme information of a very specific nature is available at this site devoted exclusively to this important medical subject. The database at this Web site provides access to enzyme information by EC (Enzyme Commission) number, enzyme class, description, chemical compound, and cofactor. There is an accompanying user manual for the enzyme database as well.

Infobiotech ⚙ ⚙ ⚙

http://www.cisti.nrc.ca/ibc/home.html

Infobiotech is a collaboration of government, academic, and private sector resources. This Canadian-based site provides general information, resources, and links to both Canadian and non-Canadian sites. In addition, it offers a large list of related sites providing current information on advances in the biotech industry.

International Food Information Council ⚙ ⚙ ⚙

http://ificinfo.health.org

The International Food Information Council collects and disseminates scientific information on food safety, nutrition, and health by working with experts to help translate research findings into understandable and useful information for opinion leaders and consumers. This site provides information and news on emerging technologies in the food industry. Resources available through this site include publications, recent news articles, government guidelines and regulations, and links to other resources on the Internet.

MedWebPlus: Biotechnology ⊙ ⊙ ⊙
http://www.medwebplus.com/subject/Biotechnology.html

MedWebPlus contains an extensive guide to online resources in biotechnology and a wide variety of other fields. The site catalogs hundreds of Internet resources containing many forms of information on the biotech industry. In addition, links are provided to journals, online publications, and recent articles of interest. Vast amounts of information are provided at this site, and links are kept current.

National Center for Biotechnology Information (NCBI) ⊙ ⊙ ⊙
http://www.ncbi.nlm.nih.gov

A collaborative effort produced by the National Library of Medicine and the National Institutes of Health, NCBI is a national resource for molecular biology information. The Center creates public databases, conducts research in computational biology, develops software tools for analyzing genome data, and disseminates biomedical information in an effort to improve the understanding of molecular processes affecting human health and disease. In addition to conducting and cataloging its own research, NCBI tracks the progress of important research projects worldwide. The site provides access to public molecular databases containing genetic sequences, structures, and taxonomy; literature databases; catalogs of whole genomes; tools for mining genetic data; teaching resources and online tutorials; and data and software available to download. Research performed at NCBI is also discussed at the site.

Recombinant Capital ⊙ ⊙ ⊙
http://www.recap.com

This online magazine provides analysis of the biotechnology industry. This is a good resource for those seeking to invest in companies on the forefront of the rapidly growing biotech industry. Although much of the information presented here is from a financial perspective, the site gives a good overview of the entire industry and provides daily news updates. The progress of developing technology can be closely monitored via this site.

World Wide Web Virtual Library: Biotechnology ⊙ ⊙ ⊙
http://www.cato.com/biotech

This is an excellent directory of sites in the field of Biotechnology. This site catalogs hundreds of reviewed links, including publications, educational resources, general information, and government links. There is also a rating system used by the editor of the site to point out links of specific importance.

12.4 **Chronic Pain Management**

American Academy of Pain Management (AAPM) ☼ ☼ ☼

http://www.aapainmanage.org

The American Academy of Pain Management is the largest multidisciplinary pain society and largest physician-based pain society in the United States, providing credentials to practitioners in the area of pain management. This site provides information about AAPM and its activities, resources for finding a professional program in pain management, accreditation and Continuing Medical Education (CME) resources, and a membership directory for locating a pain management professional. It also provides good general information on pain management and a listing of relevant links. Access to the National Pain Data Bank is available at the site, containing statistics on various pain management therapies based on an outcomes measurement system. The site is divided into two sections with information tailored to the needs of patients and healthcare professionals.

Back and Body Care ☼ ☼

http://www.backandbodycare.com

Produced by physical therapists, this site is a good starting point for consumers seeking an overview of the causes and treatments chronic pain. It provides general information in the areas of back, neck, arm, and wrist pain. The site lists possible causes of chronic problems, treatments and exercises, and preventive measures. A search engine for locating a local, qualified physical therapist is featured at the site.

Pain.com ☼ ☼ ☼

http://www.pain.com/index.cfm

This site is an excellent resource for seeking information on pain and pain management, and contains a great deal of information for the specific needs and interests of health professionals and patients. It offers an online pain journal, articles about recent advances and news in pain management, medical forums and chat rooms, and an extensive list of other Web-based resources.

Pain Net, Inc. ☼ ☼

http://www.painnet.com

Pain Net, Inc. provides visitors with useful information and links on pain control and prevention. Patients can find information on new treatments as well as a listing of pain management practitioners categorized by state. Doctors can search a database of important links and organizations, and can list their practice in the public information directory.

12.5 **Clinical Practice Management**

Cut to the Chase ○ ○ ○ (free registration)
http://www.cuttothechase.com

Healthcare management information for physicians is available at this site, including articles about practice management issues, career development resources, publications and software sources, information about other products and services related to healthcare management, and links to sites offering additional healthcare management resources. Free site registration is required for access to these resources.

Guide to Clinical Preventive Services ○ ○ ○
http://158.72.20.10/pubs/guidecps

This guide is a comprehensive online reference source covering recommendations for clinical practice on 169 preventive interventions, including screening tests, counseling interventions, immunizations, chemoprophylactic regimens, and other preventive medical tools. Sixty (60) target conditions are discussed in the report.

Health Services/Technology Assessment Text (HSTAT) ○ ○ ○
http://text.nlm.nih.gov

This electronic resource for physicians provides access to consumer brochures, evidence reports, reference guides for clinicians, clinical practice guidelines, and other full-text documents useful in making healthcare decisions. Users can download documents from the site, access general information about the system, and browse links to additional sources for information. Searches can be comprehensive or limited to specific databases within the HSTAT system, and users can also search by keyword.

InfoMedical.com v3.0—The Medical Business Search Engine ○ ○ ○
http://www.InfoMedical.com

This engine allows users to search for companies, news, and press releases from submitted sites in the following categories: companies, distributors, products, organizations, services, and World Wide Web resources.

Martindale's Health Science Guide ○ ○ ○
http://www-sci.lib.uci.edu/~martindale/HSGuide.html

An all-encompassing site for physician resources, including clinical practice and research information, this Web service offers access to teaching files, medical cases, multimedia courses and textbooks, tutorials, and other databases. There is information on different medical disciplines including Bioscience, Chemistry, Nursing, Dental Medicine, Pharmacology, Public Health, and Biotechnology.

MDGateway ⊙ ⊙

http://www.mdgateway.com

Described as an Internet "onramp for physicians busy in clinical practice," this site offers health news articles and information on clinical, professional, and personal resources. Clinical resources include links to clinical applications, medications information, practice guidelines, and patient education literature. Professional links are available with respect to coding and billing information, resources for creating and maintaining a medical practice, medical societies, and sources for medical meetings/Continuing Medical Education information. Personal finance information is also found at the site.

MedConnect ⊙ ⊙ ⊙

http://www.medconnect.com

Important medical resources at MedConnect include literature reviews, cases of the month, featured articles, journal clubs, Board reviews, free MEDLINE access, and teaching files discussing ECGs, x-rays, and CAT scans. This information is presented in separate journals of emergency medicine, pediatrics, managed care, and primary care.

MedPlanet ⊙ ⊙ ⊙

http://www.medplanet.com

Visitors to this site can search medical product classified advertisements, including surgical, anesthesia, monitoring, critical care, imaging, and laboratory equipment. The site also provides links to medical equipment manufacturers, dealers, and financing agencies. Users can add their own classified ads and include links to Web sites of equipment and product suppliers.

Medsite.com ⊙ ⊙ ⊙

http://www.medsite.com

This site describes itself as an e-services portal for the medical community. Services provided include books, medical software, and supplies at discounted prices; financial resources; a scheduling tool geared for medical professionals; and free e-mail accounts. The service requires free registration.

National Guideline Clearinghouse (NGC) ⊙ ⊙ ⊙

http://www.guideline.gov/index.asp

Four hundred and seventy-nine evidence-based clinical practice guidelines are offered at this indispensable site. Visitors can browse for guidelines by disease or condition or search for guidelines by keyword. Topical categories include immunologic, viral, endocrine, musculoskeletal, respiratory tract, urologic and male genital, nutritional and metabolic, otorhinolaryngologic, occupational, neonatal, eye, parasitic, nervous system, obstetric and gynecologic, skin and connective tissue, hemic and lymphatic, digestive system, and cardiovascular diseases, bacterial infections and mycoses, injuries, poisonings, and neoplasms.

Online Clinical Calculator ⚙ ⚙ ⚙

http://www.intmed.mcw.edu/clincalc.html

Directed at clinical practitioners, this site offers useful analytical tools and clinical formulas for a variety of medical purposes, including body surface calculations, heart disease risk, ingested substance blood level, pregnancy due date, weights and measures, and other subjects.

Online Directory of Medical Software ⚙ ⚙

http://www.healthcarecomputing.com/onlindir.html

This directory provides the names, addresses, telephone numbers, and e-mail or Web site information for each of the state medical boards. Physicians can contact a board for information on licensing in that state or for other information regarding medical regulation or standards.

PDR.net ⚙ ⚙ ⚙ (some features fee-based)

http://www.PDR.net

PDR.net is a medical and healthcare Web site created by the Medical Economics Company, publisher of healthcare magazines and directories including the PDR (Physicians' Desk Reference). The site has specific areas and content for physicians, pharmacists, physician assistants, nurses, and consumers. Access to the full-text reference book is free for U.S.-based MDs, DOs and PAs in full-time practice. There is a fee for other users of this service, but most of the site's features are free.

Physician's Guide to the Internet ⚙ ⚙ ⚙

http://www.physiciansguide.com

This site contains a directory of Web sites for physicians. Features include physician lifestyle resources, such as sites offering suggestions on stress relief; news items; clinical practice resources, including access to medical databases and patient education resources; and postgraduate education and new physician resources. Other resources include links to sites selling medical books, products, and services for physicians; links to Internet search tools; and Internet tutorials.

Practice Management Information Corporation ⚙ ⚙

http://medicalbookstore.com/arm.htm

This site provides an opportunity for physicians to order books that offer information on topics that relate to the management of a private medical practice. Books on medical coding and reimbursement are also available.

State Medical Boards Directory ◎ ◎

http://www.fsmb.org/members.htm

This directory provides the names, addresses, telephone numbers, and e-mail or Web site information for each of the state medical boards. Physicians can contact a Board for information on licensing in that state or for other information regarding medical regulation or standards.

12.6 **Genetics**

Frontiers in Clinical Genetics ◎ ◎ ◎

http://www.frontiersingenetics.com/main.htm

Presented by The George Washington University Medical Center, this site offers lectures on various genetics topics presented on the Web via Real Audio. Directed at physicians requiring CME credit, the lectures assume a good deal of prior knowledge of genetics. There is also a listing of links to related sites. Lectures are archived for a period of two years to permit future study and reference.

GeneClinics ◎ ◎ ◎

http://www.geneclinics.org

GeneClinics is a knowledge base of expert-authored, up-to-date information relating genetic testing to the diagnosis, management, and counseling of individuals and families with inherited disorders. Indexed articles are of a specific and technical nature intended for use by healthcare professionals. The site also includes an extensive listing of disease profiles that is continuously updated.

Genetics Revolution at Time.com ◎ ◎

http://www.pathfinder.com/time/daily/special/genetics/index.html

This article from Time.com tracks the progress of the rapid advances in genetic technology. The site gathers a great deal of up-to-date information and offers links to a number of additional related Web-based resources.

Genetics Virtual Library ◎ ◎ ◎

http://www.ornl.gov/TechResources/Human_Genome/genetics.html

This site contains a comprehensive listing of links to major Web sites on specific topics in genetics. Links are subdivided by organism, providing genetics information on many animals, from transgenic mice to humans. Brief descriptions are provided for many links.

Institute for Genomic Research (TIGR) ☉ ☉ ☉

http://www.tigr.org

The Institute for Genomic Research is a not-for-profit research institute with interests in structural, functional, and comparative analysis of genomes and gene products in viruses, eubacteria, archaea, and eukaryotes. Information on recent advances in genetics and continuing research projects in the area of human genomics, an extensive searchable database of previous research, and links to other genome centers worldwide are available at this site.

Kyoto Encyclopedia of Genomes and Genetics (KEGG) ☉ ☉ ☉

http://www.genome.ad.jp/kegg

The Kyoto Encyclopedia of Genes and Genomes (KEGG) attempts to computerize current knowledge of molecular and cellular biology in terms of information pathways consisting of interacting molecules or genes, and also provides links to gene catalogs produced by genome sequencing projects. Information indexed at this site ranges from basic genetic information to extremely technical descriptions of molecular pathways. Also provided is a listing of links to other major Internet sites containing information relevant to genetic research.

Molecular Genetics Jump Station ☉ ☉ ☉

http://www.horizonpress.com/gateway/genetics.html

This site provides a comprehensive listing of Web-based resources for geneticists. Sites indexed here are technical in nature and intended for investigators. Resources include links to molecular biology, microbiology, and genetics jump sites (containing catalogs of links); sites containing protocols on laboratory techniques; journals and other online publications, news groups, and mail lists; institutes and organizations; conferences and meetings announcements; commercial sites; and sources for ordering technical books. The site is sponsored by Beckman, Horizon Scientific Press, *Journal of Molecular Microbiology and Biotechnology,* and MWG-Biotech.

National Center for Biotechnology Information: Online Mendelian Inheritance in Man (OMIM) ☉ ☉ ☉

http://www.ncbi.nlm.nih.gov/Omim

Dr. Victor A. McKusick, a researcher at Johns Hopkins, and his colleagues have authored this database of human genes and genetic disorders. The database was developed for the World Wide Web by the National Center for Biotechnology Information. Reference information, texts, and images are found through the site, as well as links to the Entrez database of MEDLINE articles and sequence information. Visitors can search the OMIM Database, OMIM Gene Map, and OMIM Morbid Map (a catalog of cytogenetic map locations organized by disease) from the site. Information on the OMIM numbering system, details on creating links to OMIM, site updates, OMIM statistics, information on citing OMIM in literature, and the OMIM gene list are all found at the site. Links are available to allied resources, and the complete text of OMIM and gene maps can be downloaded from the site.

National Human Genome Research Institute (NHGRI) ◎ ◎ ◎
http://www.nhgri.nih.gov

The National Human Genome Research Institute supports the NIH component of the Human Genome Project, a worldwide research effort designed to analyze the structure of human DNA and determine the location of the estimated 50,000–100,000 human genes. The NHGRI Intramural Research Program develops and implements technology for understanding, diagnosing, and treating genetic diseases. The site provides information about NHGRI, the Human Genome Project, grants, intramural research, policy and public affairs, workshops and conferences, and news items. Resources include links to the Institute's Ethical, Legal, and Social Implications Program, and the Center for Inherited Disease Research. The site also provides genetic resources for investigators, a glossary of genetic terms, and a site search engine.

Office of Genetics and Disease Prevention ◎ ◎ ◎
http://www.cdc.gov/genetics

Created by the Centers for Disease Control and Prevention, this site offers access to current information on the impact of human genetic research and the Human Genome Project on public health and disease prevention. The site provides general information, indexes recent articles, lists events and training opportunities, and offers an extensive listing of links to other resources. Users can search the site by keyword and access the Human Genome Epidemiology Network (HuGENet), a global collaboration of individuals and organizations committed to the development and dissemination of population-based epidemiologic information on the human genome.

Primer on Molecular Genetics ◎ ◎ ◎
http://www.ornl.gov/hgmis/publicat/primer/intro.html

The United States Department of Energy presents an excellent resource for those seeking basic background information on genetics and genetic research at this site. Discussions at the site include an introduction to genetics, DNA, genes, chromosomes, and the process of mapping the human genome. Mapping strategies, genetic linkage maps, and various physical maps are available, as well as links to mapping and sequence databases and a glossary of terms. The site also summarizes the predicted impact of the Human Genome Project on medical practice and biological research.

University of Kansas Medical Center: Genetics Education Center ◎ ◎ ◎
http://www.kumc.edu/gec

Links are available at this address to Internet resources for educators interested in human genetics and the Human Genome Project. Sites are listed by topic, including the Human Genome Project, education resources, networking, genetic conditions, booklets and brochures, genetics programs and other resources, and glossaries. Lesson plans are offered both by the University of Kansas and other sources at the site. A description of different careers in genetics are also available. This site is an excellent tool for finding useful genetics Internet resources for nonprofessionals and educators.

12.7 Geriatrics

Administration on Aging: Resource Directory for Older People ○ ○ ○
http://www.aoa.dhhs.gov/aoa/dir/intro.html

The National Institute on Aging and the Administration on Aging has compiled this directory of resources, serving older people and their families, health and legal professionals, social service providers, librarians, researchers, and others interested in the field of aging. The directory includes names of organizations, addresses, telephone numbers (including toll-free numbers), and links to Internet sites, when available. Visitors can search the directory by keyword or view the entire table of contents from this address.

American Geriatrics Society (AGS) ○ ○ ○ (some features fee-based)
http://www.americangeriatrics.org/index.html

A national nonprofit association of geriatrics health professionals, research scientists, and other concerned individuals, the American Geriatrics Society is dedicated to "improving the health, independence, and quality of life for all older people." The site offers a description of the Society, adult immunization information, AGS news, conference and other events notices, legislation news, career opportunities, directories of geriatrics health care services in managed care, position statements, educational, and practice guidelines, awards information, and other professional education resources. Patient education resources, a selected bibliography in geriatrics, links to related organizations and government sites, surveys, and a site search tool are also found at this address.

12.8 Grants and Award Guides

Foundation Center ○ ○ ○
http://fdncenter.org

The Foundation Center provides direct, hot links to thousands of grant-making organizations, including foundations, corporations, and public charities, along with a search engine to enable the user to locate sources of funding in specific fields. In addition, the site provides listings of the largest private foundations, corporate grant makers, and community foundations. There is also information on funding trends, a newsletter, and grant-seeker orientation material. More than 900 grant-making organizations are accessible through this useful site.

National Institutes of Health (NIH): Funding Opportunities ◎ ◎ ◎

http://grants.nih.gov/grants

Funding opportunities for research, scholarship, and training are extensive within the federal government. At this site for the National Institutes of Health, there is a Grants Page with information about NIH grants and fellowship programs, information on Research Contracts containing information on Requests for Proposals (RFPs), Research Training Opportunities in biomedical areas, and an NIH Guide for Grants and Contracts. The latter is the official document for announcing the availability of NIH funds for biomedical and behavioral research and research training policies. Links are provided to major divisions of NIH that have additional information on specialized grant opportunities.

National Science Foundation (NSF) Grants & Awards ◎ ◎ ◎

http://www.nsf.gov/home/grants.htm

Because approximately 20% of the federal support to academic institutions for basic research comes from the National Science Foundation, this site is an important source of information for award opportunities, programs, application procedures, and other vital information. Forms and agreements may be downloaded as well, and regulations and policy guidelines are set forth clearly.

Polaris Grants Central ◎ ◎

http://polarisgrantscentral.net

For the grant seeker, this site provides resources that are available from numerous organizations pertaining to grant identification and application. There are books and publications on grant sources, descriptions of grant information providers, clearing-houses for grant information, federal contacts, grant training materials, and resources on disk or CD-ROM. Within the site, useful sections provide "Tips and Hints" on writing grant proposals, "Grants News" from different government agencies and other organizations, "Scholarships or Grants to Individuals," and information on grant workshops.

Society of Research Administrators (SRA) GrantsWeb ◎ ◎ ◎

http://sra.rams.com/cws/sra/resource.htm

The Society of Research Administrators has created an extremely useful grant information site, with extensive links to government resources, general resources, private funding, and policy/regulation sites. The site section devoted to U.S., Canadian, and other international resources provides links to government agency funding sources, the commerce business daily, the Catalog of Federal Domestic Assistance, scientific agencies, research councils, and resources in individual fields, such as health, education, and business. Grant-application procedures, regulations, and guidelines are provided throughout the site, and extensive legal information is provided through links to patent, intellectual property, and copyright offices. Associations providing funding and grant information are also listed, with direct links.

12.9 Imaging and Pathology

Center For Biomedical Imaging Technology ⊙ ⊙ ⊙
http://www.cbit.uchc.edu/index.html

Current research performed by the Center for Biomedical Imaging Technology is presented at this site in the form of medical imaging examples accomplished by the Center. A short tutorial on the classification of MR images, videos, and abstracts on light microscopy of living cells, and the structure and function of the endoplasmic reticulum are available through links at the site.

Center For Human Simulation ⊙ ⊙ ⊙
http://www.uchsc.edu/sm/chs

This site provides a browser to view cross sections from any part of the bodies from the Visible Human Project. Also included are images, animations, videos, and 3-D polygonal models of various parts of the human anatomy that were created using new imaging technology.

CT Is Us ⊙ ⊙ ⊙
http://www.ctisus.org

The CT (computed tomography) site offers information on medical imaging with a specific focus on spiral CT and 3D imaging. Images of the body and various medical conditions are organized by region, and information on Continuing Medical Education (CME) courses, teaching files, medical illustrations, and a 3D vascular atlas are all available at the site.

Digital Imaging Center ⊙ ⊙ ⊙
http://info.med.yale.edu/library/imaging

This Web site, provided by Cushing/Whitney Medical Library of Yale University, serves as a starting point for help on the various resources available through the Digital Imaging Center, including a digital camera, computer resource lab, color printers, scanners, and digital video editing capabilities. Resources at this site are most useful to visitors with access to the Cushing/Whitney Medical Library Digital Imaging Center.

Dr. Morimoto's Image Library of Radiology ◎ ◎ ◎

http://www.osaka-med.ac.jp/omc-lib/noh.html

This site provides users with access to images and videos collected by Dr. Morimoto, Department of Radiology, Osaka National Hospital. Images were scanned and stored with JPEG, GIF format, and movies with QuickTime format. Visitors can download the images freely but need permission for redistribution. Ultrasonographic anatomy images related to the liver, pancreas, and bile duct include an illustration of portal anatomy, normal bile duct, tumor of liver hilum, bile duct cancer, pancreatic cancer, esophageal varix, and obstructive jaundice. Heart and major vessels images include a normal heart, major vessels of the body, and abdominal aortic aneurysm. Head images include a surface image of human head and an image of an arachnoid cyst. Images related to the kidney and urinary tract include that of a renal cell carcinoma.

Health On the Net (HON) Foundation ◎ ◎ ◎

http://www.hon.ch/Media/anatomy.html

This site provides links to radiological and surgical images on the Internet. Images are available of the abdomen, ankle, arm, full body, brain, elbow, eye, foot, hand, head, heart, hilum, hip, kidney, knee, leg, liver, lung, muscle, neck, pancreas, pelvis, shoulder, skin, skull, teeth, thorax, trachea, blood vessels, and wrist.

Integrated Medical
Curriculum Human Anatomy ◎ ◎ ◎ (free registration)

http://www.imc.gsm.com

An extensive database of images can be easily accessed for educational purposes. The site covers Human Anatomy, Microscopic Anatomy, Radiologic Anatomy, Cross-Sectional Anatomy, as well as essentials of Human Physiology, essentials of Immunology, and Clinical Pharmacology. A simple, free registration is required.

Medical i-Way ◎ ◎ ◎

http://www.largnet.on.ca/oldlargnet

Medical i-Way demonstrates pathology through the use of medical imaging. A separate section is devoted to each anatomical group, with a list of specific pathologies available for view. Details of each image include case history, diagnosis, image findings, and descriptions of similar cases. Users can also find images through a keyword index.

Medical Images on the Web ◎ ◎ ◎

http://www.unmc.edu/library/medimag.html

Eleven links are available at this address to Internet sources for medical images. All links are accompanied by short descriptions of resources at the site.

Mudi-Muse Biomedical Imaging and Processing ◎ ◎ ◎
http://www.expasy.ch/LFMI

The MultiDimensional-MultiSensor/MultiModality Biomedical Imaging and Processing Web site provides examples and applications of different techniques used in biomedical imaging. Multidimensional, multimodality, and multi-sensor applications are described in detail with specific examples of medical applications, and discussions of new developments in this growing field are available.

National Library of Medicine (NLM) New Visible Human Project ◎ ◎ ◎
http://www.nlm.nih.gov/research/visible/visible_human.html

The Visible Human Project, devoted to the creation of complete, anatomically detailed, three-dimensional representations of the normal male and female human bodies, is an outgrowth of the National Library of Medicine's 1986 Long Range Plan. The Project has recently completed acquisition of transverse CT, MR, and cryosection images of representative male and female cadavers. The site describes the Visible Human Data Set and how to obtain data, and provides links to primary contractors for the Project, a sampler of images and animations from the project, and links to articles and other press releases discussing the Project. Applications and tools for viewing images are discussed, and links to sources of images and animations are provided. This site is also available in Spanish.

Neurosciences on the Internet: Images ◎ ◎ ◎
http://www.neuroguide.com/neuroimg.html

Internet sites are found through this address offering resources relating to human neuroanatomy and neuropathology, neuroscience images and methods, medical imaging centers, medical illustration, medical imaging indexes, and neuroanatomy atlases of animals.

Normal Radiologic Anatomy ◎ ◎
http://www.vh.org/Providers/TeachingFiles/NormalRadAnatomy/Text/RadM1title.html

This site provides visitors with X-Ray, CT, MR, and ultrasound images of the head and neck, thorax, abdomen, pelvis, upper extremity, and lower extremity. Images are labeled to identify normal anatomic structures.

PERLjam Online/Medical Images, Including Neuroanatomy ◎ ◎ ◎
http://erl.pathology.iupui.edu

This site is an online version of the PERLjam CD-ROM of pathology, histology, and laboratory medicine resources distributed to Indiana University School of Medicine students. The Indiana University School of Medicine Pathology Educational Resources Laboratory provides general and systemic pathology, histology, laboratory medicine, and dermatology images at this site. Images are categorized by organ system.

Three-Dimensional Medical Reconstruction ◎ ◎ ◎

http://www.crd.ge.com/esl/cgsp/projects/medical

Three-dimensional (3-D) reconstruction technology and medical imaging was employed to make short videos showing various sections of the human anatomy at this site. Information on the Visible Human Project and several short videos on this topic, surgical planning, and virtual endoscopy are also available.

University of Illinois College of Medicine
at Urbana, Champaign—The Urbana Atlas of Pathology ◎ ◎ ◎

http://www.med.uiuc.edu/PathAtlasf/framer2/path3.html

The site provides an extremely comprehensive collection of images sectioned into general, cardiovascular, endocrine, pulmonary, and renal pathology. The general pathology section includes images of the kidney, heart, spleen, thyroid, testis, cervix, small intestine, lung, artery, pancreas, liver, lymph nodes, brain, colon, skin, mesentery, joints, uterus, and peritoneal cavity.

University of Iowa College Of Medicine—
Division of Physiological Imaging Department Of Radiology ◎ ◎ ◎

http://everest.radiology.uiowa.edu

This site describes work done by the Division of Physiological Imaging of the University of Iowa College of Medicine. This group is dedicated to the research and advancement of medical imaging technology. Within the Web site are examples of medical imaging, selected papers on the field, descriptions of new technology and projects, and a list of links to related sites.

Visible Human Slice and Surface Server ◎ ◎ ◎

http://visiblehuman.epfl.ch

This site provides a viewer that enables the user to see images of planar and curved surfaces from the bodies of the Visible Human Project.

12.10 Medical Informatics

AMA Electronic Medical Systems & Coding ◎ ◎ ◎

http://www.ama-assn.org/med-sci/cpt/oems.htm

The American Medical Association plays a key role in the field of medical informatics. This site provides information on coding and medical information systems relative to the transmission of computerized patient and claims information. There are also links for electronic medical records, telemedicine, electronic data exchange, national uniform claim standards, and administrative simplification legislation.

American Medical Association (AMA): Coding and Medical Information Systems ◎ ◎ ◎

http://www.ama-assn.org/med-sci/cpt/cpt.htm

This site provides information on the AMA's new current procedural terminology (CPT) information services, the resource-based relative value scale, and electronic medical systems, including systems for storing electronic medical records, telemedicine resources, and electronic data interchange. Information is also available on the National Uniform Claim Committee and Administrative Simplification Legislation.

American Medical Informatics Association (AMIA) ◎ ◎ ◎

http://www.amia.org

With the proliferation of medical information, the growth of medical research, the development of medical information systems, and the creation of management systems for computerized patient data, the medical informatics field has grown substantially. This leading association provides its own organization, meeting, policy, and information access features, and also provides links to other organizations in the informatics field. Major themes of the AMIA are privacy and confidentiality of medical records, public policy development for legislation in the field, conferences of medical informatics professionals, and the issuance of papers and publications covering various aspects of the medical information field.

Medical Informatics Resources from Health Network ◎ ◎

http://www.healthwave.com

A dozen U.S. and international centers and medical departments dealing with Medical Informatics can be accessed from this central listing (click on Professional Medicine, Medical Informatics), including centers at Oregon Health Sciences University, Stanford, Columbia, and at European institutions. There are also articles, directories, and discussion group links for further resources on Medical Informatics.

12.11 Patent Searches

Introduction

The following sites provide easy access to patent information for medical researchers and healthcare professionals interested in learning about the latest techniques, therapies, products, and drugs.

Intellectual Property Network ◎ ◎ ◎

http://www.patents.ibm.com

Ideal for physicians and researchers with an interest in patents, this IBM service offers a searchable database of patent information, titles and abstracts, and inventors and companies. The database brings up patents on any topic by typing in the subject, along with inventor information, dates of filing, application numbers, and an abstract of the patent.

U.S. Patent and Trademark Office   ◎ ◎ ◎

http://www.uspto.gov/patft/index.html

Access to the database of the U.S. Patent and Trademark Office is available through this site, for detailed searching of patents by number, inventor, and topic. There are both a full-text database and a bibliographic database.

13. STUDENT RESOURCES

13.1 Fellowships and Residencies

Accreditation Council for Graduate Medical Education (ACGME) ⊙ ⊙ ⊙
http://www.acgme.org

The ACGME reviews and accredits residency programs, establishes standards of performance, and provides a process to consider complaints and possible investigations by the Council. The site offers information about ACGME, meetings, workshops, institutional reviews, contact details, links to residency review committees, and a listing of accredited programs.

AMA's Fellowship and Residency
Electronic Interactive Database Access (FREIDA) Online System ⊙ ⊙ ⊙
http://www.ama-assn.org/physdata/datacoll/datacoll.htm

Operated as a service of the American Medical Association (AMA), the FREIDA System provides online access to a comprehensive database of information on approximately 7,500 graduate medical educational programs accredited by the Accreditation Council for Graduate Medical Education (ACGME). FREIDA enables the user to search this comprehensive database and offers other services, including label printing for mailing purposes.

Educational Commission for Foreign
Medical Graduates (ECFMG) ⊙ ⊙ ⊙
http://www.ecfmg.org

The Educational Commission for Foreign Medical Graduates, through its certification program, "assesses the readiness of graduates of foreign medical schools to enter residency or fellowship programs in the United States that are accredited by the Accreditation Council for Graduate Medical Education (ACGME)." The site is a very useful source of information for foreign students to learn about testing and examination dates, clinical skills required, and available publications to review requirements for applications.

Electronic Residency Application Service ⊙ ⊙ ⊙
http://www.aamc.org

The Association of American Medical Colleges (AAMC) provides this application service for students. It transmits residency applications, recommendation letters, Dean's letters, transcripts, and other supporting credentials from medical schools to residency program directors via the Internet. At present, the service covers Obstetrics and Gynecology, Pediatrics, Surgery, and Psychiatry. The system allows tracking of an application 24 hours a day via a special document tracking system.

National Residency Matching Program (NRMP) ☺ ☺ ☺

http://nrmp.aamc.org/nrmp/index.htm

The NRMP is a mechanism for the matching of applicants to programs according to the preferences expressed by both parties. This is an extremely useful site and service, which last year placed over 20,000 applicants for postgraduate medical training positions into 3,500 residency programs at 700 teaching hospitals in the United States. The applicants and residency programs evaluate and rank each other, producing a computerized pairing of applicants to programs, in ranked order. This process provides applicants and program directors with a uniform date of appointment to positions in March, eliminating decision pressure when options are unknown. The site offers information about the service, contact details, publications, and forms for registration. Prospective residents can register with the service for a fee and access the directory of programs.

Residency Page ☺ ☺ ☺

http://www.Webcom.com/~wooming/residenc.html

The Residency Page Web site provides an online listing of medical residencies organized by specialty. Program directors can access resumes of residency applicants, and prospective residents can review documents related to residency matching programs and publications offering advice on obtaining a position.

13.2 Medical School Web Sites

American Universities ☺ ☺ ☺

http://www.clas.ufl.edu/CLAS/american-universities.html

All American university home pages are listed at this site.

Gradschools.com ☺ ☺ ☺

http://www.gradschools.com/noformsearch.html

Sponsored by several universities and other teaching institutions, Gradschools.com offers a listing of graduate programs nationwide. Programs are found by indicating a specific area of study. A directory of distance learning programs is also available.

Medical Education ☺ ☺ ☺

http://www.meducation.com/schools.html

Accredited medical schools are listed, with links, at this site.

Medical Schools ⊙ ⊙ ⊙
http://www.scomm.net/~greg/med-ed/schools.html
This medical site provides direct links to all of the medical schools of U.S. and Canada accredited by the AAMC. These include hundreds of medical school Web sites in the United States and elsewhere.

13.3 Medical Student Resources

American Medical Women's Association (AMWA) ⊙ ⊙ ⊙
http://www.amwa-doc.org
A national association, the AMWA provides information and services to women physicians and women medical students, and promotes women's health and the professional development of women physicians. Resources include news, discussions of current issues, events, conferences, online publications, fellowship and residency information accessed through FREIDA, general information and developments from AMA staff members, advocacy activities, a listing of AMWA continuing education programs, and links to sites of interest. A variety of topics related to women's health are discussed at the site.

Association of American Medical Colleges (AAMC) ⊙ ⊙ ⊙
http://www.aamc.org
This nonprofit Association committed to the advancement of academic medicine consists of American and Canadian medical schools, teaching hospitals and health systems, academic and professional societies, and medical students and residents. News, membership details, publications and other information resources, meeting and conference calendars, medical education Internet resources, research findings, and discussions related to health care are all found at the site. Employment opportunities at the AAMC are also listed.

IMpact: The Internal Medicine Newsletter for Medical Students ⊙ ⊙ ⊙
http://www.acponline.org/journals/impact/impmenu.htm
This online newsletter focuses on different medical specialties with each issue, and includes full-text articles of interest to physicians and medical students. The newsletter is produced by the American College of Physicians—American Society of Internal Medicine (ACP-ASIM). Students can apply for free membership in the ACP-ASIM if they are currently enrolled in medical school.

Medical Books at Amazon.com ○ ○ ○

http://www.abcba.com/books/medical.htm

This site allows users to search by medical topic or keyword for medical textbooks. Dictionaries, encyclopedias, and Physician's Desk References on different subjects may be ordered through the site.

Medical Student Section of the AMA ○ ○ ○

http://www.ama-assn.org/ama/pub/category/0,1120,14,FF.html

The Medical Student Section of the American Medical Association (AMA) is dedicated to representing medical students, improving medical education, developing leadership, and promoting activism for the health of America. The site offers information about the section, current issues and advocacy activities, business issues of the section, chapter information, and leadership news. Special interest groups within the section include those for residents, young physicians, organized staff, students, international medical graduates, and senior physicians.

Medical Student Web Site ○ ○ ○

http://www.medicalstudent.com

This is an excellent, current site for medical students, describing itself as "a digital library of authoritative medical information for all students of medicine." It contains an extensive medical textbook section organized by discipline, patient simulations, consumer health information, access to MEDLINE and medical journals online, continuing education sources, board exam information, medical organizations, and Internet medical directories.

Stanford MedWorld ○ ○ ○

http://www-med.stanford.edu/medworld/home

MedWorld, sponsored by the Stanford Medical Alumni Association, offers information for students, patients, physicians, and the healthcare community. Resources include case reports and global rounds, links to quality medical sites and MEDLINE, doctor diaries and medical news, and newsgroups and discussion forums. Visitors can access Stanford's medical search engine, MEDBOT, to simultaneously utilize many Internet medical search engines.

Student Doctor Network: The Interactive Medical Student Lounge ○ ○ ○

http://www.medstudents.net

This is an excellent site for medical students with interests in all medical specialties as well as all aspects of the medical community. The site provides information on applying to medical school, financial aid, internships and residencies, medical chat rooms, databases, discussions of educational issues, links to online journals, news, updates, and broadcasts. In addition, the site provides access to discounts on medical equipment and books, the purchase and sale of used medical texts, medical software and medical CD-ROMs. Students can access medical reference material, medical school sites, medical search engines, student groups, externships, foreign residencies, and medical missions abroad.

14. PATIENT EDUCATION AND PLANNING

14.1 Patient Resources

Introduction

Patient information regarding various medical conditions and health issues can be obtained at any of the general medical search engines that are included. Below are listings of health Web sites accessible through the well-known search engines, as well as other sites that cover wide-ranging topics of interest to patients.

Allexperts.com ○ ○

http://www.allexperts.com/browse.asp?Meta=24

Allexperts.com is a free online question and answer service. A message board and many frequently asked questions are present. Available medical topics are listed alphabetically, and users can choose a specific "volunteer expert" to contact after reading short biographies and descriptions of specialty areas.

allHealth.com ○ ○ ○

http://www.allhealth.com

Resources at this site include a site search engine; a drug database; information on specific conditions; weight management information; and special information centers devoted to seniors', women's, and men's health, pediatrics, mental health, sexual health, alternative medicine, asthma, headaches, smoking cessation, HIV/AIDS, heartburn, and family health. Physician directories for home and when traveling, elder care directories, interactive health calculators, an online newsletter, research information, chat forums, and news articles are also provided.

America Online (AOL) ○ ○

http://www.aol.com/timesavers/health.html

Sponsored by America Online, this site is a useful medical information source for the general public. The user can search for a disease; use a symptom analyzer; learn about rare illnesses; obtain advice; find support groups; and research topics on health, medicine, and wellness.

American Academy of Family Physicians Health Information Page ○ ○ ○

http://familydoctor.org

This site allows visitors to search information by keyword or category, and is written and reviewed by the physicians and patient education professionals at the Academy of Family Physicians.

American Medical Association (AMA): Health Insight ◎ ◎ ◎

http://www.ama-assn.org/consumer.htm

Information for consumers at this site includes medical news; detailed information on a wide range of conditions; general health topic discussions; family health resources for children, adolescents, men, and women; interactive health calculators; healthy recipes; and general safety tips. Specific pages are devoted to comprehensive resources related to HIV/AIDS, asthma, migraines, and women's health. Patients will find this site an excellent source for accurate, useful health information. American Medical Association information at this site includes a directory of advisory board members and contact information for the Association.

BestDoctors.com ◎ ◎ (free registration)

http://www.bestdoctors.com

Best Doctors' Inc. provides information and searching services for superior medical care to major insurers, managed care companies, self-insured corporations, foreign governments, and individuals. The site provides visitors with news, feature articles from a participating doctor, drug information, general information, and suggested sites relating to over 40 health topics. Contact information, employment details, a directory of the company's medical advisory board, rating information on medical Web sites, news and events information, contact information for a physician referral service, and answers relating to recent Internet health-related rumors are all found at the site. Registered users can ask health questions, participate in chat forums, and gain access to medical newsletters.

Boston University Medical Center— Community Outreach Health Information System ◎ ◎ ◎

http://www.bu.edu/cohis

This site provides the general public with an excellent resource for health information. A wide range of health topics are discussed at the site, including AIDS/HIV, infectious diseases, sexually transmitted diseases, cancer, blood and heart diseases, nutrition, smoking cessation, domestic violence, teen pregnancy, and alcohol and substance abuse. More specific topics are also listed. Visitors can submit health questions and access a physician directory.

Columbia University College of Physicians and Surgeons Complete Home Medical Guide ◎ ◎ ◎

http://cpmcnet.columbia.edu/texts/guide

Patients will consider this site an excellent resource for healthcare information. Topics include receiving proper medical care, the correct use of medications, first aid and safety, preventative medicine, and good nutrition. Chapters containing more specific information on health concerns for men, women, and children; disorders; infectious diseases; mental and emotional health; and substance abuse are also available.

Combined Health Information Database (CHID) ◎ ◎ ◎

http://chid.nih.gov

The Combined Health Information Database (CHID) is produced by several agencies of the federal government offering a searchable file of health promotion publications, education materials, and program descriptions. The site offers simple and detailed search options, and users can also indicate specific search criteria, including date and language of the publication. Availability and ordering information is provided for the resources included. Site updates are performed quarterly.

DiscoveryHealth.com ◎ ◎ ◎

http://www.discoveryhealth.com/DH/ihtIH?t=20707&st=20707&r=WSDSC000

In association with InteliHealth, this site from the makers of the Discovery Channel offers consumer health resources. News items, feature articles and reports, a site search engine, links to health reference materials, chat forums, a forum for asking health questions, and descriptions of recent research advances are all found at this site. Visitors can learn interesting health facts and access information specific to men, women, senior citizens, children, mental health, and health in the workplace. Nutrition, fitness, and weight management tools are also available at this site.

DoctorDirectory: HealthNews Directory ◎ ◎

http://www.doctordirectory.com/HealthNews/Directory/Default.asp

In addition to daily news and a national directory of doctors listed by state, this site contains links to resources related to various health topics, including AIDS, allergies/asthma, alternative medicine, cancer, children's health, clinical trials, cosmetic surgery, dentistry, diabetes, women's health, geriatrics, healthcare companies, insurance, and other subjects.

drkoop.com ◎ ◎ ◎

http://www.drkoop.com

This site provides patients and the general public with an excellent source for current health information. Free registration and e-mail newsletters, site search engines, health news, chat topics, general information about clinical trials, and a drug interaction search tool are some of the most useful features. Please note that some sections of the site offering specific information are sponsored by pharmaceutical products, i.e., a company producing a smoking cessation medication sponsors a section designed to help users quit.

Family Village—
A Global Community of Disability-Related Resources ⊙ ⊙ ⊙
http://www.familyvillage.wisc.edu/index.htmlx

This site provides the general public with cataloged information about a wide range of disorders and disabilities. Chat room links and other networking resources, support and medical resources, technology/products links, recreation programs, research programs, publications, and educational resources for children are all found at this comprehensive patient support site.

Health-Center.com ⊙ ⊙
http://site.health-center.com/default.htm

This site contains a variety of links to fact sheets on family issues, senior citizen related topics, general wellness topics, mental health information, and medications. There are also links to professional resources, including postings of online continuing education resources.

HealthAnswers.com ⊙ ⊙ ⊙
http://www.healthanswers.com

This site provides the general public with informational resources on a wide range of health topics, including senior health, pregnancy, alternative medicine, diseases, and healthy lifestyle tips. Partners include the American Academy of Pediatrics, the Center for Pharmacy, the National Health Council, the National Transplant Society, Reuters Health News, and other national groups and information resources.

HealthCentral.com ⊙ ⊙ ⊙
http://www.healthcentral.com/home/home.cfm

News items, feature columns, quizzes and polls, a doctor's column, drug and herb information, health profiles and assessment tools, online shopping, and medical reference materials are all available at this useful site. Information centers offer specific resources on "hot topics," alternative medicine, fitness, life issues, wellness, consumer health, health improvement, such as weight loss and smoking cessation, and medical conditions.

HealthlinkUSA ⊙ ⊙ ⊙
http://www.healthlinkusa.com

At this site, links to many general health sites are listed in alphabetical order by topic or disorder. Interested persons can access links to specific health issues or browse for sites by medical category.

HealthWorld Online ◎ ◎ ◎

http://www.healthy.net

A subject map appears at the beginning of this site indicating the many aspects of the health and medical world covered by numerous links. There is a topical site search engine, access to publications through MEDLINE at the National Library of Medicine, information on specific diseases and alternative therapies, a referral network, a global calendar, and information on wellness, fitness, and nutrition.

InteliHealth: Home to Johns Hopkins Health Information ◎ ◎ ◎

http://www.intelihealth.com/IH/ihtIH?t=408&st=408&r=WSIHW000

This comprehensive site offers consumers tips on healthy living, information, and other resources on specific conditions, a site search engine for specific information, health news by topic, special reports, an online newsletter, pharmaceutical drug information, and an online store offering health items for the home. Conditions and health topics discussed at the site include allergy, arthritis, asthma, babies, cancer, caregivers, childhood, diabetes, digestive, fitness, headache, heart, mental health, pregnancy, vitamin and nutrition, and weight management. Links are available to other sites offering consumer health resources.

Johns Hopkins Medical Institutions (InfoNet) ◎ ◎ ◎

http://infonet.welch.jhu.edu/advocacy.html

A database of patient advocacy groups is housed at this site. Telephone contact information and links to an associated Web site is offered for most organizations. A search tool is available to find groups for specific disorders.

KidsHealth.org ◎ ◎ ◎

http://kidshealth.org/index2.html

This site, created by the Nemours Foundation Center for Children's Health Media, provides expert health information about children from before birth through adolescence. Specific sections target kids, teens, and parents, with age-appropriate information and language.

Mayo Health ◎ ◎ ◎

http://www.mayohealth.org/index.htm

Visitors to this informative site will find answers to patient questions, news and articles on featured topics, registration details for e-mail alerts of site updates, and site search engines for health information and prescription drug information. Specific information centers are devoted to allergy and asthma, Alzheimer's disease, cancer, children's health, digestive health, heart health, general medicine, men's and women's health, and nutrition. A library of answers to health questions, a glossary of medical terms, and a forum for asking specific questions are also available at the site.

MDAdvice.com ⊙ ⊙

http://www.mdadvice.com

In addition to containing links to informative fact sheets on a variety of health topics (arranged alphabetically), this site provides detailed information on pharmaceuticals, medicine in the news, information on health centers, expert advice, and chat rooms.

Med Help International ⊙ ⊙ ⊙

http://www.medhelp.org

This all-encompassing site describes itself as "the largest online consumer health information resource with tens of thousands of entries." It includes a medical search engine, library access and doctor forums, medical and health news, and support groups.

MedicineNet ⊙ ⊙ ⊙

http://www.medicinenet.com

An efficient and thorough source of information on hundreds of diseases and medical conditions, MedicineNet enables the user to click on subjects in an alphabetical list. The site's medical content is produced by Board certified physicians and allied health professionals. Topics include diseases and treatments, procedures and tests, a pharmacy section, a medical dictionary, first aid information, and a list of poison control centers.

Mediconsult.com, Inc. ⊙ ⊙ ⊙

http://www.mediconsult.com

Mediconsult provides medical news and information on a variety of topics, including cancer, chronic pain, eating disorders, and migraines. The information at the site is drawn from journals, research centers, and other sources, and is subject to a rigorous clinical review process. Specific sections are devoted to health issues relevant to women, men, seniors, children, and caregivers. Additional resources include a medical directory of disease information, drug information, fitness and nutrition discussions, a question and answer forum, and live chat events.

MEDLINEplus ⊙ ⊙ ⊙

http://www.nlm.nih.gov/medlineplus

This site is a source for information on various diseases and health topics for the public, featuring a directory of links divided into categories such as health topics, dictionaries, other directories, organizations, and publications. The site links to MEDLINE, either through PubMed or the Internet Grateful Med.

National Women's Health Information Center (NWHIC) ◎ ◎ ◎

http://www.4woman.org

This searchable site offers lists of publications and organizations for information on a wide range of women's health topics. There are also links to resources for special groups, journals, FAQs, news items and affiliated organizations, as well as information about the NWHIC itself.

NetWellness ◎ ◎ ◎ (some features fee-based)

http://www.netwellness.org

NetWellness is a Web-based consumer health information service with one of the largest groups of medical and health experts who answer consumer questions on the Web. Developed by the University of Cincinnati Medical Center, The Ohio State University, and Case Western Reserve University, over 200 health faculty answer questions on over 40 topics. Responses are usually provided within two to three days. Users can also search archives of articles.

New York Online Access to Health (NOAH) ◎ ◎ ◎ (some features fee-based)

http://www.noah.cuny.edu

This site is offered as a public resource by many providers, including hospitals, institutes, foundations, research centers, and city and state agencies. Users can access information concerning a wide range of health topics, including diseases, mental health, nutrition, and links to patient resources. A site-based search engine is available. A health information database containing abstracts and articles from selected health-related periodicals is only available to users accessing the site from specific institutions, including the New York Public Library branches.

OnHealth.com ◎ ◎ ◎

http://www.onhealth.com/ch1/index.asp

Visitors to this site can search for health information by keyword or condition, access news and reports, ask health questions, and find many useful information resources related to specific topics, such as smoking cessation, pharmaceutical drugs, alternative medicine, vitamins and minerals, and first aid. Chat forums, information on live chat events, physician and medical center directories, online shopping opportunities, and interactive health assessment tools are all found at this site.

Prevention Magazine Online ◎ ◎ ◎

http://www.healthyideas.com

Prevention Magazine offers resources for healthier living at this site. Health tools include a calorie calculator, exercise and weight loss information, recipes, vitamin and herb information, and tips on skin care. Online newsletters and stores, chat forums, and subscription details for the magazine are available, as well as resource centers offering specific information on health conditions, men's and women's health, and pediatrics. Links are also found to women.com for specific women's resources.

Psci-com   ☺ ☺ ☺

http://www.psci-com.org.uk

Psci-com is described as "a gateway to public understanding of science and science communication information on the Internet." The site offers a searchable catalog of Internet resources selected and cataloged by the Wellcome Trust for the benefit of the UK public.

Quackwatch   ☺ ☺ ☺

http://www.quackwatch.com

Quackwatch is a nonprofit corporation combating "health-related frauds, myths, fads, and fallacies." The group investigates questionable health claims, answers consumer inquiries, distributes publications, reports illegal marketing, generates consumer-protection lawsuits, works to improve the quality of health information on the Internet, and attacks misleading Internet advertising. Operation costs are generated solely from the sales of publications and individual donations. Sister sites, Chirobase and MLM Watch, offer a consumer's guide to chiropractors and a skeptical guide to multilevel marketing. Information for cancer patients includes alerts of questionable alternative health treatments, a discussion of how questionable practices may harm cancer patients, and other related discussions. Cancer prevention information alerts are also posted. Visitors to the site can purchase publications, read general information about questionable medical practices, and read information about specific questionable products and services. Links to government agencies and other sites providing information about health fraud are available at this important site.

Thrive   ☺ ☺ ☺

http://www.thriveonline.com

Thrive Online offers information resources in the areas of general medicine, fitness, sexuality, nutrition, serenity and mental wellness, and weight. Users can find information by choosing from a list of medical conditions, or employ search capabilities by keyword or in question form.

University of California (UC), Davis Medical Center Patient Care   ☺ ☺ ☺

http://www.pcs.ucdmc.ucdavis.edu

This site contains information about patient care services at UC Davis Medical Center as well as a list of health resources on the Internet. Specific resources include topics in patient care, education, and epidemiology and infection control.

Virtual Hospital:
University of Iowa Health Care ◎ ◎ ◎ (some features fee-based)

http://www.vh.org

The Virtual Hospital is a service of the University of Iowa, providing patients and healthcare professionals with a digital library of health information. The library contains hundreds of books and brochures on health related issues, and also provides physicians with Continuing Medical Education resources. The site provides information about the departments at the University of Iowa hospitals, a link to the Virtual Children's Hospital, Continuing Medical Education information, and resource sections for patients and healthcare providers. Two sections are restricted to University of Iowa students, faculty, and affiliates.

Yahoo! ◎ ◎ ◎

http://www.yahoo.com

A reliable source of information in most fields, Yahoo offers a Health Section covering diseases, medical topics, patient information, fitness, and other health topics. It is a good place to start for a patient seeking general information.

14.2 Support Groups

Ask NOAH About: Support Groups ◎ ◎ ◎

http://www.noah.cuny.edu:8080/support1.html

This directory of Web sites and other resources includes links to other directories, general health sites, toll-free telephone numbers, face-to-face support groups, support organizations, newsgroups, mailing lists, chat forums, and other online support resources. Visitors can browse listings by type of resource or by specific medical conditions.

Support-Group.com ◎ ◎ ◎

http://www.support-group.com

Support-Group.com allows people with health, personal, and relationship issues to share their experiences through bulletin boards and online chats, and provides plenty of links to support-related information on the Internet. The A to Z listing offers hundreds of connections to disease-related support, bereavement assistance, marriage and family issue groups, and women's/men's issues, to name a few. The Bulletin Board Tracker lists the most recent messages and provides a complete cross-reference of topics. By visiting the Support-Group.com Chat Schedule page, dates, times, and group facilitators for upcoming chat events can be viewed. Users have the option of participating in real time Chat Groups via Internet Relay Chat or JavaChat using a Java-capable Web browser. Complete instructions are available at the Web site.

14.3 **Medical Planning**

Blood Bank Information

America's Blood Centers ⊛ ⊛
http://www.americasblood.org

America's Blood Centers are found in 46 states and collect approximately 47% of the U.S. blood supply. This site provides contact information for each of this organization's centers.

American Association of Blood Banks ⊛ ⊛ ⊛
http://www.aabb.org

This site provides a contact list for each state on locating and arranging blood donation, including information on storing blood for an anticipated surgery or emergency (autologous blood transfusion). It also answers general questions about blood and blood transfusion.

Caregiver Resources

Caregiver Network ⊛ ⊛ ⊛
http://www.caregiver.on.ca/content_main.html

This resource center, based in Canada, offers support, advice, seminars, and information for caregivers of the elderly and chronically ill. Text excerpts from an educational video program are available, and visitors can order the video series online. A caregiver resource guide offers telephone numbers and other contact information for government agencies, organizations, service providers, support agencies, publications, and periodicals. Suggested book and video lists and links to related Internet resources are available.

Caregiver Survival Resources ⊛ ⊛
http://www.caregiver911.com

Maintained by professionals in the field of caregiving, this site offers bulletin boards, forums for questions, telephone numbers for related organizations, and links to government agencies and other sites for additional information searches. Visitors can access a list of suggested publications, read book excerpts, and books online from the site.

National Family Caregivers Association (NFCA) ◎ ◎

http://www.nfcacares.org

The NFCA is national organization offering education, information, support, public awareness campaigns, and advocacy to American caregivers. The address discusses caregiving and provides statistics, a survey report, news, an informational pamphlet, a reading list, caregiving tips, and contact details. Caregivers will find this site a source of support, encouragement, and information.

Chronic and Terminal Care Planning

American Association for
Retired Persons (AARP): Basic Facts about Reverse Mortgages ◎ ◎ ◎

http://www.aarp.org/hecc/basicfct.html

This fact sheet within the AARP Web site describes reverse mortgages, including eligibility requirements, how reverse mortgages work, what a borrower receives from the mortgage, typical payments, and contact details for information on other programs or services not involving a loan against the home.

Chronic Pain Solutions ◎ ◎ ◎

http://www.chronicpainsolutions.com

Chronic Pain Solutions is a quarterly guide for chronic pain sufferers linking traditional and natural medical care. The site contains the online newsletter, contact and home subscription details, an online store for ordering therapeutic products, and biographies of contributing writers.

Consumer Guide to Viatical Settlements ◎ ◎

http://www.nvrnvr.com/guide.html

This online booklet, *Every Question You Need To Ask Before Selling Your Life Insurance Policy,* is provided by National Viator Representatives, a viatical settlement information source, advisor, and broker. Users can access the publication online, download the document, or order a hard copy at 1-800-932-0050.

Living Will and Values History Project ◎ ◎

http://www.euthanasia.org/lwvh.html

This site offers a Living Will package and Values History document, both available for download free-of-charge. Users can also receive hard copies for a nominal charge. The site also contains an extensive list of links to related sites.

Living Wills ⚙ ⚙

http://www.kepro.org/Bene_LivingWill.htm

Prepared by the Pennsylvania Medical Society, this site answers questions for the average patient regarding the development and use of a living will. It also provides a link to a free sample copy of a living will that can be completed and signed by individuals to be placed in their medical record.

National Chronic Care Consortium ⚙ ⚙ (some features fee-based)

http://www.ncccresourcecenter.org/index.html

The National Chronic Care Consortium is dedicated to transforming the delivery of chronic care services. Members of this group strive to make the delivery of chronic care more efficient and cost effective. The site provides information on conferences, contact details, and links to related sites. Members can take part in the Alzheimer's Project Developmental Group Discussion at the site and access other services.

Organ Donation ⚙ ⚙ ⚙

http://www.organdonor.gov

This government site answers frequently asked questions, dispels myths, and presents facts about organ donation. Visitors can download and print a donor card, and find links to related organizations on the Internet.

U.S. Living Will Registry ⚙ ⚙ ⚙

http://www.uslivingwillregistry.com

This free service electronically stores advance directives and makes them available directly to hospitals by telephone. Registration materials are available to download online or by calling 1-800-LIV-WILL.

USAhomecare.com ⚙ ⚙ ⚙

http://www.USAhomecare.com

USAhomecare.com is a consumer-oriented home care (home health and hospice) site. The site provides answers to common questions, a bookstore, links to related sites, news, contact information, and a directory of agencies offering home care or hospice services.

Directing Healthcare Concerns and Complaints

Congress.org ⚙ ⚙ ⚙

http://congress.org/main.html

This site offers a Capital directory, including members of Congress, the Supreme Court, state governors, and the White House. Users can also find comments on members of Congress by associations and advocacy groups, determine a bill's status through the site's search engine, send messages to Congress members, and find local congressional representatives.

Families USA ○ ○ ○
http://www.familiesusa.org

Families USA is a national nonprofit, nonpartisan organization dedicated to the achievement of high-quality, affordable health, and long-term care for all Americans. The site offers a clearinghouse of information on Medicaid, Medicare, and General Managed Healthcare. Assistance and advice is provided on choosing an HMO, how to tell if a health policy or plan is good, and who to address if you have a healthcare complaint. Within the site, at www.familiesusa.org/medicaid/state.htm, a state-specific healthcare information guide is provided. This directory includes phone numbers to every state's Department of Insurance, which allows users to obtain reports on plans and information on complaint ratios.

Joint Commission of
Accreditation of Healthcare Organizations (JCAHO) ○ ○
http://www.jcaho.org/news/nb189.html

The JCAHO site lists a toll-free complaint hotline for patients, their families, and caregivers to express concerns about the quality of care at accredited healthcare organizations at this site. (The toll-free U.S. telephone number is 1-800-994-6610. The hotline is staffed between 8:30 a.m. and 5 p.m., central time, during weekdays.) The site also describes a mechanism for transmitting complaints via e-mail.

Medicare Rights Center (MRC) ○ ○ ○
http://www.medicarerights.org

Medicare Rights Center is a national, nonprofit organization focused to ensure that seniors and people with disabilities on Medicare have access to quality, affordable healthcare. The site offers information on specific MRC programs, news, consumer publications, information on professional membership, and details on the Initiative for the Terminally Ill on Medicare. Visitors can also subscribe for a fee to a biweekly newsletter delivered by fax.

Quality Improvement Organizations ○ ○
http://www.qio.org

This site contains a directory of Peer Review Organizations (PRO) listed by state. These organizations monitor the care given to Medicare patients. Each state has a PRO that can decide whether care given to Medicare patients is reasonable, necessary, provided in the most appropriate setting, and meets standards of quality generally accepted by the medical profession. Peer Review Organizations can also be contacted to investigate beneficiary complaints.

State Insurance Commissioners ⚙ ⚙ ⚙

http://www.dtonline.com/insur/inlistng.htm

Deloitte and Touche Financial Counseling Services offers the addresses and phone numbers of each state's insurance commissioner at this site.

Elder and Extended Care

Administration on Aging ⚙ ⚙ ⚙

http://www.aoa.dhhs.gov

This site provides resources for seniors, practitioners, and caregivers, including news on aging, links to Web sites on aging, statistics about older people, consumer fact sheets, retirement and financial planning information, and help finding community assistance for seniors.

American Association for Retired Persons (AARP) ⚙ ⚙ ⚙

http://www.aarp.org

This nonprofit group is dedicated to the needs and rights of elderly Americans. Topics discussed at the site include caregiver support, community and volunteer organizations, Medicare, Medicaid, help with home care, finances, health and wellness, independent living, computers and the Internet, and housing options. Benefits and discounts provided to members are described, reference and research materials are available, and users can search the site by keyword.

American Association of Homes and Services for the Aging (AAHSA) ⚙ ⚙ ⚙

http://www.aahsa.org

This Association represents nonprofit organizations providing health care, housing, and services to the elderly. The site offers tips for consumers and family caregivers on choosing facilities and services, notices of upcoming events, press releases, fact sheets, an online bookstore, and links to sponsors, business partners, an international program, and other relevant sites.

Eldercare Locator ⚙ ⚙ ⚙

http://www.aoa.dhhs.gov/aoa/pages/loctrnew.html

The Eldercare Locator is a nationwide, directory assistance service designed to help older persons and caregivers locate local support resources for aging Americans. This site helps senior citizens find community assistance and Medicaid information. Interested parties can also contact the Eldercare Locator toll free at 1-800-677-1116.

Extendedcare.com ⚙ ⚙ ⚙ (some features fee-based)

http://www.elderconnect.com/asp/default.asp

This address offers information on choosing an extended care provider, a "Geriatric Library" of information resources, a glossary of terms related to extended care, a forum for asking questions of a participating physician, and information on over 60,000 care providers. Visitors can search for care providers by type of care and zip code, subscribe to an e-mail newsletter, and read archived newsletters and press releases. A tool for assessing an individual's care needs is also available. A professional section is available to users associated with registered hospitals.

**Insure.com: Answers to Seniors'
Health Insurance Questions (on Medicare and Medicaid)** ⚙ ⚙ ⚙

http://www.insure.com/health/ship.html

This site provides the phone number to each state's Health Insurance Advisory Program (SHIP). SHIP is a federally funded program found in all states under different names, helping elderly and disabled Medicare and Medicaid recipients understand their rights and options for healthcare. Services include assistance with bills, advice on buying supplement policies, explanation of rights, help with payment denials or appeals, and assistance in choosing a Medicare health plan.

End of Life Decisions

**American Medical Association: Education
for Physicians on End-of Life Care (EPEC)** ⚙ ⚙ ⚙ (free registration)

http://www.ama-assn.org/ethic/epec/index.htm

Supported by a grant from the Robert Wood Johnson Foundation, EPEC is a two-year program designed to educate physicians nationwide on "the essential clinical competencies in end-of-life care." Visitors will find an overview of the project's purpose, design, and scope, a call for EPEC training conference applications, previous conference details, a mailing list, and an annotated list of educational resource materials. Users must complete a free registration process to view educational materials.

Before I Die ⚙ ⚙ ⚙

http://www.pbs.org/wnet/bid

This address presents the Web companion to a public television program exploring the medical, ethical, and social issues associated with end-of-life care in the United States. Personal stories, a bulletin board, a glossary of terms, contact details for important support sources and organizations, and suggestions on forming a discussion group are available at the site. A program description, viewer's guide, outreach efforts and materials, and credits for the program are also provided.

CareOfDying.org: Supportive Care of the Dying ⊚ ⊚ ⊚
http://www.careofdying.org

This site is presented by a coalition of 13 Catholic healthcare associations and the Catholic Health Association, advocating for an improvement in supportive care for persons with life-threatening illnesses and their caregivers. Assessment tools available at the site include patient, family caregiver, bereaved family, and professional questionnaires, and a tool assessing competency. A quarterly newsletter, research report, and hints for conducting focus groups are also available. Links are listed to related resources, including information on an upcoming PBS end-of-life series, hosted by Bill Moyers.

Choice in Dying ⊚ ⊚
http://www.choices.org

Services offered by Choice in Dying include advance directives, counseling for patients and families, professional training, advocacy, and publications. Membership details, press releases, news, information on end-of-life issues, an online newsletter, state-specific advance directive documents, and a petition for end-of-life care are all found at this site. Visitors can also order publications and videos, and access links to related sites.

Decisions Near the End of Life ⊚ ⊚
http://www.edc.org/CAE/Decisions/dnel.html

Decisions Near the End of Life is a Continuing Medical Education program helps professional staff and patients of hospitals and nursing homes improve the way ethical decisions are made. The site describes typical program attendees, goals, format, leadership training, institutional profiles developed by the program, on-site programs, program components, and Continuing Medical Education credit details.

End of Life: Exploring Death in America ⊚ ⊚ ⊚
http://www.npr.org/programs/death

National Public Radio's "All Things Considered" presents transcripts of a recent series on death and dying and other resources at this excellent site. Contact information and links to valuable organizations and other support sources, a bibliography of important publications, texts related to death, dying, and healing, and a forum for presenting personal stories are found at this address.

George Washington University: Toolkit of Instruments to Measure End of Life ⊚ ⊚ ⊚
http://www.gwu.edu/~cicd/toolkit/toolkit.htm

Toolkits assessing the quality of end-of-life care are available at this address, providing healthcare institutions with information to "assess, improve, and enhance care for dying patients and their loved ones." Visitors can download a chart review instrument, surrogate questionnaires, and a patient questionnaire. Resources at the site assess quality of life, pain and other symptoms, depression and emotional symptoms, functional status, survival time and aggressiveness of care, continuity of care, spirituality, grief, caregiver and family experience, and patient and family member satisfaction with the quality of care.

Last Acts ◎ ◎ ◎
http://www.lastacts.org

Designed to improve end-of-life care, Last Acts is devoted to "bring end-of-life issues out in the open and to help individuals and organizations pursue the search for better ways to care for the dying." The site presents information on Last Acts activities, a newsletter, press releases, and discussion forums. Links are available to details of recent news headlines, sites offering additional information resources, grant-making organizations, and a directory of Robert Wood Johnson Foundation end-of-life grantees.

Project on Death in America: Transforming the Culture of Dying ◎ ◎ ◎
http://www.soros.org/death

The Project on Death and Dying in America supports initiatives in research, scholarship, the humanities, and the arts in transforming the American culture and experience of dying and bereavement. The Project also promotes innovations in care, public education, professional education, and public policy. Information is presented on the Project's Faculty Scholars Program, Professional Initiatives in Nursing, Social Work, and Pastoral Care, Arts and Humanities Initiative, Public Policy Initiative, Legal Initiative, and Community Initiative. Other resources described at the site include Grantmakers Concerned with Care at the End of Life, media resources, and other publications offered by the Project.

Hospice and Home Care

American Academy of Hospice and Palliative Medicine (AAHPM) ◎ ◎ ◎
http://www.aahpm.org

This national nonprofit organization is comprised of physicians "dedicated to the advancement of hospice/palliative medicines, its practice, research, and education". Academy details, contact information, news, press releases, position statements, events and meetings notices, employment listings, and links to related sites are found at this address. Publications, Continuing Medical Education opportunities, and conference tapes are also available.

Growth House, Inc. ✪ ✪ ✪

http://www.growthhouse.org

Growth House, Inc. offers a comprehensive resource for hospice and home care information at this site. General information, a listing of local hospice providers, online book reviews, and an index of reviewed resources for end-of-life care are available at the site.

Hospice Association of America (HAA) ✪ ✪ ✪

http://www.hospice-america.org

Serving the needs of the most seriously ill patients with cancer and other diseases, the HAA offers a full menu of information about the field of hospice care, as well as a directory of home care and hospice state associations. Each localized association listing offers the name of the executive director, the address, telephone, fax, and e-mail contact.

Hospice Foundation of America ✪ ✪ ✪

http://www.hospicefoundation.org

The Hospice Foundation of America offers a range of books and training services for hospice professionals and the general public. The Web site provides general information on hospice and specific types of grief management. There is also a listing of other Web resources and useful literature for both the healthcare provider and the patient.

Hospice Net ✪ ✪ ✪

http://www.hospicenet.org

Hospice Net is dedicated to helping patients and families facing life-threatening illnesses. The site contains a listing of useful articles, FAQ sheets, caregiver information, and a listing of well-chosen links to other major Web resources.

HospiceWeb ✪ ✪ ✪

http://www.hospiceweb.com/index.htm

This site contains general information, a listing of frequently asked questions, discussion board, hospice locator, and an extensive list of links to valuable sites. Links to other hospice organizations are categorized by state.

National Association for Home Care (NAHC) ✪ ✪ ✪ (some features fee-based)

http://www.nahc.org

NAHC is a trade association representing more than 6,000 home care agencies, hospices, and home care aide organizations. The site offers news and Association announcements, a newsletter on pediatric home care, links to affiliates, international employment listings, legislative and regulatory information, statistics and technical papers, and directories of related state associations. Visitors can access a home care and hospice search tool for finding local service providers, and a consumer section offers information on choosing a home care provider, including descriptions of agencies providing home care, tips for finding information about agencies, and discussions of services, payment, patients' rights, accrediting agencies, and state resources. One section is restricted to members.

National Hospice Organization (NHO) ◎ ◎ ◎

http://www.nho.org

The oldest and largest nonprofit public benefit organization devoted exclusively to hospice care, the NHO offers a comprehensive site providing information on all aspects of hospice care for the seriously and terminally ill, along with a state-by-state and city-by-city guide to hospice organizations in the United States. For each listing of a hospice facility, there is a telephone number and contact person.

Medical Insurance and Managed Care

Agency for Healthcare Research and Quality (AHRQ): Checkup On Health Insurance Choices ◎ ◎ ◎

http://www.ahcpr.gov/consumer/insuranc.htm

This discussion of health insurance choices informs consumers on topics including why individuals need insurance, sources of health insurance, group and individual insurance, making a decision of coverage, and managed care. Types of insurance described at the site include fee-for-service and "customary" fees, health maintenance organizations, preferred provider organizations, Medicaid, Medicare, disability insurance, hospital indemnity insurance, and long-term care insurance. The site also includes a checklist and worksheet to determine features important to an individual when choosing insurance. A glossary of terms is available for reference.

American Association of Health Plans Online ◎ ◎ ◎

http://www.aahp.org/menus/index.cfm?CFID=221345&CFTOKEN=11327695

Located in Washington, D.C., the American Association of Health Plans represents more than 1,000 HMOs, PPOs, and other network-based plans. The site offers information on government and advocacy activities, public relations materials, reports and statistics, selected bibliographies listed by subject, information on services and products, conference details, and training program information. Consumer resources include information on choosing a health plan, descriptions of different types of health plans, women's health resources, and fact sheets about health plans. Users can search each specific area of the site for information by keyword.

drkoop.com Insurance Center ◎ ◎ ◎
http://www.drkoop.com/hcr/insurance

This area of drkoop.com features an interactive Plan Profiler and Policy Chooser to help determine what type of plan is right for an individual consumer. An insurance library, glossary of insurance terms, and health insurance news updates are featured at the site.

Employer Quality Partnership (EQP) ◎ ◎
http://www.eqp.org

This site provides a guide to employees in selecting and understanding healthcare plans, provides assistance to employers in evaluating healthcare plans, and also guides employers on ways to improve the quality of their health plans. The site was developed by EQP, a volunteer coalition of employer organizations interested in promoting positive change in the healthcare marketplace and in educating employees regarding their employer-based healthcare plans.

Glossary of Managed Care and Organized Healthcare Systems Terms ◎ ◎ ◎
http://www.uhc.com/resource/glossary.html

Users will find and extensive list of managed care and organized healthcare terms and acronyms defined at this site.

Healthcare Financing Administration ◎ ◎ ◎
http://www.hcfa.gov

This federal site provides a wealth of information on Medicare and Medicaid for both patients and healthcare professionals. It covers the basic features of each program and discusses laws, regulations, and statistics about federal healthcare programs. Information is also provided at the state level (state Medicaid), providing a list of sites with important state information.

Joint Commission of Accreditation of Healthcare Organizations (JCAHO) ◎ ◎ ◎
http://www.jcaho.org

The Joint Commission of Accreditation of Healthcare Organizations evaluates and accredits nearly 18,000 healthcare organizations and programs. Quality Check, a service offered by the Commission, allows consumers to check ratings and evaluations of accredited organizations at the site. Information is available for the general public, employers, healthcare purchasers, and unions; the international community; and healthcare professionals and organizations. The site also contains information on filing complaints, career opportunities, news, and links to related sites.

Managed Care Glossary ◎ ◎ ◎

http://mentalhelp.net/articles/glossary.htm

To be used for professional training purposes or as a general information source, this managed care glossary contains a continuously updated compilation of new terminology related to managed care with additional items in the field of information technology continuously being added. Physician and other healthcare professionals may want to bookmark this site to ensure a more complete understanding of modern health maintenance and preferred provider organization structure and service delivery.

Medical Insurance Resources ◎

http://www.nerdworld.com/trees/nw1654.html

This site offers a large index of medical insurance resources on the Internet. Links are provided to major insurance companies, and other related sites. Each link is accompanied by a brief explanation of what can be found at that particular site.

Medicare ◎ ◎ ◎

http://www.medicare.gov

The Health Care Financing Administration (HCFA) administers Medicare, the nation's largest health insurance program, which covers 39 million Americans. This site answers Medicare questions regarding eligibility, additional insurance, Medicare amounts, and enrollment. Consumer information includes answers to frequently asked questions on Medicare and helps regarding health plan options. Those interested in additional information can call 1-800-MEDICARE to receive additional help in organizing Medicare health options.

National Committee for Quality Assurance (NCQA) ◎ ◎ ◎

http://www.ncqa.org/Pages/Main/index.htm

The National Committee for Quality Assurance (NCQA) is a private, nonprofit organization dedicated to assessing and reporting on the quality of managed healthcare plans. These activities are accomplished through accreditation and performance measurement of participating plans. Almost half the HMOs in the nation, covering three-quarters of all HMO enrollees, are involved in the NCQA accreditation process. A set of more than 50 standardized performance measures called the Health Plan Employer Data and Information Set (HEDIS), is used to evaluate and compare health plans. The NCQA Web site allows the user to search the accreditation status list. The search results will include the accreditation status designation and a summary report of the strengths and weaknesses of the plan entered. NCQA accreditation results allow users to evaluate healthcare plans in such key areas as quality of care, member satisfaction, access, and service.

Quotesmith.com ◎ ◎ ◎

http://www.quotesmith.com

Visitors to this site can access current quotes for individual, family, and small group medical plans. Instant quotes on dental and term life insurance are also available.

U.S. News and World Report: America's Top HMOs ◎ ◎ ◎

http://www.usnews.com/usnews/nycu/health/hetophmo.htm

This site helps consumers to rate their managed care plan by ranking HMOs by state. Other useful tools include an HMO glossary, a medical dictionary, a best hospitals finder, and a list of the 40 highest rated HMOs in the United States. Fitness tips, articles related to HMOs, and a forum for answering health professionals are all found at this site.

Yahoo! Life and Health Insurance Center ◎ ◎ ◎

http://insurance.yahoo.com/life.html

The Yahoo insurance center is an excellent starting point for locating insurance information. Yahoo provides answers to frequently asked questions, a glossary of common terms, and quick estimates on the cost of a health insurance policy. An extensive list of links to related sites and a list of current articles of interest are available.

14.4 Nutrition and Physical Wellness

American Dietetic Association ◎ ◎ ◎ (fee-based)

http://www.eatright.org

The American Dietetic Association presents an ideal site for consumers, students, and dietetic professionals. This site has information on nutrition resources, government affairs, current issues and publications, job opportunities, and a public relations team to answer media questions. Users can contact other dietitians through the site. A search engine and a site map are provided to ease in the searching process. There are also links to consumer education and public policy sites; dietetic associations and networking groups; dietetic practice groups; food; food service and culinary organizations; and medical, health, and other professional organizations.

AOL's Health Webcenter ◎ ◎ ◎

http://www.aol.com/webcenters/health/diet.adp

AOL's Health Webcenter contains well-organized links to a variety of health related sites organized by topic. The site focuses on consumer needs, providing information on topics including illness and treatment; fitness and sports medicine; health and beauty; and women's, men's, children's, and seniors health. A health assessment and drug information search tool, vitamin guide, pregnancy calendar, calorie counter, and body-mass calculator are additional features of the site.

Arbor Nutrition Guide ☺ ☺ ☺

http://www.netspace.net.au/%7Ehelmant/search.htm

The Arbor Nutrition Guide covers all areas of nutrition including applied and clinical nutrition. The site provides links to information on dietary guidelines, special diets, sports nutrition, individual vitamins and minerals, and cultural nutrition. There are also links relating to food science, such as food labeling in other countries, food regulation, food additives, science journals, phytochemistry, and other related topics.

Austin Nutritional Research ☺ ☺ ☺

http://www.realtime.net/anr/referenc.html

This megasite provides links to various organizations and institutions worldwide regarding health and nutrition. Sites include those of professional organizations, research centers, and alternative therapy sources.

Health Resource Links ☺ ☺ ☺

http://www.rxmed.com/healthresourcelinks.html

This site provides links to many professional health-related associations and government agencies. Prescribing information, patient handouts, travel health resources, employment opportunities, medical supply resources, and investment information are all included at this comprehensive site.

International Food Information Council ☺ ☺ ☺

http://ificinfo.health.org

The International Food Information Council presents resources at this site including current issues, up to date information for the media, food safety and nutrition facts, and extensive links to government affairs and agencies. The site also serves as a reference tool for educators, and provides users with a site search engine for locating specific information.

Nutrition & Health Linkstation ☺ ☺ ☺

http://www.amazingstocks.com/nutrition/

The Nutrition & Health Linkstation provides links to recipes, discussion groups, nutrient analysis programs, and energy calculators. The site also offers direct searches of government health organizations, associations, national health research pages, world health research pages, and pharmacy and medicine sites.

Public Health Nutritionists' Home Page ⊙ ⊙ ⊙

http://Weber.u.washington.edu/~phnutr/Internet/nutrlist.html

The Public Health Nutritionists' Home Page is an extensively compiled site for public health and nutrition organized by the School of Public Health and Community Medicine at the University of Washington. This site provides access to many resources, including applied nutrition, cardiovascular disease, food security, vegetarianism, growth charts, breast feeding and infant feeding. Access to the UNICEF gopher server is available to learn more about the United Nations program. Information on educational programs and newsletters are also available.

ThinkQuest Library of Entries ⊙ ⊙ ⊙

http://library.thinkquest.org/library/list.cgi?c=HEALTH_%26_SAFETY

Click on "Food and Nutrition" at this site to access in-depth information for adults, teens, and children on food and nutrition. The links provide access to information on RDA, BMI, personal caloric needs, eating out, specific sites for teens, and general information on more specific health and nutrition topics.

Tufts University Nutrition Navigator ⊙ ⊙ ⊙

http://navigator.tufts.edu

This site, presented by the Center on Nutrition Communication, School of Nutrition Science and Policy at Tufts University, is an up-to-date, rated guide to other nutrition sites. It provides information on general nutrition for parents, kids, women, health professionals, and journalists. One section is devoted to sites providing information about special dietary needs. A search engine is provided at the site for more specific resources.

U.S. Department of Agriculture (USDA) Nutrient Values ⊙ ⊙

http://www.rahul.net/cgi-bin/fatfree/usda/usda.cgi

Visitors can utilize the search engine housed at this site to find the recommended daily allowance (RDA) nutrient values of over 5,000 food items for three different serving sizes in men averaging 174 pounds, and women averaging 138 pounds, between the ages of 25 and 50.

U.S. Department of Health and Human Services (HHS) ⊙ ⊙ ⊙

http://www.dhhs.gov

The Department of Health and Human Services (HHS) is the United States government's principal agency for protecting the health of all Americans and providing essential human services, especially for those who are least able to help themselves. HHS Operating Divisions include National Institutes of Health, Food and Drug Administration, Centers for Disease Control and Prevention, Agency for Toxic Substances and Disease Registry, Indian Health Service, Health Resources and Services

Administration, Substance Abuse and Mental Health Services Administration, and the Agency for Health Care Policy and Research. This site provides news and public affairs information related to HHS, a site search engine, and notices of new site features.

University of Pennsylvania Library ⚙ ⚙ ⚙
http://www.library.upenn.edu

The University of Pennsylvania Library presents an informative site containing information on health disciplines and topics. The site provides access to databases as well as lists of associations, government organizations, and other search tools. Links to alternative medicine sites are also available.

14.5 Online Drug Stores

Corner Drugstore Specialties ⚙ ⚙
http://www.cornerdrug.com

Corner Drugstore Specialties provides customers with a catalog of pharmacy products that includes nonprescription drugs, vitamins, personal care items, and other products typically found in a convenience store or pharmacy.

CVS Pharmacy ⚙ ⚙ ⚙
http://www.cvs.com

This site offers customers a way to order prescription and nonprescription drugs along with other pharmacy items. The prescription section offers an extensive description of the purpose of the drug, side effects, precautions, drug interactions, and other prescribing information. All prescription orders are verified by the pharmacy and will be sent by either the U.S. Postal Service or UPS. Non-prescription drugs, vitamins, first aid, home care, and personal care items are also available.

Drug Emporium ⚙ ⚙
http://www.drugemporium.com

This Web site offers customers a wide variety of products including over-the-counter medicine, personal care items, vitamins, and electronics. Prescription medicine is also available. New patients must register by filling out an online form and provide a way to contact their doctors for prescription information. Prescriptions are processed by a registered pharmacist. Orders are shipped via UPS and shipping costs are added to the bill.

Drugstore.com ◎ ◎ ◎
http://www.drugstore.com

As one of the first online drugstores, Drugstore.com has developed an extensive and informative site that provides prescription and nonprescription medicine, personal care products, vitamins, and other products. There are also articles on solutions to some health and beauty problems, an opportunity to ask a Drugstore.com pharmacist questions, and opinions on products from customers.

Home Pharmacy ◎ ◎
http://www.homepharmacy.com

Home Pharmacy is an online drugstore that provides a variety of healthcare products at a relatively low cost. Products can be sent by standard shipping or by Federal Express.

Merck-Medco Managed Care Online ◎ ◎ ◎
http://www.merck-medco.com

An online pharmacy, the Merck-Medco site provides information on member services; a newsletter, *Optimal Health* with current health news; medication information and articles for healthy aging; client and provider services, including a list of selected FDA-approved prescription medications; a newsroom containing news releases on Merck-Medco and prescription drug-care; and important drug-related consumer announcements.

Online Drugstore.com ◎ ◎
http://www.onlinedrugstore.com

Prescription products at a low cost can be ordered from this service by phone, mail, or e-mail. Visitors can compare prices offered by competitors, access a list of products, and find a more detailed description of the service.

Planet Rx ◎ ◎ ◎
http://www.planetrx.com

Planet Rx, one of the first online drugstores, offers customers a variety of products and information resources. Prescription and nonprescription drugs, personal care items, beauty and spa products, and medical supplies are available. The site also offers articles on health problems and possible treatments, and opinions on products from customers.

Safeweb Medical ◎ ◎
http://drugstore.virtualave.net

The Safeweb Medical Web site provides selected popular prescription drugs and online consultations. The customer receives orders 24–48 hours after doctors approve a prescription.

Self Care ✪ ✪ ✪

http://www.selfcare.com

This Web site has sections for beauty and spa items, nonprescription drugs and medicinal supplies, alternative therapies, nutrition and fitness products, and home care merchandise. Descriptions of products are also available. Orders are sent by standard shipping, priority air delivery, or express air delivery.

Verified Internet Pharmacy Practice Sites (VIPPS) Program ✪ ✪ ✪

http://www.nabp.net/vipps/intro.asp

The Verified Internet Pharmacy Practice Sites (VIPPS) Program of the National Association of Boards of Pharmacy (NABP) was developed in 1999 out of public concern for the safety of pharmacy practices on the Internet. This site contains a menu with links providing information on the criteria for VIPPS certification; a VIPPS list (which includes the pharmacy name and Web site address); VIPPS definitions; and links to Web sites of state boards of pharmacy, state medical boards, federal agencies, and professional organizations.

15. WEB SITE AND TOPICAL INDEX

M

Q

References

1. Feiger A, Kiev A, Shrivastava RK, *et al.* Nefazodone versus sertraline in outpatients with major depression: focus on efficacy, tolerability, and effects on sexual function and satisfaction. *J Clin Psychiatry.* 1996;57(suppl 2):53-62.
2. Data on file, Medical Affairs Department, Bristol-Myers Squibb Company.
3. Baldwin DS, Hawley CJ, Abed RT, *et al.* A multicenter double-blind comparison of nefazodone and paroxetine in the treatment of outpatients with moderate-to-severe depression. *J Clin Psychiatry.* 1996;57(suppl 2):46-52.
4. Feiger AD, Bielski RJ, Bremner J, *et al.* Double-blind, placebo-substitution study of nefazodone in the prevention of relapse during continuation treatment of outpatients with major depression. *Int Clin Psychopharmacol.* 1999;14:19-28.
5. Feighner J, Targum SD, Bennett ME, *et al.* A double-blind, placebo-controlled trial of nefazodone in the treatment of patients hospitalized for major depression. *J Clin Psychiatry.* 1998;59:246-253.
6. Robinson DS, Roberts DL, Smith JM, *et al.* The safety profile of nefazodone. *J Clin Psychiatry.* 1996;57(suppl 2):31-38.
7. Lian J, McQuade R, Jody D. Nefazodone treatment of depression requires less use of concomitant anxiolytic and sedative/hypnotic drugs. Presented at American Psychiatric Association annual meeting; 1997.
8. Rush AJ, Armitage R, Gillin JC, *et al.* Comparative effects of nefazodone and fluoxetine on sleep in outpatients with major depressive disorder. *Biol Psychiatry.* 1998;44:3-14.
9. Gillin JC, Rapaport M, Erman MK, *et al.* A comparison of nefazodone and fluoxetine on mood and on objective, subjective, and clinician-rated measures of sleep in depressed patients: a double-blind, 8-week clinical trial. *J Clin Psychiatry.* 1997;58:185-192.
10. Armitage R, Yonkers K, Cole D, *et al.* A multicenter, double-blind comparison of the effects of nefazodone and fluoxetine on sleep architecture and quality of sleep in depressed outpatients. *J Clin Psychopharmacol.* 1997;17:161-168.

SERZONE® **Rx only**
(nefazodone hydrochloride) Tablets

BRIEF SUMMARY

SERZONE® (nefazodone hydrochloride) Tablets

INDICATIONS AND USAGE: SERZONE (nefazodone hydrochloride) is indicated for the treatment of depression.

CONTRAINDICATIONS: Coadministration of terfenadine, astemizole, cisapride, or pimozide with SERZONE is contraindicated (see **WARNINGS** and **PRECAUTIONS** sections). SERZONE is contraindicated in patients with known hypersensitivity to nefazodone or other phenylpiperazine antidepressants. The coadministration of triazolam and nefazodone causes a significant increase in the plasma level of triazolam (see **WARNINGS** and **PRECAUTIONS** sections), and a 75% reduction in the initial triazolam dosage is recommended if the two drugs are to be given together. Because not all commercially available dosage forms of triazolam permit a sufficient dosage reduction, the coadministration of triazolam and SERZONE should be avoided for most patients, including the elderly.

WARNINGS: ***Potential for Interaction with Monoamine Oxidase Inhibitors:*** **In patients receiving antidepressants with pharmacological properties similar to nefazodone in combination with a monoamine oxidase inhibitor (MAOI), there have been reports of serious, sometimes fatal, reactions. For a selective serotonin reuptake inhibitor, these reactions have included hyperthermia, rigidity, myoclonus, autonomic instability with possible rapid fluctuations of vital signs, and mental status changes that include extreme agitation progressing to delirium and coma. These reactions have also been reported in patients who have recently discontinued that drug and have been started on an MAOI. Some cases presented with features resembling neuroleptic malignant syndrome. Severe hyperthermia and seizures, sometimes fatal, have been reported in association with the combined use of tricyclic antidepressants and MAOIs. These reactions have also been reported in patients who have recently discontinued these drugs and have been started on an MAOI. Although the effects of combined use of nefazodone and MAOI have not been evaluated in humans or animals, because nefazodone is an inhibitor of both serotonin and norepinephrine reuptake, it is recommended that nefazodone not be used in combination with an MAOI, or within 14 days of discontinuing treatment with an MAOI. At least 1 week should be allowed after stopping nefazodone before starting an MAOI.** ***Interaction with Triazolobenzodiazepines:*** Interaction studies of nefazodone with two triazolobenzodiazepines, i.e., triazolam and alprazolam, metabolized by cytochrome P4503A4, have revealed substantial and clinically important increases in plasma concentrations of these compounds when administered concomitantly with nefazodone. **Triazolam:** When a single oral 0.25-mg dose of triazolam was coadministered with nefazodone (200 mg BID) at steady state, triazolam half-life and AUC increased 4-fold and peak concentrations increased 1.7-fold. Nefazodone plasma concentrations were unaffected by triazolam. ***Coadministration of nefazodone potentiated the effects of triazolam on psychomotor performance tests.*** If triazolam is coadministered with SERZONE, a 75% reduction in the initial triazolam dosage is recommended. Because not all commercially available dosage forms of triazolam permit sufficient dosage reduction, coadministration of triazolam with SERZONE should be avoided for most patients, including the elderly. In the exceptional case where coadministration of triazolam with SERZONE may be considered appropriate, only the lowest possible dose of triazolam should be used (see **CONTRAINDICATIONS** and **PRECAUTIONS** sections). **Alprazolam:** When alprazolam (1 mg BID) and nefazodone (200 mg BID) were coadministered, steady-state peak concentrations, AUC and half-life values for alprazolam increased by approximately 2-fold. Nefazodone plasma concentrations were unaffected by alprazolam. If alprazolam is coadministered with SERZONE, a 50% reduction in the initial alprazolam dosage is recommended. No dosage adjustment is required for SERZONE.***Potential Terfenadine, Astemizole, Cisapride, and Pimozide Interactions:*** **Terfenadine, astemizole, cisapride, and pimozide are all metabolized by the cytochrome P450 3A4 (CYP3A4) isozyme, and it has been demonstrated that ketoconazole, erythromycin, and other inhibitors of CYP3A4 can block the metabolism of these drugs, which can result in increased plasma concentrations of parent drug. Increased plasma concentrations of terfenadine, astemizole, cisapride, and pimozide are associated with QT prolongation and with rare cases of serious cardiovascular adverse events, including death, due principally to ventricular tachycardia of the torsades de pointes type. Nefazodone has been shown *in vitro* to be an inhibitor of CYP3A4. Consequently, it is recommended that nefazodone not be used in combination with either terfenadine, astemizole, cisapride, or pimozide (see CONTRAINDICATIONS** and **PRECAUTIONS** sections).

PRECAUTIONS: ***General:*** **Postural Hypotension:** A pooled analysis of the vital signs monitored during placebo-controlled premarketing studies revealed that 5.1% of nefazodone patients compared to 2.5% of placebo patients ($p \leq 0.01$) met criteria for a potentially important decrease in blood pressure at some time during treatment (systolic blood pressure ≤90 mmHg *and* a change from baseline of ≥ 20 mmHg). While there was no difference in the proportion of nefazodone and placebo patients having adverse events characterized as 'syncope' (nefazodone, 0.2%; placebo, 0.3%), the rates for adverse events characterized as 'postural hypotension' were as follows: nefazodone (2.8%), tricyclic antidepressants (10.9%), SSRI (1.1%), and placebo (0.8%). Thus, the prescriber should be aware that there is some risk of postural hypotension in association with nefazodone use. SERZONE should be used with caution in patients with known cardiovascular or cerebrovascular disease that could be exacerbated by hypotension (history of myocardial infarction, angina, or ischemic stroke) and conditions that would predispose patients to hypotension (dehydration, hypovolemia, and treatment with antihypertensive medication). **Activation of Mania/Hypomania:** During premarketing testing, hypomania or mania occurred in 0.3% of nefazodone-treated unipolar patients and 1.6% of bipolar patients. Activation of mania/hypomania is a known risk in a small proportion of patients with major affective disorder treated with other marketed antidepressants. As with all antidepressants, SERZONE should be used cautiously in patients with a history of mania. **Suicide:** The possibility of a suicide attempt is inherent in depression and may persist until significant remission occurs. Close supervision of high risk patients should accompany initial drug therapy. Prescriptions for SERZONE should be written for the smallest quantity of tablets consistent with good patient management in order to reduce the risk of overdose. **Seizures:** During premarketing testing, a recurrence of a petit mal seizure was observed in a patient receiving nefazodone who had a history of such seizures. In addition, one nonstudy participant reportedly experienced a convulsion (type not documented) following a multiple-drug overdose (see **OVERDOSAGE** section). Rare occurrences of convulsions (including grand mal seizures) following nefazodone administration have been reported since market introduction. A causal relationship to nefazodone has not been established (see **ADVERSE REACTIONS** section). **Priapism:** While priapism did not occur during premarketing experience with nefazodone, rare reports of priapism have been received since market introduction. A causal relationship to nefazodone has not been established (see **ADVERSE REACTIONS** section). If patients present with prolonged or inappropriate erections, they should discontinue therapy immediately and consult their physicians. If the condition persists for more than 24 hours, a urologist should be consulted to determine appropriate management. **Use in Patients with Concomitant Illness:** SERZONE has not been evaluated or used to any appreciable extent in patients with a recent history of myocardial infarction or unstable heart disease. Patients with these diagnoses were systematically excluded from clinical studies during the product's premarketing testing. Evaluation of electrocardiograms of 1153 patients who received nefazodone in 6- to 8-week, double-blind, placebo-controlled trials did not indicate that nefazodone is associated with the development of clinically important ECG abnormalities. However, sinus bradycardia, defined as heart rate ≤50 bpm and a decrease of at least 15 bpm from baseline, was observed in 1.5% of nefazodone-treated patients compared to 0.4% of placebo-treated patients ($p \leq 0.05$). Because patients with a recent history of myocardial infarction or unstable heart disease were excluded from clinical trials, such patients should be treated with caution. In patients with cirrhosis of the liver, the AUC values of nefazodone and HO-NEF were increased by approximately 25%. ***Laboratory Tests:*** There are no specific laboratory tests recommended. ***Drug Interactions:*** **Drugs Highly Bound to Plasma Protein:** Because nefazodone is highly bound to plasma protein (see **CLINICAL PHARMACOLOGY** section, **Pharmacokinetics** subsection, of the full prescribing information), administration of SERZONE to a patient taking another drug that is highly protein bound may cause increased free concentrations of the other drug, potentially resulting in adverse events. Conversely, adverse effects could result from displacement of nefazodone by other highly bound drugs. **CNS-Active Drugs:** *Monoamine Oxidase Inhibitors* — See **WARNINGS** section. *Haloperidol* — When a single oral 5-mg dose of haloperidol was coadministered with nefazodone (200 mg BID) at steady state, haloperidol apparent clearance decreased by 35% with no significant increase in peak haloperidol plasma concentrations or time of peak. This change is of unknown clinical significance. Pharmacodynamic effects of haloperidol were generally not altered significantly. There were no changes in the pharmacokinetic parameters for nefazodone. Dosage adjustment of haloperidol may be necessary when coadministered with nefazodone. *Lorazepam* — When lorazepam (2 mg BID) and nefazodone (200 mg BID) were coadministered to steady state, there was no change in any pharmacokinetic parameter for either drug compared to each drug administered alone. Therefore, dosage adjustment is not necessary for either drug when coadministered. *Triazolam/Alprazolam* — See **CONTRAINDICATIONS** and **WARNINGS** sections. *Alcohol* — Although nefazodone did not potentiate the cognitive and psychomotor effects of alcohol in experiments with normal subjects, the concomitant use of SERZONE and alcohol in depressed patients is not advised. *Buspirone* — In a study of steady-state pharmacokinetics in healthy volunteers, coadministration of buspirone (2.5 or 5 mg BID) with nefazodone (250 mg BID) resulted in marked increases in plasma buspirone concentrations (increases up to 20-fold in C_{max} and up to 50-fold in AUC) and statistically significant decreases (about 50%) in plasma concentrations of the buspirone metabolite 1-pyrimidinylpiperazine. With 5-mg BID doses of buspirone, slight increases in AUC were observed for nefazodone (23%) and its metabolites hydroxynefazodone (17%) and mCPP (9%). The side effect profile for subjects receiving buspirone 2.5 mg BID and nefazodone 250 mg BID was similar to that for subjects receiving either drug alone. Subjects receiving buspirone 5 mg BID and nefazodone 250 mg BID experienced side effects such as lightheadedness, asthenia, dizziness, and somnolence. If the two drugs are to be used in combination, a low dose of buspirone (e.g., 2.5 mg BID) is recommended. Subsequent dose adjustment of either drug should be based on clinical assessment. *Pimozide*—See **CONTRAINDICATIONS, WARNINGS,** and **PRECAUTIONS**: *Pharmacokinetics of Nefazodone in 'Poor Metabolizers' and Potential Interaction with Drugs that Inhibit and/or Are Metabolized by Cytochrome P450 Isozymes. General Anesthetics* — Little is known about the potential for interaction between nefazodone and general anesthetics; therefore, prior to elective surgery, SERZONE should be discontinued for as long as clinically feasible. *Other CNS-Active Drugs* — The use of nefazodone in combination with other CNS-active drugs has not been systematically evaluated. Consequently, caution is advised if concomitant administration of SERZONE and such drugs is required. **Cimetidine**: When nefazodone (200 mg BID) and cimetidine (300 mg QID) were coadministered for one week, no change in the steady-state pharmacokinetics of either nefazodone or cimetidine was observed compared to each dosed alone. Therefore, dosage adjustment is not necessary for either drug when coadministered. **Cardiovascular-Active Drugs:** *Digoxin* — When nefazodone (200 mg BID) and digoxin (0.2 mg QD) were coadministered for 9 days to healthy male volunteers (n = 18) who were phenotyped as CYP2D6 extensive metabolizers, C_{max}, C_{min} and AUC of digoxin were increased by 29%, 27%, and 15%, respectively. Digoxin had no effects on the pharmacokinetics of nefazodone and its active metabolites. Because of the narrow therapeutic index of digoxin, caution should be exercised when nefazodone and digoxin are coadministered; plasma level monitoring for digoxin is recommended. *Propranolol* —The coadministration of nefazodone (200 mg BID) and propranolol (40 mg BID) for 5.5 days to healthy male volunteers (n = 18), including 3 poor and 15 extensive CYP2D6 metabolizers, resulted in 30% and 14% reductions in C_{max} and AUC of propranolol, respectively, and a 14% reduction in C_{max} for the metabolite, 4-hydroxypropranolol. The kinetics of nefazodone, hydroxynefazodone, and triazole-dione were not affected by coadministration of propranolol. However, C_{max}, C_{min}, and AUC of m-chlorophenylpiperazine were increased by 23%, 54%, and 28%, respectively. No change in initial dose of either drug is necessary, and dose adjustments should be made on the basis of clinical response. *HMG-CoA Reductase Inhibitors* — When single 40-mg doses of simvastatin or atorvastatin, both substrates of CYP3A4, were given to healthy adult volunteers who had received SERZONE 200 mg BID for 6 days, approximately 20-fold increases in plasma concentrations of simvastatin and simvastatin acid and 3-4-fold increases in plasma concentrations of atorvastatin and atorvastatin lactone were seen. These effects appear to be due to the inhibition of CYP3A4 by SERZONE because, in the same study, SERZONE had no significant effect on the plasma concentrations of pravastatin, which is not metabolized by CYP3A4 to a clinically significant extent. There have been rare reports of rhabdomyolysis involving patients receiving the combination of SERZONE and either simvastatin or lovastatin, also a substrate of CYP3A4 (see **ADVERSE REACTIONS: Postintroduction Clinical Experience** section). Rhabdomyolysis has been observed in patients receiving HMG-CoA reductase inhibitors administered alone (at recommended dosages) and in particular, for certain drugs in this class, when given in combination with inhibitors of the CYP3A4 isozyme. Caution should be used if SERZONE is administered in combination with HMG-CoA reductase inhibitors that are metabolized by CYP3A4, such as simvastatin, atorvastatin, and lovastatin, and dosage adjustments of these HMG-CoA reductase inhibitors are recommended. Since metabolic interactions are unlikely between SERZONE and HMG-CoA reductase inhibitors that undergo little or no metabolism by the CYP3A4 isozyme, such as pravastatin or fluvastatin, dosage adjustments should not be necessary. **Cyclosporine:** There have been rare reports of increased serum cyclosporine levels (up to seven times higher) in patients receiving SERZONE and cyclosporine concomitantly. Since cyclosporine is a substrate of CYP3A4 and nefazodone is known to inhibit this enzyme, monitoring of serum cyclosporine levels is recommended when the two agents are coadministered. **Pharmacokinetics of Nefazodone in 'Poor Metabolizers' and Potential Interaction with Drugs that Inhibit and/or Are Metabolized by Cytochrome P450 Isozymes:** *CYP3A4 Isozyme* —Nefazodone has been shown *in vitro* to be an inhibitor of CYP3A4. This is consistent with the interactions observed between nefazodone and triazolam, alprazolam, buspirone, atorvastatin, and simvastatin, drugs metabolized by this isozyme. Consequently, caution is indicated in the combined use of nefazodone with any drugs known to be metabolized by the CYP3A4. In particular, the combined use of nefazodone with triazolam should be avoided for most patients, including the elderly. The combined use of nefazodone with terfenadine, astemizole, cisapride, or pimozide is contraindicated (see **CONTRAINDICATIONS** and **WARNINGS** sections). *CYP2D6 Isozyme* —A subset (3% to 10%) of the population has reduced activity of the drug-metabolizing enzyme CYP2D6. Such individuals are referred to commonly as "poor metabolizers" of drugs such as debrisoquin, dextromethorphan, and the tricyclic antidepressants. The pharmacokinetics of nefazodone and its major metabolites are not altered in these "poor metabolizers." Plasma concentrations of one minor metabolite (mCPP) are increased in this population; the adjustment of SERZONE (nefazodone hydrochloride) dosage is not required when administered to "poor metabolizers." Nefazodone and its metabolites have been shown *in vitro* to be extremely weak inhibitors of CYP2D6. Thus, it is not likely that nefazodone will decrease the metabolic clearance of drugs metabolized by this isozyme. *CYP1A2 Isozyme*—Nefazodone and its metabolites have been shown *in vitro* not to inhibit CYP1A2. Thus, metabolic interactions between nefazodone and drugs metabolized by this isozyme are unlikely. **Electroconvulsive Therapy (ECT):** There are no clinical studies of the combined use of ECT and nefazodone. *Carcinogenesis, Mutagenesis, Impairment of Fertility.* **Carcinogenesis.** There is no evidence of carcinogenicity with nefazodone. The dietary administration of nefazodone to rats and mice for 2 years at daily doses of up to 200 mg/kg and 800 mg/kg, respectively, which are approximately 3 and 6 times, respectively, the maximum human daily dose on a mg/m² basis, produced no increase in tumors. **Mutagenesis:** Nefazodone has been shown to have no genotoxic effects based on the following assays: bacterial mutation assays, a DNA repair assay in cultured rat hepatocytes, a mammalian mutation assay in Chinese hamster ovary cells, an *in vivo* cytogenetics assay in rat bone marrow cells, and a rat dominant lethal study. **Impairment of Fertility:** A fertility study in rats showed a slight decrease in fertility at 200 mg/kg/day (approximately three times the maximum human daily dose on a mg/m² basis) but not at 100 mg/kg/day (approximately 1.5 times the maximum human daily dose on a mg/m² basis). *Pregnancy: Teratogenic Effects— Pregnancy Category C:* Reproduction studies have been performed in pregnant rabbits and rats at daily doses up to 200 and 300 mg/kg, respectively (approximately 6 and 5 times, respectively, the maximum human daily dose on a mg/m² basis). No malformations were observed in the offspring as a result of nefazodone treatment. However, increased early pup mortality was seen in rats at a dose approximately 5 times the maximum human dose, and decreased pup weights were seen at this and lower doses when dosing began during pregnancy and continued until weaning. The cause of these deaths is not known. The no-effect dose for rat pup mortality was 1.3 times the human dose on a mg/m² basis. There are no adequate and well-controlled studies in pregnant women. Nefazodone should be used during pregnancy only if the potential benefit justifies the potential risk to the fetus. *Labor and Delivery:* The effect of SERZONE on labor and delivery in humans is unknown. *Nursing Mothers:* It is not known whether SERZONE (nefazodone hydrochloride) or its metabolites are excreted in human milk. Because many drugs are excreted in human milk, caution should be exercised when SERZONE is administered to a nursing woman. *Pediatric Use:* Safety and effectiveness in individuals below 18 years of age have not been established. *Geriatric Use:* Over 500 elderly (≥65 years) individuals participated in clinical studies with nefazodone. No unusual adverse age-related phenomena were identified in this cohort of elderly patients treated with nefazodone. Due to the increased systemic exposure to nefazodone seen in single dose studies in elderly patients (see **CLINICAL PHARMACOLOGY** section, **Pharmacokinetics** subsection, of the full prescribing information), treatment should be initiated at half the usual dose, but titration upward should take place over the same range as in younger patients (see **DOSAGE AND ADMINISTRATION** section of the full prescribing information). The usual precautions should be observed in elderly patients who have concomitant medical illnesses or who are receiving concomitant drugs.

ADVERSE REACTIONS: *Associated with Discontinuation of Treatment:* Approximately 16% of the 3496 patients who received SERZONE in worldwide premarketing clinical trials discontinued treatment due to an adverse experience. The more common (≥1%) events in clinical trials associated with discontinuation and considered to be drug related included: nausea, dizziness, insomnia, asthenia, and agitation. *Incidence in Controlled Trials:* **Commonly Observed Adverse Events in Controlled Clinical Trials:** The most commonly observed adverse events associated with the use of SERZONE (incidence of 5% or greater) and not seen at an equivalent incidence among placebo-treated patients were: somnolence (25% vs 14%), dry mouth (25% vs 13%), nausea (22% vs 12%), dizziness (17% vs 5%), constipation (14% vs 8%), asthenia (11% vs 5%), lightheadedness (10% vs 3%), blurred vision (9% vs 3%), confusion (7% vs 2%), and abnormal vision (7% vs 1%). The following adverse events occurred at an incidence of 1% or more in patients treated with SERZONE dosed at ranges of 300 mg to 600 mg/day and were more frequent than in the placebo groups in 6- to 8-week placebo-controlled trials. **Body as a Whole:** headache, asthenia, infection, flu syndrome, chills, fever, neck rigidity. **Cardiovascular:** postural hypotension, hypotension. **Dermatological:** pruritus, rash. **Gastrointestinal:** dry mouth, nausea, constipation, dyspepsia, diarrhea, increased appetite, nausea and vomiting. **Metabolic:** peripheral edema, thirst. **Musculoskeletal:** arthralgia. **Nervous:** somnolence, dizziness, insomnia, lightheadedness, confusion, memory impairment, paresthesia, vasodilatation, abnormal dreams, concentration decreased, ataxia, incoordination, psychomotor retardation, tremor, hypertonia, libido decreased. **Respiratory:** pharyngitis, cough increased. **Special Senses:** blurred vision, abnormal vision, tinnitus, taste perversion, visual field defect. **Urogenital:** urinary frequency, urinary tract infection, urinary retention, vaginitis, breast pain. Events for which the SERZONE incidence was equal to or less than placebo included the following: abdominal pain, pain, back pain, accidental injury, chest pain, neck pain, palpitation, migraine, sweating, flatulence, vomiting, anorexia, tooth disorder, weight gain, edema, myalgia, cramp, agitation, anxiety, depression, hypesthesia, CNS stimulation, dysphoria, emotional lability, sinusitis, rhinitis, dysmenorrhea, dysuria. Studies show a clear dose dependency for some of the more common adverse events associated with SERZONE use. **Vital Sign Changes:** (See PRECAUTIONS section, Postural Hypotension Subsection.) **Weight Changes:** In a pooled analy-

sis of placebo-controlled premarketing studies, there were no differences between nefazodone and placebo groups in the proportions of patients meeting criteria for potentially important increases or decreases in body weight (a change of ≥ 7%). **Laboratory Changes:** Pooled analysis revealed a statistical trend between nefazodone and placebo for potentially important decrease in hematocrit, ie, 2.8% of nefazodone patients compared to 1.5% of placebo patients (0.05 < p ≤ 0.10). **ECG Changes:** Pooled analysis revealed a statistically significant difference between nefazodone and placebo for sinus bradycardia, ie, 1.5% of nefazodone patients compared to 0.4% of placebo patients (p < 0.05). *Other Events Observed During the Premarketing Evaluation of SERZONE:* During its premarketing assessment, multiple doses of SERZONE were administered to 3496 patients. Events are categorized by body system and listed in order of decreasing frequency according to the following definitions: frequent adverse events are those occurring on one or more occasions in at least 1/100 patients (only those not already listed in the tabulated results from placebo-controlled trials appear in this listing); infrequent adverse events are those occurring in 1/100 to 1/1000 patients; rare events are those occurring in fewer than 1/1000 patients. **Body as a Whole** — *Infrequent:* allergic reaction, malaise, photosensitivity reaction, face edema, hangover effect, abdomen enlarged, hernia, pelvic pain, and halitosis. *Rare:* cellulitis. **Cardiovascular System** — *Infrequent:* tachycardia, hypertension, syncope, ventricular extrasystoles, and angina pectoris. *Rare:* AV block, congestive heart failure, hemorrhage, pallor, and varicose vein. **Dermatological System** —*Infrequent:* dry skin, acne, alopecia, urticaria, maculopapular rash, vesiculobullous rash, and eczema. **Gastrointestinal System** — *Frequent:* gastroenteritis. *Infrequent:* eructation, periodontal abscess, abnormal liver function tests, gingivitis, colitis, gastritis, mouth ulceration, stomatitis, esophagitis, peptic ulcer, and rectal hemorrhage. *Rare:* glossitis, hepatitis, dysphagia, gastrointestinal hemorrhage, oral moniliasis, and ulcerative colitis. **Hemic and Lymphatic System** — *Infrequent:* ecchymosis, anemia, leukopenia, and lymphadenopathy. **Metabolic and Nutritional System** — *Infrequent:* weight loss, gout, dehydration, lactic dehydrogenase increased, SGOT increased, and SGPT increased. *Rare:* hypercholesteremia and hypoglycemia. **Musculoskeletal System** — *Infrequent:* arthritis, tenosynovitis, muscle stiffness, and bursitis. *Rare:* tendinous contracture. **Nervous System** — *Infrequent:* vertigo, twitching, depersonalization, hallucinations, suicide attempt, apathy, euphoria, hostility, suicidal thoughts, abnormal gait, thinking abnormal, attention decreased, derealization, neuralgia, paranoid reaction, dysarthria, increased libido, suicide, and myoclonus. *Rare:* hyperkinesia, increased salivation, cerebrovascular accident, hyperesthesia, hypotonia, ptosis, and neuroleptic malignant syndrome. **Respiratory System**—*Frequent:* dyspnea and bronchitis. *Infrequent:* asthma, pneumonia, laryngitis, voice alteration, epistaxis, hiccup. *Rare:* hyperventilation and yawn. **Special Senses** —*Frequent:* eye pain. *Infrequent:* dry eye, ear pain, abnormality of accommodation, diplopia, conjunctivitis, mydriasis, keratoconjunctivitis, hyperacusis, and photophobia. *Rare:* deafness, glaucoma, night blindness, and taste loss. **Urogenital System**—*Frequent:* impotence.ᵃ *Infrequent:* cystitis, urinary urgency, metrorrhagia,ᵃ amenorrhea,ᵃ polyuria, vaginal hemorrhage,ᵃ breast enlargement,ᵃ menorrhagia,ᵃ urinary incontinence, abnormal ejaculation,ᵃ hematuria, nocturia, and kidney calculus. *Rare:* uterine fibroids enlarged,ᵃ uterine hemorrhage,ᵃ anorgasmia, and oliguria.ᵃAdjusted for gender.

Postintroduction Clinical Experience: Postmarketing experience with SERZONE has shown an adverse experience profile similar to that seen during the premarketing evaluation of nefazodone. Voluntary reports of adverse events temporally associated with SERZONE have been received since market introduction that are not listed above and for which a causal relationship has not been established. These include: Rare occurrences of convulsions (including grand mal seizures) and priapism (see **PRECAUTIONS** section); Rare reports of rhabdomyolysis involving patients receiving the combination of SERZONE and lovastatin or simvastatin (see PRECAUTIONS section); Rare reports of liver necrosis and liver failure, in some cases leading to liver transplantation and/or death.

DRUG ABUSE AND DEPENDENCE: *Controlled Substance Class:* SERZONE (nefazodone hydrochloride) is not a controlled substance. However, evaluate patients carefully for a history of drug abuse and follow such patients closely, observing them for signs of misuse or abuse of SERZONE (e.g., development of tolerance, dose escalation, drug-seeking behavior). **OVERDOSAGE:** In premarketing clinical studies, seven patients ingested from 1000 mg to 11,200 mg of nefazodone; commonly reported symptoms included nausea, vomiting, and somnolence. None of the patients died. Ensure an adequate airway, oxygenation, and ventilation. Monitor cardiac rhythm and vital signs. General supportive and symptomatic measures are also recommended. Induction of emesis is not recommended. Gastric lavage with a large-bore orogastric tube with appropriate airway protection, if needed, may be indicated if performed soon after ingestion, or in symptomatic patients. Activated charcoal should be administered. Due to the wide distribution of nefazodone in body tissues, forced diuresis, dialysis, hemoperfusion, and exchange transfusion are unlikely to be of benefit. No specific antidotes for nefazodone are known. In managing overdosage, consider the possibility of multiple drug involvement.

Bristol-Myers Squibb Company

Princeton, New Jersey 08543, U.S.A.

1017710A6   Revised: October 1999   Printed in U.S.A   D5-K028-K029-K030-K033